A PRACTIC

MOV

DISCORDERS

A PRACTICAL APPROACH TO
MOVEMENT
DISORDERS

Diagnosis and Management, Second Edition

Editors

HUBERT H. FERNANDEZ, MD

Head, Section of Movement Disorders
Center for Neurological Restoration
Cleveland Clinic
and
Professor of Medicine (Neurology)
Cleveland Clinic Lerner College of Medicine
Case Western Reserve University

ANDRE G. MACHADO, MD, PHD

Director, Center for Neurological Restoration
Staff, Department of Neurosurgery
Associate Staff, Department of Biomedical Engineering
Associate Staff, Department of Neurosciences
Cleveland Clinic

MAYUR PANDYA, DO

Director, Comprehensive Huntington's Disease Clinic
Center for Neurological Restoration
Cleveland Clinic
and
Assistant Professor of Medicine (Psychiatry)
Cleveland Clinic Lerner College of Medicine
Case Western Reserve University

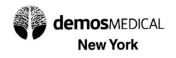

demosMEDICAL
New York

Visit our website at www.demosmedical.com

ISBN: 9781620700341
e-book ISBN: 9781617051937

Acquisitions Editor: Beth Barry
Compositor: Amnet Systems

Medicine is an ever-changing science. Research and clinical experience are continually expanding our knowledge, in particular our understanding of proper treatment and drug therapy. The authors, editors, and publisher have made every effort to ensure that all information in this book is in accordance with the state of knowledge at the time of production of the book. Nevertheless, the authors, editors, and publisher are not responsible for errors or omissions or for any consequences from application of the information in this book and make no warranty, expressed or implied, with respect to the contents of the publication. Every reader should examine carefully the package inserts accompanying each drug and should carefully check whether the dosage schedules mentioned therein or the contraindications stated by the manufacturer differ from the statements made in this book. Such examination is particularly important with drugs that are either rarely used or have been newly released on the market.

LIBRARY OF CONGRESS CATALOGING-IN-PUBLICATION DATA

Fernandez, Hubert H., author.
  A practical approach to movement disorders / Hubert H. Fernandez, Andre G. Machado, Mayur Pandya. — Second edition.
      p. ; cm.
  Preceded by A practical approach to movement disorders / Hubert H. Fernandez ... [et al.]. c2007.
  Includes bibliographical references and index.
  ISBN 978-1-62070-034-1 (print : alk. paper) — ISBN 978-1-61705-193-7 (e-book)
  I. Machado, Andre G. (Neurosurgeon), author. II. Pandya, Mayur, author. III. Title.
  [DNLM: 1. Movement Disorders—Handbooks. WL 39]
  RC376.5
  616.8′3—dc23
                                                                    2014013970

Special discounts on bulk quantities of Demos Medical Publishing books are available to corporations, professional associations, pharmaceutical companies, health care organizations, and other qualifying groups. For details, please contact:

Special Sales Department
Demos Medical Publishing, LLC
11 West 42nd Street, 15th Floor
New York, NY 10036
Phone: 800-532-8663 or 212-683-0072
Fax: 212-941-7842
E-mail: specialsales@demosmedical.com

Printed in the United States of America by Gasch Printing.
16 17 / 5 4

This book is warmly dedicated to our wives, Cecilia, Sandra, and Laura, and to our children, Annella Marie, Gabriella, Julia, Sameer, and Sara, for unconditionally supporting us in good times and bad; for providing us the strength to overcome all challenges, big and small; and most of all, for inspiring us to strive to become better men, with pride and with humility.

H. H. F.
A. G. M.
M. P.

CONTENTS

IV Surgical Approach to Movement Disorders

V Nonpharmacologic Approach to Movement Disorders

CONTRIBUTORS

Anwar Ahmed, MD
Staff, Center for Neurological Restoration
Fellowship Program Director, Section of Movement Disorders
Neurological Institute
Cleveland Clinic
Cleveland, Ohio
Neurological Approach to Tremors

Kristin Appleby, MD
Staff, Center for Neurological Restoration
Neurological Institute
Cleveland Clinic
Cleveland, Ohio
Neurological Approach to Tics

Joseph Austerman, DO
Staff, Center for Behavioral Health
Neurological Institute
Cleveland Clinic
Cleveland, Ohio
Psychiatric Issues in Tourette Syndrome

Jawad Bajwa, MD
Assistant Professor of Neurology
King Saud bin Abdulaziz University for Health Sciences
Riyadh, Saudi Arabia;
Program Director, Adult Movement Disorders and
    Neurorestoration
Clerkship Director, Neuroscience
Department of Neurology

National Neuroscience Institute
King Fahd Medical City
Riyadh, Saudi Arabia;
Adjunct Assistant Professor of Neurology
University of Florida
Gainesville, Florida
Neurological Approach to Ataxia

Amy Chan, PT, NCS
Clinical Specialist
Mellen Center for Multiple Sclerosis
Neurological Institute
Cleveland Clinic
Cleveland, Ohio
Physical and Occupational Therapy

Margo Funk, MD, MA
Staff, Center for Behavioral Health
Neurological Institute
Cleveland Clinic
Cleveland, Ohio
Approach to Conversion Disorder

Gencer Genc, MD
Fellow, Center for Neurological Restoration
Neurological Institute
Cleveland Clinic
Cleveland, Ohio;
Neurologist, Gumussuyu Military Hospital
Istanbul, Turkey
Nutritional Considerations

Justin Havemann, MD
Staff, Center for Behavioral Health
Neurological Institute
Cleveland Clinic
Cleveland, Ohio
Psychiatric Issues in Parkinson's Disease

Ilia Itin, MD
Staff, Center for Behavioral Health
Neurological Institute
Cleveland Clinic
Cleveland, Ohio
Neurological Approach to Dystonia

Thien Thien Lim, MD, MRCP (UK)
Fellow, Center for Neurological Restoration
Neurological Institute
Cleveland Clinic
Cleveland, Ohio;
Consultant, Island Hospital
Penang, Malaysia
Neurological Approach to Parkinsonism
Neurological Approach to Parkinson's Disease

Andre G. Machado, MD, PhD
Director, Center for Neurological Restoration
Neurological Institute
Cleveland Clinic
Cleveland, Ohio
Surgical Approach to Movement Disorders

Raja Mehanna, MD
Fellow, Center for Neurological Restoration
Neurological Institute
Cleveland Clinic
Cleveland, Ohio;
Assistant Professor, Department of Neurology
University of Texas Health Science Center at Houston
Houston, Texas
Neurological Approach to Sleep-Related Movement Disorders

Heather Murphy, SLP
Clinical Specialist, Mellen Center for Multiple Sclerosis
Neurological Institute
Cleveland Clinic
Cleveland, Ohio
Speech and Swallowing Therapy

Rafael Palacio Jr, MD
Fellow, Center for Neurological Restoration
Neurological Restoration
Cleveland Clinic
Cleveland, Ohio;
Chief of Clinics
Western Batangas Medical Center
Balayan, Batangas, Philippines
Getting Started: The Body Language of Movement Disorders

Mayur Pandya, DO
Staff, Center for Neurological Restoration
Director, Huntington's Disease Comprehensive Clinic
Neurological Institute
Cleveland Clinic
Cleveland, Ohio
The Psychiatric Assessment
Psychiatric Issues in Huntington's Disease

Joseph Rudolph, MD
Staff, Center for Regional Neurosciences
Neurological Institute
Cleveland Clinic
Cleveland, Ohio
Neurological Approach to Dystonia

Junaid Habib Siddiqui, MD, MRCP (UK)
Fellow, Movement Disorders
Center for Neurological Restoration
Neurological Institute
Cleveland Clinic
Cleveland, Ohio
Neurological Approach to Myoclonus

Sumeet Vadera, MD, PhD
Resident, Neurosurgery
Neurological Institute
Cleveland Clinic
Cleveland, Ohio
Surgical Approach to Movement Disorders

Ryan Walsh, MD, PhD
Staff, Lou Ruvo Center for Brain Health and Center for
    Neurological Restoration
Neurological Institute
Cleveland Clinic—Las Vegas
Las Vegas, Nevada
Neurological Approach to Chorea

PREFACE

Medicine is evolving at an unprecedented pace. Therefore, 7 years after the success of *A Practical Approach to Movement Disorders*, we felt that it was time for a second edition. Now more than ever, busy practicing clinicians need a quick guide to the diagnostic approach and to the medical, behavioral, surgical, and nonpharmacologic therapies for various movement disorders. To fill this need, we have kept the handy, paper-bound, fit-in-your-coat-pocket format and the practical yet authoritative guide to all types of movement disorders that was offered in the first edition. Our readers appreciated the expanded outline and bulleted point format with an emphasis on clinical presentation, diagnosis, workup, and management. However, we have added several new features, which we hope will increase the usefulness of this handbook for even the busiest clinician faced with a patient who has a movement disorder.

This handbook is now divided into four parts: neurological, psychiatric, surgical, and nonpharmacologic approaches to movement disorders. The first section, on the neurological approach, provides a starting point for the clinician who has a patient presenting with a movement disorder. A new chapter on sleep-related movement disorders has been added, the latest genetic discoveries have been incorporated, and the approach to Parkinson's disease is discussed in greater depth. Another new addition to this book is the section on the psychiatric approach, as almost all movement disorders manifest with behavioral and psychiatric features, which can be intimidating to even the most experienced clinicians. Emphasis is placed on the psychiatric features of Parkinson's disease, Huntington's Disease, Tourette syndrome, and conversion disorders that present with movement abnormalities. With the recent advancements in functional neurosurgery, the section on the surgical approach has been completely updated. And finally, the section on the nonpharmacologic approach acknowledges the need for a comprehensive approach to treatment that includes nutritional, physical, occupational, speech, and swallowing therapy.

Content overlap between chapters was encouraged and is intentional, to emphasize essential concepts and principles in diagnosis and treatment. Also, several disorders can present with various movement disorder phenomenologies, and these are therefore discussed in several chapters. We added more figures, flow charts, and tables that simplify approaches and summarize key findings.

We hope that this second edition, even more than the first, will help to make the assessment and treatment of the most common movement disorders less intimidating and more rewarding.

Hubert H. Fernandez
Andre G. Machado
Mayur Pandya

ACKNOWLEDGMENTS

We would like to sincerely thank Christine Moore for the editorial support she has provided, without which this book would never have been finished, and Terri O'Brian for the wonderful illustrations and figures that make this book fun to read and easy to follow.

We would also like to thank our colleagues, including the following: Michael S. Okun, Ramon L. Rodriguez, Frank M. Skidmore, Harrison N. Jones, Neila J. Donovan, John C. Rosenbek, and Keith J. Myers, who all contributed to the first edition of *Practical Approach to Movement Disorders* and whose chapters served as the foundation for this second edition.

I

Getting Started

1

THE BODY LANGUAGE OF MOVEMENT DISORDERS

Movement is controlled by a highly evolved and sophisticated system of interacting circuits in the nervous system that allow human thought to be expressed! Because of this level of sophistication, disorders affecting the control of movement may have a plethora of manifestations. The treatment of movement disorders is a subspecialty of neurology concerned with patients who move either "too much" or "too little."[1] Therefore, movement disorders are neurological syndromes in which there is either an excess of movement (*hyperkinesia*) or a paucity of voluntary and automatic movements (*hypokinesia*) that is unrelated to weakness or spasticity.[2]

■ Most, but not all, movement disorders result from some element of basal ganglia dysfunction and are sometimes termed *extrapyramidal disorders*.

■ However, movement disorders can also result from injury to the cerebral cortex, cerebellum, brainstem, spinal cord, peripheral nerves, and other elements of the central and peripheral nervous system.

PREVALENCE OF MOVEMENT DISORDERS

Movement disorders are quite common. Before the recognition of restless legs syndrome (RLS), the most common movement disorder was essential tremor (ET). The estimated prevalence rates of the most common movement disorders per 100,000 of the general population are listed in Table 1.1.[3]

APPROACH TO THE PATIENT WITH A MOVEMENT DISORDER

The approach to a patient with a movement disorder, like that to a patient with any other condition, begins with taking the *history of the illness* (Figure 1.1).

Then, the examination of a patient with a movement disorder depends on careful observation.

Table 1.1
Estimated Prevalence of the Most Common Movement Disorders
per 100,000 of the General Population

Movement Disorder	Prevalence
Restless legs syndrome	9,800
Essential tremor	415
Parkinson's disease	187
Tourette syndrome	29–1,052
Primary torsion dystonia	33
Hemifacial spasm	7.4–14.5
Blepharospasm	13.3
Hereditary ataxia	6
Huntington's disease	2–12
Wilson's disease	3
Progressive supranuclear palsy	2–6.4
Multiple systems atrophy	4.4

Source: Adapted from Ref. 3: Schrag A. Epidemiology of movement disorders. In: Jankovic J, Tolosa E, eds. *Parkinson's Disease and Movement Disorders.* 4th ed. Philadelphia, PA: Lippincott Williams & Wilkins; 2002:73–89.

■ The first task should be to determine whether the phenomenon represents too little movement (hypokinesia) or too much movement (hyperkinesia) (Figure 1.2).

■ If the patient is hyperkinetic, the next question to be answered is whether the extraneous movements are involuntary, voluntary, or "semivoluntary."

   ○ It should be noted that as a general rule, abnormal involuntary movements, including those with an organic etiology, are exaggerated by anxiety, and most diminish or disappear during sleep.[2]

HYPOKINETIC DISORDERS

Patients with hypokinetic disorders present with a paucity of symptoms and are often best observed while they are unaware that their examination has already begun. For example, patients can be observed from the time they enter the room to the moment when they reach the chair or examination table. Verbal prompting, although a standard part of examinations, may cause patients' movements to be faster (or slower) than those of their usual state.

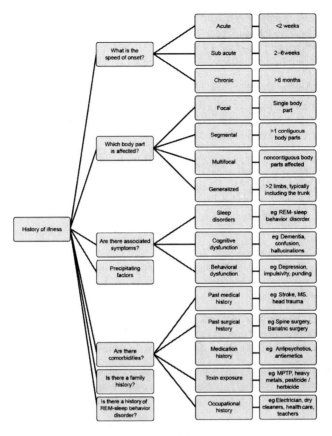

Figure 1.1
Features worth extracting from the patient's history.

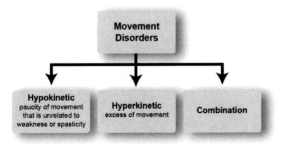

Figure 1.2
Classification of movement disorders.

Akinesia, bradykinesia, and *hypokinesia* literally mean "absence," "slowness," and "decreased amplitude" of movement, respectively. The three terms are commonly grouped together for convenience, and the conditions they describe are usually referred to collectively as *bradykinesia* (Figure 1.3).[2]

- Bradykinesia is one of the cardinal motor features of *parkinsonism.*

- These motor features are elicited during voluntary tasks and may also be seen when the automatic or "unvoluntary" movements associated with learned tasks are observed.

Parkinsonism is the most common cause of hypokinesia, but there are other, less common causes, such as cataplexy and drop attacks, catatonia, hypothyroid slowness, rigidity, and stiff muscles (Table 1.2).

Hypokinetic movements may be further subdivided into those with parkinsonian or nonparkinsonian etiologies (Figure 1.4).

Parkinsonism is the most recognized form of hypokinesia and accounts for about half of all hypokinetic movement disorders.

- It manifests as any combination of its four cardinal motor features: *resting tremor, bradykinesia* (slowness in movement), *rigidity* (stiffness), and *gait/ postural instability.*

- Not all four motor features need to be present. At least two of the cardinal features need to be present, with one of them being resting tremor or bradykinesia, before the diagnosis of parkinsonism is made.

- There are several forms of parkinsonism, which can be broadly categorized as primary, secondary, parkinson-plus, and heredodegenerative disorders (Figure 1.5).

- In general, primary parkinsonism (ie, idiopathic Parkinson's disease) is a progressive, neurodegenerative, almost "purely" parkinsonian disorder of unclear etiology. Sometimes, this diagnosis can be made only after other causes of parkinsonism have been systematically excluded. It is probably the most common form of parkinsonism.

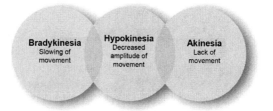

Figure 1.3
The spectrum of bradykinesia.

Table 1.2
Phenomenology of Movement Disorders

Hyperkinetic Disorders	Hypokinetic Disorders
Common	**Common**
Chorea	Parkinsonism
Dystonia	
Myoclonus	
Restless legs syndrome	
Tremor	
Tic	
Less common	**Less common**
Abdominal dyskinesia	Apraxia
Akathitic movements	Blocking (holding) tics
Ataxia/asynergia/dysmetria	Cataplexy and drop attacks
Athetosis	Catatonia, psychomotor depression,
Ballism	and obsessional slowness
Hemifacial spasm	Freezing phenomenon
Hyperekplexia	Hesitant gaits
Hypnogenic dyskinesia	Hypothyroid slowness
Jumping disorders	Rigidity
Jumpy stumps	Stiff muscles
Movement of toes and fingers	
Myokymia and synkinesis	
Myorhythmia	
Paroxysmal dyskinesia	
Periodic movements in sleep	
REM sleep behavior disorder	
Stereotypy	

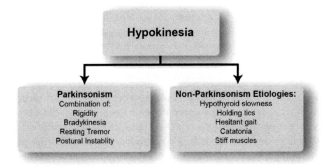

Figure 1.4
Classification of hypokinetic disorders according to the presence or absence of parkinsonism.

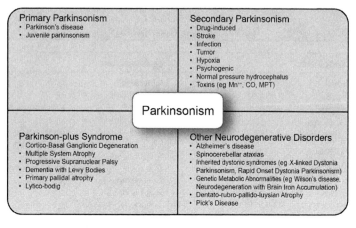

Figure 1.5
Classification of parkinsonism according to etiology.

- Secondary parkinsonism refers to parkinsonism with an identifiable cause, such as drug-induced parkinsonism (eg, by dopamine receptor blockers like antipsychotic and antiemetic drugs) or parkinsonism resulting from a stroke (vascular parkinsonism), infection (postencephalitic parkinsonism), or tumors in the basal ganglia.

- **Parkinson-plus syndromes** are progressive neurodegenerative disorders in which parkinsonism is the main but not the only feature. Examples of Parkinson-plus disorders are the following: *progressive supranuclear palsy*, often presenting with early dementia, vertical gaze palsy, and frequent falls at disease onset; *multiple system atrophy*, characteristically presenting with a lack of tremor, relatively prominent cerebellar features (eg, ataxia and incoordination), significant autonomic dysfunction (eg, urinary incontinence, erectile dysfunction, orthostatic hypotension), and pyramidal features (eg, turned-up toes and spasticity); and *corticobasoganglionic degeneration* or *corticobasal degeneration*, presenting with early dementia, cortical sensory loss, apraxia, limb dystonia, and "alien limb phenomenon" characterized by autonomous movements of a limb.

- Other neurodegenerative disorders can also present with parkinsonism. The main difference between this group of disorders and the parkinson-plus disorders is that parkinsonism is not their most prominent feature. For example, Alzheimer disease is primarily a neurodegenerative disorder of memory dysfunction, but parkinsonism can occur at the later stages of the illness.

Drop attacks are sudden falls that occur with or without a loss of consciousness. They are caused by either a collapse of postural muscle tone or an abnormal contraction of the leg muscles during ambulation or standing.

- About two-thirds of cases of drop attacks are of unclear etiology.

- Known causes include epilepsy, myoclonus, startle reactions, and structural central nervous system lesions (eg, cervical cord pathology from disk disease).

- Syncope is the most common nonneurological cause (Table 1.3).

Cataplexy is another cause of symptomatic drop attacks. Patients fall suddenly without a loss of consciousness, but with the inability to speak during an attack.

- There is often a preceding trigger, usually laughter or a sudden emotional stimulus.

- Cataplexy is one of the four cardinal features of narcolepsy, along with excessive sleepiness, sleep paralysis, and hypnagogic hallucinations (see Table 1.3).

Catatonia is a syndrome (not a specific diagnosis) that is characterized by catalepsy (development of fixed postures), waxy flexibility (retention of limbs for an indefinite period of time in the position in which they are placed), and mutism. It can also be associated with bizarre mannerisms.

- Patients remain in one position for hours and move exceedingly slowly in response to commands, but when they move spontaneously (eg, scratch themselves), they do so quickly.

- Catatonia is classically a feature of schizophrenia but can also occur with severe depression, hysterical disorders, and even organic brain disease (see Table 1.3).

Hypothyroid slowness can be mistaken for parkinsonism. Additional clues, such as decreased metabolic rate, cool temperature, bradycardia, myxedema, and a lack of the rigidity and resting tremors seen in parkinsonism, should suggest the diagnosis (see Table 1.3).

Table 1.3
Features of Other Nonparkinsonian Hypokinetic Movements

Drop Attacks	Cataplexy	Catatonia	Hypothyroid Slowness	Rigidity
• Collapse of postural muscle tone, typically without (but can be with) loss of consciousness	• Brief loss of postural muscle tone with inability to speak	• Development of fixed postures, waxy flexibility, mutism, and bizarre mannerisms	• Decreased metabolic rate • Cool temperature • Bradycardia • Myxedema	• Increased muscle tone, especially noted with slow, passive motion (ie, *not* velocity-dependent)

Rigidity is characterized by an increase in muscle tone that is especially noted during slow and passive motion. It is distinguished from spasticity (a sign of corticospinal/pyramidal tract pathology) in that it is present equally in all directions of the passive movement. Rigidity is not velocity-dependent and as such does not exhibit the "clasp-knife" phenomenon. Rigidity is almost always associated with parkinsonism but can occur independently.

HYPERKINETIC DISORDERS

To help determine the phenomenology of hyperkinetic movement disorders, evaluate features such as rhythmicity, speed, duration, and movement pattern (eg, repetitive, flowing, continual, paroxysmal, diurnal).

- Hyperkinetic movements can be described based on how they are induced (ie, stimuli, action, exercise); the complexity of the movements (complex or simple); and their suppressibility (by volitional attention or by "sensory tricks").

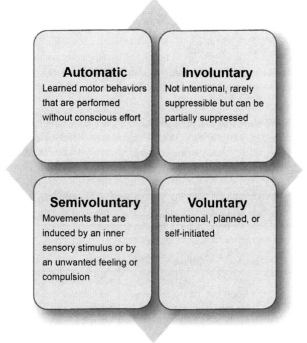

Automatic
Learned motor behaviors that are performed without conscious effort

Involuntary
Not intentional, rarely suppressible but can be partially suppressed

Semivoluntary
Movements that are induced by an inner sensory stimulus or by an unwanted feeling or compulsion

Voluntary
Intentional, planned, or self-initiated

Figure 1.6
Movement categories based on volition.

- It is also worthwhile to determine whether movements are accompanied by sensations such as restlessness or the urge to make a movement to release built-up tension.

- The description of a hyperkinetic movement disorder should always identify which body parts are involved.[2]

- As mentioned earlier, it is important to note that not all hyperkinetic movements are involuntary. Hyperkinetic (or hypokinetic) movements can be seen in four major states: *automatic, voluntary, semivoluntary* (eg, as in RLS or akathisia), and *involuntary* (Figure 1.6).

- Common hyperkinetic disorders include *RLS, dystonia, chorea, tics, myoclonus,* and *tremors* (Table 1.4).

Table 1.4 Characteristics of the Most Common Types of Hyperkinetic Disorders	
Chorea	Involuntary, irregular, purposeless, nonrhythmic, often abrupt, rapid, and unsustained movements seem to flow randomly from one body part to another; they are unpredictable in timing, direction, and distribution.
Dystonia	Both agonist and antagonist muscles of a body region contract simultaneously to produce a *twisted posture* of the limb, neck, or trunk. In contrast to chorea, dystonic movements repeatedly involve the same group of muscles. They do not necessarily flow or affect different muscle groups randomly.
Myoclonus	Sudden, brief, shocklike jerks are caused by muscular contraction (positive myoclonus) or inhibition (negative myoclonus, such as asterixis).
Restless legs syndrome	An unpleasant, crawling sensation in the legs (or arms), particularly during sitting and relaxation, is most prominent in the evening (but can also occur during the day). It disappears (or is significantly relieved) during ambulation.
Tics	Abnormal, stereotypic, repetitive movements (motor tics) or abnormal sounds (phonic tics) can be suppressed temporarily but may need to be "released" at some point. The release provides internal "relief" to the patient until the next "urge" is felt.
Tremor	An oscillatory, usually rhythmic (to-and-fro) movement of one or more body parts, such as the neck, tongue, chin, or vocal cords or a limb. The rate, location, amplitude, and constancy vary depending on the specific type of tremor. • Resting tremor • Postural/sustention tremor • Action/intention tremor

- Less common hyperkinetic movement disorders include entities such as *paroxysmal dyskinesia, stereotypies, episodic ataxia, RLS, periodic limb movements of sleep, myokymia, myorhythmia, hemifacial spasm,* and *hyperekplexia.*[1]

Chorea refers to involuntary, irregular, purposeless, nonrhythmic, abrupt, rapid, unsustained movements that seem to flow from one body part to another.

- They are unpredictable in timing, direction, and distribution.

- They can be partially suppressed, and the patient can often camouflage some of the movements by incorporating them into semipurposeful movements (termed *parakinesia*).

- An example of a movement disorder that presents primarily with chorea is Huntington's disease.

Involuntary movements that are slow, writhing, and continuous are sometimes called *athetosis.* **Athetosis** has been used in two senses: to describe a class of slow, writhing, continuous, involuntary movements and to describe the syndrome of athetoid cerebral palsy.

- Athetotic movements affect the limbs, especially distally, but can also involve the axial musculature, including that of the neck, face, and tongue.

- Athetosis is often associated with sustained contractions producing abnormal posturing. In this regard, athetosis can blend with dystonia.

- However, these involuntary movements can sometimes be faster and blend with those of chorea; the term *choreoathetosis* is then used.

- *Pseudoathetosis* refers to distal athetoid movements of the fingers and toes due to loss of proprioception.[2]

- When movements are very large in amplitude and involve primarily the proximal parts of the limbs, causing flinging and flailing limb movements, they are referred to as *ballism.*

- **Ballism** is frequently unilateral and is classically (but not solely) described as resulting from a lesion of the contralateral subthalamic nucleus.

- Athetosis, chorea, and ballism may represent a continuum of one type of hyperkinetic movement disorder and are sometimes combined (*choreoathetosis* or *chorea-ballism*) (Figure 1.7).

Dystonia is characterized by involuntary, sustained, patterned, and often repetitive contractions of opposing muscles, causing twisting movements or abnormal postures.

- In contrast to the movements of chorea, which are more random in nature, dystonic movements repeatedly involve the same group of muscles (Table 1.5). The movements appear to progress to prolonged abnormal postures.

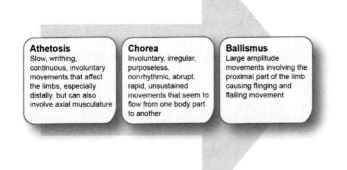

Figure 1.7
The spectrum of chorea.

Table 1.5
Classification of Dystonia Based on Distribution

Distribution	Description
Focal	Single body part (eg, blepharospasm, spasmodic torticollis, writer's cramp)
Segmental	Two or more contiguous regions of the body (eg, craniocervical dystonia or Meige syndrome)
Generalized	Trunk, legs, and other body parts (eg, idiopathic torsion dystonia)

- The abnormal posturing is caused by the simultaneous contraction or co-contraction of the agonist and antagonist group of muscles.

- Patterned involvement means that the movements affect the same muscle groups repeatedly.

- Initially, dystonia manifests mostly with voluntary action of the affected part and disappears with rest. This is called *action dystonia.*

- Dystonia can also involve distant muscle groups that are not primarily involved with the voluntary action (eg, abnormal posturing of the hands while the patient walks). This often occurs with progression of the disease and is called *overflow dystonia*. Overflow dystonia can also be seen in athetosis and dopa-induced dyskinesias.

■ Dystonia may eventually be present even during rest, as the disease progresses. Therefore, organicity of the dystonia is often questioned when the abnormal posturing occurs suddenly and is initially present at rest, rather than during action.

■ Primary dystonia usually begins as action dystonia and may persist as a kinetic or clonic dystonia. Secondary dystonia can begin with sustained postures (tonic dystonia).

■ The speed of the movement in dystonia varies widely.[2] The duration of the co-contraction contributes to the variation in the presentation of dystonia (Table 1.6).

■ A feature that is unique to dystonia is that the movements can often diminish with a tactile or proprioceptive *geste antagoniste* ("sensory trick").

○ This phenomenon can be seen as a reduction in muscle contraction when the involved body part or adjacent area is touched (or sometimes, just nearly touched).

○ Eliciting this sign suggests an organic rather than a psychogenic movement disorder.[2]

■ Tonic ocular deviation is a specific kind of dystonia. Upward tonic deviation is usually called *oculogyric crisis*. Although oculogyria is commonly associated with dopamine receptor blockers, it was initially associated with encephalitis lethargica and has been documented to occur along with other parkinsonian syndromes due to biochemical deficiencies of the monoamine pathways, such as pterin deficiency and aromatic amino acid deficiency.[2]

■ A particular form of dystonia appears when the patient is eating. The tongue is uncontrollably pushed out of the mouth during chewing. As a result, food is pushed out of the mouth and the tongue is bitten. This type

Table 1.6
Dystonic Presentations According to the Duration of Co-Contraction

Type	Description
Athetotic dystonia	Slow writhing movements with superimposed posturing
Myoclonic dystonia	Superimposed, shocklike movements or jerks in a twisted body part
Dystonic movement	Sustained for seconds
Dystonic postures	Sustained for minutes to hours
Dystonic tremors	Intermittent, usually arrhythmic tremors that are superimposed over a dystonic body part

of dystonia, termed *lingual feeding dystonia*, is almost pathognomonic for neuroacanthocytosis.[2]

Myoclonus is a sudden, brief, shocklike jerk caused by muscular contraction (positive myoclonus) or inhibition (negative myoclonus) (Table 1.7).

- The most common form of negative myoclonus is asterixis. Asterixis is commonly associated with metabolic encephalopathies. It is seen as a brief flapping of an outstretched limb.

- Myoclonus often arises from lesions elsewhere in the central nervous system and does not appear to be related primarily to any basal ganglia pathology.

- Lesions that produce myoclonus may be located in the cerebral cortex (*cortical reflex myoclonus*), brainstem (*reticular reflex myoclonus, hyperekplexia, rhythmic brainstem myoclonus, ocular myoclonus*), or spinal cord (*rhythmic segmental myoclonus, nonrhythmic propriospinal myoclonus*).

Restless legs syndrome is defined as a syndrome induced by a desire to move the legs. RLS is a very common illness.

- Although the legs are commonly involved, the same restless sensation has been described in the arms and even the trunk.

- There are two distinct types of RLS: primary (idiopathic) and secondary (Table 1.8).

- Moreover, the diagnostic criteria have been recently updated (Table 1.9).

Table 1.7
"Positive" Versus "Negative" Myoclonus

Positive Myoclonus (Muscle Contraction)	Negative Myoclonus (Muscle Inhibition)
Associated with: • Epileptic syndromes • Drugs • Metabolic disturbance • Central nervous system lesions	Associated with: • Asterixis (hepatic or renal impairment)

Table 1.8
Types of Restless Legs Syndrome

Primary	Usually a positive family history, an autosomal dominant mode of inheritance, and a high concordance rate in monozygotic twins
Secondary	Often associated with iron deficiency anemia, pregnancy, end-stage renal disease, and certain medications, such as antidepressants and dopamine antagonists

Table 1.9
Restless Legs Syndrome

Standardized Clinical Criteria for Restless Legs Syndrome
• The patient experiences a desire to move the limbs (with or without paresthesias), and the arms may be involved.
• The urge to move or the unpleasant sensation is relieved by activity, and symptoms are worse during rest or inactivity.
• The urge to move or the unpleasant sensations are partially or totally relieved by movement.
• The symptoms have a circadian variation, occurring most often in the evening or at night when the patient lies down. Patients often describe an unpleasant, crawling sensation in the legs, particularly when they are sitting and relaxing in the evening, that disappear when they are walking.

Tics consist of abnormal movements (*motor tics*) and/or abnormal sounds (*phonic tics*).

■ When both types of tics are present, occur in a person younger than 15 years of age, and are accompanied by obsessive–compulsive features, the designation of *Tourette syndrome* is commonly applied.

■ Tics frequently vary in severity over time, and patients can have remissions and exacerbations.

■ Motor and phonic tics can be simple (eg, a grunt) or complex (eg, a phrase or full sentence). Most of the time tics are repetitive or stereotypic.

■ They can be suppressed temporarily but will need to be "released" at some point to provide internal "relief" to the patient until the next "urge" is felt.

■ Examples include shoulder shrugging, head jerking, blinking, twitching of the nose, touching other people, head shaking with shoulder shrugging, kicking of the legs, obscene gesturing, grunting, and throat clearing.

Tremors are oscillatory, usually rhythmic, to-and-fro regular movements affecting one or more body parts, such as the limbs, neck, tongue, chin, or vocal cords.

■ The rate, location, amplitude, and constancy vary depending on the specific type of tremor (Table 1.10).

■ Tremors can be present at rest (*resting tremor*), while a posture is held (*postural tremor*), or during actions like writing and pouring water (*intention* or *kinetic tremor*).

Table 1.10
Phenomenologic Classification of Tremors

Types of Tremor		
Resting	Tremors are evident when the affected body part is supported against gravity (and often diminish or disappear during voluntary movement).	
Action	Tremors are evident during voluntary movement.	
	Different types of action tremor:	
	Postural	Evident during maintenance of an antigravity posture, such as keeping the arms in an outstretched horizontal position
	Kinetic	Evident when the voluntary movement starts (*initial tremor*), during the course of the movement (*dynamic tremor*), or as the affected body part approaches the target (*terminal tremor*)
	Task-specific	Evident or exacerbated only while a certain task is performed (eg, handwriting tremor, voice tremor)
	Position-specific	Evident while a certain posture is maintained
	Isometric	Evident during voluntary muscular contraction without a change in the position of the body part

Table 1.11
Classification of Hyperkinesia Based on Duration and Repetitiveness

Paroxysmal (Sudden and Intermittent)	Continual (Repetitive)	Continuous (Nonstop)
Tics	Ballism	Abdominal dyskinesia
Paroxysmal kinesigenic dyskinesia	Chorea	Athetosis
Paroxysmal nonkinesigenic dyskinesia	Dystonic movements	Tremors
	Myoclonus, arryhthmic	Dystonic postures
Paroxysmal tremor	Akathitic moaning	Minipolymyoclonus
Paroxysmal ataxia		Myoclonus, rhythmic
Hypnogenic dystonia		Tardive stereotypy
Stereotypies		Myokymia
Akathitic movements		Tic status
Jumpy stumps		Moving toes/fingers
		Myorhythmia

The various types of hyperkinesia can also be described in terms of the suddenness and duration of their presentation (Table 1.11). *Paroxysmal dyskinesia* episodes are often sudden and end abruptly. Movements are *continual* if they appear as recurring episodes, whereas *continuous* episodes are nonstop and nonrepetitive.

Table 1.12
Less Common Types of Hyperkinesia

Akathisia	A feeling of inner, general restlessness that is reduced or relieved by moving about
Hemifacial spasm	Unilateral facial muscle contractions that may be either clonic (continual, rapid, brief, repetitive) or tonic (prolonged, sustained spasms) interrupted by periods of quiescence
Painful legs/moving toes	Toes (unilateral or bilateral) are in continual flexion–extension with some lateral motion; usually associated with deep pain in the leg
Jumpy stumps	Involuntary, chaotic movements of the remaining stump (amputated limb)
Belly dancer's dyskinesia	Abnormal movements of the abdominal wall resulting in movement of the umbilicus (usually associated with trauma)
Stereotypy	Coordinated movements that are repeated continually and identically (usually in patients with tardive dyskinesia, schizophrenia, intellectual disability, or autism)
Myorhythmia	Low-frequency, continuous, patterned, relatively rhythmic movement that occurs during rest but may persist during activity
Hyperekplexia	Excessive motor response or jump in response to unexpected auditory and sometimes somesthetic and visual stimuli

Table 1.13
Hyperkinetic Disorders Classified Based on Speed of Movements (Fast Versus Slow)

Fastest	Intermediate	Slowest
Minipolymyoclonus	Chorea	Moving toes/fingers
Myoclonus	Ballism	Myorhythmia
Hyperekplexia	Jumpy stumps	Akathitic movements
Hemifacial spasm	Tardive stereotypy	

Finally, some movement disorders are not as common but still noteworthy (Table 1.12).

USEFUL CLUES IN IDENTIFYING MOVEMENT DISORDERS

Hyperkinetic disorders can be further classified based on the speed of the movements (Table 1.13), their amplitude (Table 1.14), and their response to voluntary control (Tables 1.15 and 1.16).[1]

Table 1.14
Hyperkinetic Disorders Based on Amplitude of Movements (Large Versus Small)

Large	Medium	Small
Ballism	Chorea and all others	Minipolymyoclonus

Note: Tremors may present with a large, medium, or small amplitude.

Table 1.15
Classification of Hyperkinetic Movements Based on Force Required to Overcome Them

Difficult to Overcome	Intermediate	Easy to Overcome
Stiff-person syndrome Jumpy stump	Dystonia	Resting tremor Postural tremor Chorea

Table 1.16
Suppressible and Nonsuppressible Forms of Dyskinesia

Suppressible	Stereotypies > tics, akathitic movements > chorea > ballism > dystonia > tremor > moving toes
Nonsuppressible	Hemifacial spasm, minipolymyoclonus, myoclonus, hyperekplexia, myorhythmia, moving toes/fingers

Hyperkinetic movements can also be described in terms of their relation to sleep. Most movement disorders disappear or diminish during sleep. Some persist, and a few appear only during sleep (Table 1.17).

Hyperkinetic movements can also be described in terms of their relationship to voluntary movement. Some types of hyperkinesia appear only when a limb is at rest, and others appear only during active limb movement. Patients with the latter are asymptomatic while at rest in a supine or sitting position. Several types appear regardless of whether or not there is voluntary movement (Table 1.18).

Several conditions manifest with a combination of types of hyperkinesia. The phenomenology of the movements is difficult to classify under any one particular description. This phenomenon is usually seen in a few conditions, which are listed in Table 1.19.

Dyskinetic movements can also be associated with characteristic symptoms that can help focus the differential diagnosis (Table 1.20). These may require

Table 1.17
Hyperkinesia Classified According to Level of Sensorium

Appears During Sleep and Disappears on Awakening	Persists During Sleep	Diminishes During Sleep
Hypnogenic dyskinesias Periodic movements in sleep REM sleep behavior disorder	Secondary palatal myoclonus Ocular myoclonus Spinal myoclonus Oculofaciomasticatory myorhythmia Moving toes Myokymia Neuromyotonia (Isaacs syndrome) Severe dystonia Severe tics	All others

Table 1.18
Hyperkinesia in Relation to State of Activity

At Rest Only (Disappears With Action)	With Action Only	At Rest and Continues With Action
Akathitic movements Paradoxical dystonia Resting tremor (but can reemerge with posture holding) Restless legs Orthostatic tremor (only while subject is standing still)	Ataxia Action dystonia Action myoclonus Orthostatic tremor Tremor (postural, action, intention) Task-specific tremor Task-specific dystonia	Abdominal dyskinesia Athetosis Chorea Dystonia Jumpy stumps Minipolymyoclonus Moving toes/fingers Myoclonus Myokymia Pseudodystonia Tics

Table 1.19
Diseases Presenting With the Phenomenology of More Than One Movement Disorder

Disease	Phenomenology
Psychogenic movement disorders	Myoclonus, dystonia, chorea, tremor
Tardive syndromes	Dystonia (typically retrocollis, opisthotonus, sometimes blepharospasm); chorea (typically oral–lingual–buccal); akathisia; myoclonus; tics

continued

Table 1.19 (cont.)
Diseases Presenting With the Phenomenology of More Than One Movement Disorder

Disease	Phenomenology
Neuroacanthocytosis	Chorea (with characteristic food propulsion during eating), dystonia, akathisia, tics
Wilson's disease	Tremor (sometimes characteristically described as "wing beating"), parkinsonism, dystonia, and sometimes chorea
Dentatorubropallidoluysian atrophy (DRPLA)	Cerebellar ataxia, choreoathetosis, dystonia, rest and postural tremor, parkinsonism
Huntington's disease	Chorea, dystonia, motor impersistence, dysarthria, parkinsonism (in juvenile Huntington's disease), sometimes myoclonus, tics
X-linked dystonia parkinsonism	Dystonia (typically seen early in the disease), parkinsonism (more prominent later in the disease)
Spinocerebellar ataxia (SCA) types 1, 2, 3, 17	Ataxia, parkinsonism, dystonia (SCA type 3), chorea (SCA types 1, 2, 3)
Rapid-onset dystonia parkinsonism	Dystonia, parkinsonism
Myoclonus–dystonia syndrome	Myoclonus, dystonia (alcohol-responsive)

Table 1.20
Dyskinesia With Various Characteristic Associated Findings

Associated Findings	Etiology
Dyskinesia with vocalizations	Huntington's disease Neuroacanthocytosis Cranial dystonia
Dyskinesia with self-mutilation	Lesch-Nyhan syndrome Neuroacanthocytosis Tourette syndrome Psychogenic movement disorders
Dyskinesia with complex movements	Stereotypies Tics Psychogenic movement disorders
Dyskinesia with a sensory component	Akathisia Painful legs/moving toes syndrome Restless legs syndrome

continued

Table 1.20 (cont.)
Dyskinesia With Various Characteristic Associated Findings

Associated Findings	Etiology
Dyskinesia of ocular movements	Oculogyric crises Opsoclonus Ocular myoclonus Ocular myorhythmia Ocular dysmetria Nystagmus
Dyskinesia with epilepsy	Myoclonus epilepsy with ragged red fibers Kearns-Sayre syndrome Infantile myoclonus epilepsy Infantile convulsions and choreoathetosis syndrome Anti-N-methyl-d-aspartate (NMDA) receptor encephalitis Leigh disease Dentatorubropallidoluysian atrophy (DRPLA) Huntington's disease–like 2 and 3 Neuroacanthocytosis Encephalopathy
Dyskinesia with neuropathy	Fragile X–associated tremor/ataxia syndrome Neuroacanthocytosis Riley-Day syndrome Machado-Joseph disease (spinocerebellar ataxia 3)
Dyskinesia with gastrointestinal symptoms	Sandifer syndrome Celiac disease Gluten hypersensitivity
Dyskinesia with dementia	Huntington's disease Lafora disease Creutzfeldt-Jakob disease Hashimoto encephalitis
Dyskinesia that responds to alcohol intake	Essential tremor Alcohol-responsive myoclonus syndrome

a longer period of observation. Being aware of these symptoms and including them in the description of the phenomenology may help in narrowing the etiology.

Finally, the differential diagnosis for a *pediatric* patient presenting with a movement disorder can be different from that for an adult patient. Table 1.21 lists some of the disorders to consider when a pediatric patient presents with a hyperkinetic disorder.

Table 1.21
Differential Diagnoses to Consider in a Pediatric Patient With a Movement Disorder

Hyperkinetic Disorder	Differential Diagnosis
Chorea	Sydenham chorea Huntington's disease Wilson's disease Fahr disease Pantothenate kinase–associated neurodegeneration (PKAN) Ramsay Hunt syndrome (dentatorubral atrophy) Neuroaxonal dystrophy Lesch-Nyhan syndrome Pelizaeus-Merzbacher syndrome Metabolic: hyper- and hypothyroidism, hyper- and hypoparathyroidism Drugs: phenytoin, phenothiazines, lithium, amphetamine Toxins: mercury, carbon monoxide
Dystonia	Huntington's disease Wilson's disease Fahr disease PKAN Ceroid lipofuscinosis Sea-blue histiocytosis Leigh disease GM1/GM2 gangliosidosis Dystonia musculorum deformans Dopamine-responsive dystonia Tumors Trauma Encephalitis
Ataxia (acute)	Acute cerebellar ataxia Occult neuroblastoma Traumatic posterior fossa hematoma, subdural/epidural Fisher variant of Guillain-Barré syndrome Basilar migraine Metabolic: maple syrup urine disease, Hartnup pyruvate decarboxylase deficiency, arginosuccinic aciduria, hypothyroidism Acute intermittent familial ataxia Childhood multiple sclerosis/Schilder disease Leigh disease
Ataxia (chronic)	Cerebellar hypoplasia Arnold-Chiari malformation Dandy Walker syndrome Cerebral palsy

continued

Table 1.21 (cont.)
Differential Diagnoses to Consider in a Pediatric Patient With a Movement Disorder

Hyperkinetic Disorder	Differential Diagnosis
	Tumors: medulloblastoma, cerebellar astrocytoma
	Spinocerebellar ataxias
	Friedreich ataxia
	Roussy-Levy form (hereditary motor sensory neuropathy type 1)
	Ataxia telangiectasia
	Bassen-Kornzweig syndrome
	Refsum disease
	Metachromatic leukodystrophy
	Tay-Sachs disease
	Maple syrup urine disease
Myoclonus	Wilson's disease
	PKAN
	Lafora body disease
	Ceroid lipofuscinosis
	Ramsay Hunt syndrome (dyssynergia cerebellaris myoclonica)
	Ataxia telangiectasia
	Subacute sclerosing panencephalitis
	Herpes simplex virus infection
	Herpes zoster
	HIV infection
	Metabolic: hypoglycemia, uremia, hepatic failure, hyponatremia
	Hypoxia
	Bismuth toxicity

REFERENCES

1. Frucht SJ, Fahn S. A brief introduction to movement disorders. In: Frucht SJ, Fahn S, eds. *Movement Disorder Emergencies: Diagnosis and Treatment.* Totowa, NJ: Humana Press; 2005:1–8.
2. Fahn S, Jankovic J, Hallett M. Clinical overview and phenomenology of movement disorders. In: Fahn S, Jankovic J, Hallett M, eds. *Principles and Practice of Movement Disorders.* 2nd ed. Edinburgh, United Kingdom: Elsevier Saunders; 2011:1–35.
3. Schrag A. Epidemiology of movement disorders. In: Jankovic J, Tolosa E, eds. *Parkinson's Disease and Movement Disorders.* 4th ed. Philadelphia, PA: Lippincott Williams & Wilkins; 2002:73–89.

II

Neurological Approach to
Movement Disorders

2

TREMORS

Tremor is defined as a rhythmic, involuntary, oscillating movement of a body part occurring in isolation or as part of a clinical syndrome. In clinical practice, characterization of tremor is important for etiologic consideration and treatment. Common types include resting tremor, postural tremor, kinetic tremor, intention tremor, and task-specific tremor.

PATHOPHYSIOLOGY

The pathophysiology of tremor is not fully understood. However, four basic mechanisms are linked to the production of tremor.[1,2] It is likely that combinations of these mechanisms produce tremor in different disease states (Figure 2.1).

- *Mechanical oscillations* of the limb can occur at a particular joint; this mechanism applies in cases of *physiologic tremor*.

- *Reflex oscillation* is elicited by afferent muscle spindle pathways and is responsible for stronger tremors by synchronization. This mechanism is a possible cause of tremor in hyperthyroidism or other toxic states.

- *Central oscillators* are groups of cells in the central nervous system in the thalamus, basal ganglia, and inferior olives. These cells have the capacity to fire repetitively and produce tremor. *Parkinsonian tremors* may originate in the basal ganglia, and *essential tremors* may originate within the inferior olives and thalamus.

- Abnormal functioning of the cerebellum can produce tremor. Positron emission tomography studies have shown cerebellar activation in almost all forms of tremor.[3]

Two neuronal pathways are of particular importance in the production of tremor (Figure 2.2).[4]

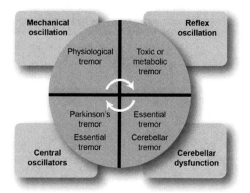

Figure 2.1
Pathophysiology of different etiologies of tremor.

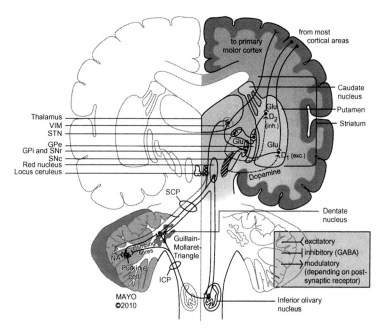

Figure 2.2
Schematic and simplified synopsis of the brain regions and pathways involved in tremorogenesis. See text for details. D1, dopamine receptor type 1; D2, dopamine receptor type 2; exc., excitatory; GABA, gamma-amino butyric acid; Glu, glutamate; GPe, external globus pallidus; GPi, internal globus pallidus; ICP, inferior cerebellar peduncle; inh., inhibitory; SCP, superior cerebellar peduncle; SNc, substantia nigra, pars compacta; SNr, substantia nigra, pars reticulata; STN, subthalamic nucleus; VIM, ventrointermediate nucleus of thalamus.

From Ref. 4: Puschmann A, Wszolek ZK. Diagnosis and treatment of common forms of tremor. Semin Neurol 2011;31(1), 65–77, with permission.

- One is the corticostriatothalamocortical loop through the basal ganglia. This pathway maintains the ongoing pattern of movement.

- The other pathway connects the red nucleus, inferior olivary nucleus, and dentate nucleus, forming the "Guillain-Mollaret triangle." This pathway is involved in fine-tuning the precision of voluntary movements.

CLASSIFICATION (Figure 2.3)

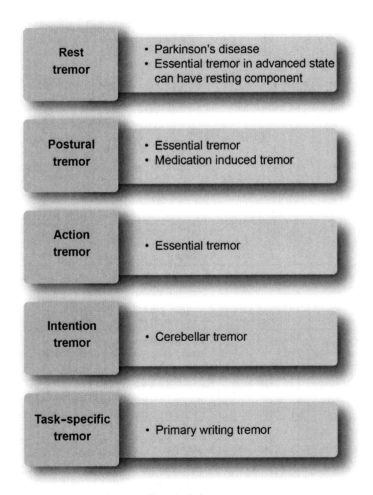

Rest tremor
- Parkinson's disease
- Essential tremor in advanced state can have resting component

Postural tremor
- Essential tremor
- Medication induced tremor

Action tremor
- Essential tremor

Intention tremor
- Cerebellar tremor

Task-specific tremor
- Primary writing tremor

Figure 2.3
Classification of tremors.

RESTING TREMOR. Resting tremor occurs when the affected extremity is at complete rest and diminishes with movement of the affected body part.

POSTURAL TREMOR. Postural tremor occurs when the affected limb is held in sustention against gravity.

ACTION OR KINETIC TREMOR. Action or kinetic tremor occurs during voluntary movement.

INTENTION TREMOR. Intention (or terminal) tremor manifests as a marked increase in tremor amplitude during the terminal portion of a targeted movement.

TASK-SPECIFIC TREMOR. Task-specific tremor emerges during a specific activity. An example of this type is primary writing tremor.

CLINICAL DISORDERS (Table 2.1)

Table 2.1
Tremor Characteristics by Condition

Diagnosis	Predominant Tremor	Remarks
Parkinson's disease	Resting	Associated symptoms include rigidity, bradykinesia, and postural instability. Usually an elderly patient (> 50 y) with asymmetric onset, 4–6 Hz.
Essential tremor	Postural and kinetic	Usually symmetric, responds to alcohol, bimodal age at onset (teens, > 50 y), 4–10 Hz.
Cerebellar tremor	Intention	Postural component may be present, other cerebellar features on examination. Unilateral or bilateral depending on location of lesion, 2–4 Hz.
Holmes tremor	Rest, postural, and intention	Seen in multiple sclerosis and traumatic brain injury, 2–5 Hz.
Dystonic tremor	Postural and intention	Abnormal posture of affected limb may be observed, variable frequency, 4–8 Hz.
Enhanced physiologic tremor	Postural	Check for metabolic disorders (thyroid, diabetes, renal failure, liver disease) or tremor-inducing drugs, 8–12 Hz.
Orthostatic tremor	Postural, in the legs, upon standing	Usually occurs when patient stands up, improves with ambulation and sitting, 15–18 Hz.
Palatal tremor	Postural	1–6 Hz.
Neuropathic tremor	Postural and kinetic	In association with neuropathy, 5–9 Hz.
Wilson's disease	Resting, postural, or action	All tremor types are possible; "wing-beating tremor" usually manifests later. Should be considered in any movement disorder in a patient < 50 y.

Physiologic Tremor

Physiologic tremor is a very-low-amplitude, fine tremor (6–12 Hz) that is barely visible to the eye.

- It is present in every normal person while a posture or movement is being maintained.

- The neurological examination is often nonfocal in patients with physiologic tremor.

Enhanced Physiologic Tremor

Enhanced physiologic tremor is a high-frequency, low-amplitude, visible tremor that occurs primarily when a specific posture is maintained.

- Drugs and toxins induce this form of tremor. The suspected mechanism is mechanical activation at the muscular level. Signs and symptoms of drug toxicity or other side effects may or may not be present.

- Trigger conditions include hyperthyroidism, liver disease, benzodiazepine withdrawal, lithium, valproate, calcium channel blockers, anxiety, and hypoglycemia, among other conditions.

- Tremor symptoms can improve after the discontinuation of the causative agents or management of the underlying problem.

Parkinson's Disease

Parkinson tremor (see also Chapter 4 and Table 2.2) is often characterized by a low-frequency resting tremor typically seen as a *pill-rolling tremor*. Some patients may have postural and action tremors as well. Resting tremors may also be observed in other parkinsonian syndromes.

- Parkinson tremors occur in association with other symptoms, such as micrographia, slowness (bradykinesia), and muscle rigidity.

- A characteristic feature of the symptoms in Parkinson's disease (PD) is the asymmetric nature of the symptoms, especially early in the disease.

- The characteristic frequency associated with this tremor is 4 to 6 Hz. Tremors can emerge during posture (reemergent tremor when it occurs a few seconds after the hands have been held in sustention) and action.

- The areas most commonly affected include the hands, legs, chin, and jaw.

- Patients sometimes complain of the sensation of "internal tremors" that are not visible externally.

Table 2.2
Characteristics of Parkinsonian Versus Essential Tremor

Characteristic	Essential Tremor	Parkinson Tremor
Tremor type	Postural and action tremors	Resting tremor
Age	All age groups	Older age (> 60 y)
Family history	Positive in > 60% of patients	Usually negative
Alcohol response	Often beneficial	Not beneficial
Tremor onset	Usually bilateral	Unilateral in about 80%
Muscle tone	Normal	Cogwheel rigidity
Facial expression	Normal	Decreased
Gait	Normal	Decreased arm swing
Tremor latency during hand sustention	None or shorter: 1–2 sec	Longer, sometimes up to 8–9 sec

Essential Tremor

Essential tremor (ET) (Table 2.2) is the most common type of tremor disorder in the general population.

- The characteristic tremors seen in ET are postural and action tremors, with a frequency between 4 and 8 Hz. Most patients have a symmetric onset of their tremor.

- In familial ET, the mode of inheritance is autosomal dominant, with incomplete penetrance.

  ○ A positive family history is reported by 50% to 70% of patients with ET.

- The tremor worsens during eating, drinking, and writing.

- Drinking alcohol may temporarily help to alleviate ET.

- The most hands, head, and voice are most commonly affected, but tremors can also be seen in the legs, trunk, and face.

- Mild resting tremor can sometimes develop in patients with long-standing ET.

- The tremor in ET is exacerbated by conditions such as stress, exercise, fatigue, caffeine, and certain medications, and it improves with relaxation and alcohol.

- Other associated symptoms can include mild gait difficulty, manifested as tandem walking.

- Some patients with ET have decreased hearing.

- Several tremor conditions are believed to be variants of essential tremor, including the following:

  - Task-specific tremor (eg, primary writing tremor)

  - Isolated voice tremor

  - Isolated chin tremor

Cerebellar Tremor

Cerebellar tremor is a slow-frequency tremor, between 3 and 5 Hz. It occurs during the execution of a goal-directed (intentional) movement.

- The amplitude usually increases with the movement and as the intended target is approached, and the tremor can be associated with a postural component.

- Signs and symptoms of cerebellar dysfunction may be present, including ataxia, dysmetria, dysdiadochokinesia, and dysarthria.

- Another tremor with a cerebellar etiology is titubation, better described as a slow-frequency "bobbing" motion of the head or trunk.

- It is usually seen in conditions such as multiple sclerosis, hereditary ataxia syndromes, brainstem stroke affecting cerebellar pathways, and traumatic brain injury.

  Unfortunately, these tremors are highly disabling and very difficult to treat.

Holmes Tremor

Holmes tremor or *rubral tremor* designates a combination of rest, postural, and action tremors due to midbrain lesions in the vicinity of the red nucleus.

- This type of tremor is irregular and of low frequency (2–4 Hz).

- Signs of ataxia and weakness may be present.

- Common causes include cerebrovascular accident and multiple sclerosis, with a possible delay of 2 weeks to 2 years in tremor onset and the occurrence of lesions.

- The tremor is disabling and resistant to treatment.

Dystonic Tremor

As the name implies, dystonic tremor is a tremor that occurs in a body region affected by dystonia.

- It presents as a postural/action tremor with irregular amplitudes and frequencies.

- An example of this tremor is the dystonic, *no-no* or *yes-yes* head tremor associated with spasmodic torticollis. This tremor tends to be irregular or arrhythmic and may improve with a "sensory trick" (*geste antagoniste*), superimposed on abnormal neck posturing, in contrast to the rhythmic head tremor seen in ET.

Neuropathic Tremor

Neuropathic tremors are mostly postural or action tremors that occur in the setting of a peripheral neuropathy.

- They are more commonly associated with demyelinating neuropathies of the dysgammaglobulinemic type.[5]

- The tremor frequency is often described as between 3 and 6 Hz in the hand and arm muscles.

- The exact etiology of this tremor is unknown.

Palatal Tremor

Palatal tremors (see also Chapter 7) are brief, rhythmic, involuntary, low-frequency movements of the soft palate.
　　Palatal tremors are classified in two forms:

- *Symptomatic palatal tremor* is believed to arise from a lesion of the brainstem or cerebellum (within the Guillain-Mollaret triangle), resulting in a rhythmic contraction of the levator veli palatini. Movement of the edge of the palate is appreciated.

- *Essential palatal tremor* is not associated with central nervous system (CNS) lesions and is a result of the rhythmic contractions of the tensor veli palatini, often associated with an ear click. Movement of the roof of the palate is also seen.

Drug-Induced Tremors

Types of tremors induced by drugs include enhanced physiologic tremor, rest tremor, and action tremor. The signs and symptoms of drug-induced tremors depend on the drug used and on a patient's predisposition to its side effects. Some drugs cause extrapyramidal side effects manifesting as bradykinesia, rigidity, and tremor. Table 2.3 lists drugs that can induce tremor.

Table 2.3
List of Potential Toxins and Drugs Inducing Tremor

Toxins	Drugs
Alcohol	Adrenalin
Arsenic	Antiarrhythmics (amiodarone)
Carbon monoxide	Antidepressants
Cyanide	Caffeine
Cytostatics (vincristine, doxorubicin, cytosine arabinoside, ifosfamide)	Calcitonin
Dichlorodiphenyltrichloroethane (DDT)	Cocaine
Dioxins	Dopamine
Immunosuppressants (cyclosporin A)	Lithium
Kepone	Metoclopramide
Lead	Mexiletine, procainamide
Lindane	Neuroleptics
Manganese	Perhexiline
Mercury	Reserpine
Naphthalene	Steroids
Nicotine	Tetrabenazine
Phosphor	Theophylline
Toluene	Valproate
Thyroid hormones	

Source: Adapted from Refs. 6–8.

Hysterical Tremors

Also known as *psychogenic tremors*, hysterical tremors usually present a challenge in any neurological practice.

- Psychogenic tremors usually have an irregular frequency and are associated with sudden onsets and remissions.

- The frequency and amplitude may vary and diminish or disappear with distraction; a "coactivation sign" may be observed, and other somatization history may be present.

Orthostatic Tremor

Orthostatic tremor is tremor mostly confined to the legs that will occur upon standing and will subside with walking and sitting.

- There is no problem during sitting or lying down;
- The tremor rate is between 13 and 18 Hz (via electromyography [EMG]).
- Treatment includes low-dose clonazepam or primidone.

Tremor in Wilson's disease

All tremor types can be seen in Wilson's disease. This diagnosis should be considered for any patient with a movement disorder presenting before the age of 50 years.

- Resting and postural tremors are most common.
- The classic "wing-beating tremor" is not typically seen early in the disease, and it may be refractory to medication.
- Ataxia, parkinsonism, dysarthria, dystonia, and risus sardonicus are also common neurological manifestations.
- Wilson's disease is often accompanied by liver disease and psychiatric manifestations (eg, depression, anxiety, psychosis).

EVALUATION OF THE PATIENT WITH TREMOR

Once the history has been reviewed (ie, once the patient history of the neuropathy, drug use, and toxic exposure and the family history of tremors have been obtained), one should proceed with the physical examination (Table 2.4 and Figure 2.4).

Diagnostic Testing

A laboratory workup is not necessary for most patients with tremor. However, in some patients, a focused workup may be helpful (Table 2.5).

Treatment

PARKINSON'S DISEASE. The resting tremor in PD usually responds to dopaminergic therapy (dopamine agonists, levodopa) and anticholinergic agents (Table 2.6).

- Levodopa is the most efficacious medication, sometimes resulting in dramatic tremor suppression. It may be combined with dopamine agonists or anticholinergic agents in patients with resistant tremors.

Table 2.4
Clinical Examination of the Tremulous Patient

Technique	Examination Technique	Findings
Observe	What is the affected body region? Is there an abnormal body posture? Does the tremor occur at rest, or is it associated with purposeful movement? Are there leg tremors?	• Assess degree of disability; if head tremors only, consider spasmodic torticollis. • Suggests a dystonic tremor. Tremor at rest suggests PD. • Tremor with posture/intention suggests ET or other disorders. • If the tremors occur only with standing, orthostatic tremor is the most likely diagnosis; resting tremor with sitting is more suggestive of PD.
	Is there a masked facies? Is there reduced amplitude of movement? Is there voice tremor? Is there a shuffling gait?	• A masked facies or shuffling gait suggests parkinsonism. • Assess with finger taps, hand and arm movements; presence of bradykinesia suggests parkinsonism. • Suggestive of ET and dystonia; also seen in other conditions, but less pronounced. • Suggestive of parkinsonism.
Examine	With the patient keeping the extremities at rest, distract the patient by asking him or her to perform serial sevens.	• This maneuver may provoke the emergence of resting tremors (facilitation), suggestive of PD.
	Examine extremities in the postural position (hands in front with arms outstretched, parallel to the floor). Finger-to-nose testing.	• Postural tremors suggest ET; fast-frequency tremors may suggest exaggerated physiologic tremors; delay in tremors may suggest reemergent tremors, seen in PD. • Intention tremors and ataxia suggest cerebellar or Holmes tremors. • Intention tremors on their own suggest ET. • Intention tremors with dystonia suggest dystonic tremors.
	Examine for rigidity and bradykinesia, decreased arm swing.	• Presence of these suggests PD or any parkinsonian syndrome
	Examine for task-specific tremor by asking patient to write.	• Tremors manifest only during handwriting (primary writing tremor).

continued

Table 2.4 (cont.)
Clinical Examination of the Tremulous Patient

Technique	Examination Technique	Findings
	Examine for orthostatic tremor by asking patient to stand up and put both hands on leg.	• Orthostatic tremors are sometimes better felt with hands on the legs and may not be visible.
Stance/gait	Casual gait	• Shuffling suggests parkinsonian syndromes. • Wide-based gait suggests the presence of ataxia, seen with cerebellar tremor. • Freezing of gait suggests parkinsonian disorders. • Abnormal body postures suggest dytonia.
	Tandem gait	• Abnormalities may be seen in ET.
Speech evaluation	Prepared text may be helpful (eg, "The Rainbow Passage"). See Appendix.	• Altered articulation of words. • Abnormal fluency. • Slowed speech. • "Scanning dysarthria": words are broken into syllables. • Voice tremors.

Abbreviations: ET, essential tremor; PD, Parkinson's disease.

▦ For patients with disabling tremors not responding to usual doses, the dose can be escalated as tolerated. Side effects from medications are usually the limiting factor.

▦ For the patient who continues to have disabling, medication-refractory tremors despite comprehensive trials of medication, or for the patient who cannot tolerate medications because of side effects, functional neurosurgery is an option.[9] PD tremors have shown significant improvement with lesioning procedures (eg, thalamotomy) or with deep brain stimulation (of the thalamus, globus pallidus, or subthalamic nucleus).[10,11]

ESSENTIAL TREMOR. Propranolol and primidone are the preferred first-line treatments for essential tremor, alone or in combination (Table 2.7).

▦ There is often a better response for hand tremors than for voice and head tremors.

▦ The dose range for propranolol is from 10 to 60 mg divided 3 times per day, and for the long-acting formulation the range is 60 to 320 mg 1 or 2 times per day. Propranolol is relatively contraindicated in patients with asthma, diabetes, or cardiac arrhythmias.

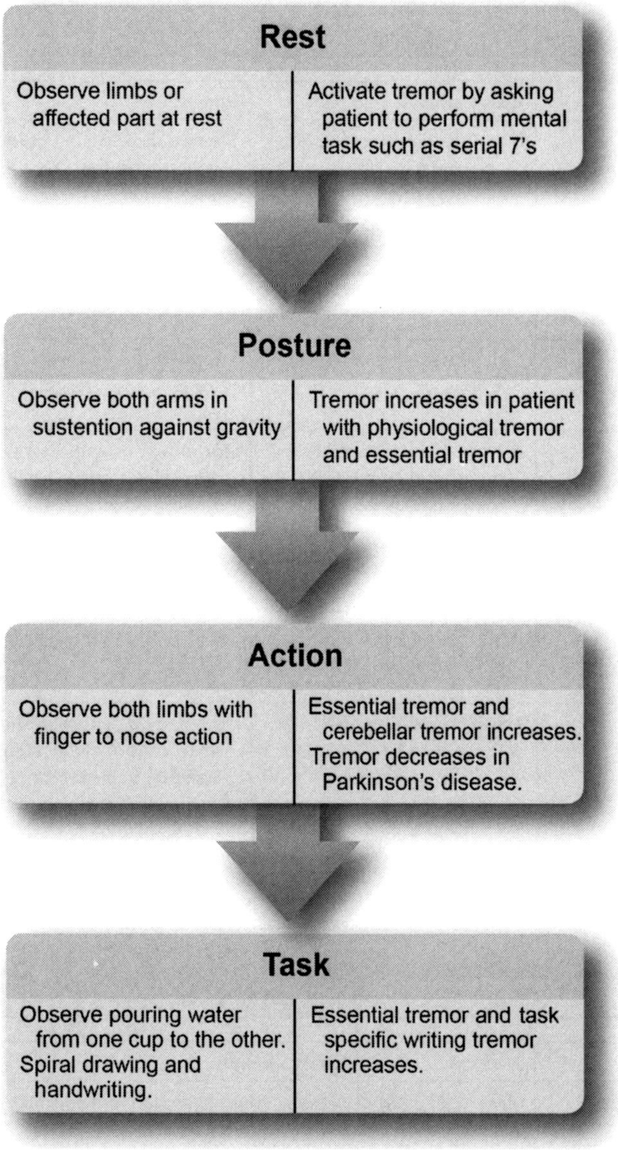

Figure 2.4
Sequence of examination for tremor.

Table 2.5
Diagnostic Workup for Tremor

Test	Recommendations	Comments
Thyroid function tests	If hypo/hyperthyroid, treat as neccesary.	Thyroid disorders, in particular hyperthyroidism, are associated with tremors.
Liver function studies	Screen for liver disease.	Hepatic encephalopathy may be associated with tremors.
Complete chemistry	Correct metabolic disturbances as necessary.	Uremia may induce tremors.
Serum ceruloplasmin	Usually obtained in patients < 50 y.	Twenty-four-hour urine collection for copper excretion is also recommended.
Toxicology screen	Assess for drug-induced tremors, illicit drug use, toxic etiology (mercury, lead, other).	Drug abuse or withdrawal (eg, ethanol withdrawal) may be associated with tremors.
Drug levels	Antiepileptic agents, immunosuppressants.	Common examples are cyclosporine, valproate.
MRI of the brain	Assess for structural, demyelinating, vascular lesions.	Cerebellar lesions for cerebellar tremors.
FP-CIT SPECT scan (DaTscan)	Assess for dopaminergic loss.	Differentiate parkinsonism (results in an abnormal DaTscan) from essential tremor or drug-induced tremor (results in a normal DaTscan).

Table 2.6
Pharmacologic Treatment Options for the Patient With Newly Diagnosed Parkinson's disease

Drug	Dose Range	Potential Side Effects
Carbidopa/ levodopa	300–1,200 mg/d	Nausea, vomiting, sedation, hallucinations
Ropinirole	8–24 mg/d	Nausea, vomiting, sedation, hallucinations, sleep attacks, impulse control disorder
Pramipexole	1.5–4.5 mg/d	Nausea, vomiting, sedation, hallucinations, sleep attacks, impulse control disorder

continued

Table 2.6 (cont.)
Pharmacologic Treatment Options for the Patient With Newly Diagnosed Parkinson's disease

Drug	Dose Range	Potential Side Effects
Rotigotine patch	6–8 mg/d	Nausea, vomiting, sedation, hallucinations, sleep attacks, impulse control disorder
Trihexyphenidyl	3–15 mg/d	Confusion, sedation, hallucinations, dry mouth, bladder retention
Benztropine	1–6 mg/d	Confusion, sedation, hallucinations, dry mouth, bladder retention
Amantadine	200–400 mg/d	Confusion, hallucinations, dry mouth, bladder retention, livedo reticularis, leg edema
Selegiline	5 mg 2 times per day (breakfast and lunch)	Confusion, hallucinations, insomnia
Rasagiline	0.5–1.0 mg/d	Confusion, hallucinations

Note: See also Chapter 3.

Table 2.7
Pharmacologic Therapy for Essential Tremor

Medication	Dosage[a]	Potential Side Effects
Propranolol	10–60 mg divided 2 or 3 times daily	Contraindicated in cardiac arrhythmias, diabetes, and pulmonary disorders. Watch for hypotension and depression.
Propranolol LA (long-acting formulation)	60–320 mg 1 or 2 times daily	Same as above.
Primidone	50–750 mg divided 3 times daily or given at bedtime	Sedation, nausea, dizziness, confusion.
Gabapentin (Neurontin)	900–2,400 mg divided 3 times daily	Leukopenia, somnolence, dizziness, ataxia
Topiramate	Up to 400 mg/d	Paresthesias, anorexia, difficulty with concentration, kidney stones.
Clonazepam	0.5–6 mg/d	Drowsiness.

[a]Slow titration schedules are recommended for all the above medications to reduce the incidence of side effects.

Source: Adapted from Refs. 14, 16.

- The recommended dose range for primidone is 50 to 750 mg divided 3 times per day. Primidone is associated with drowsiness, nausea, dizziness, and confusion.

- If monotherapy with primidone or propranolol is not beneficial, the two agents may be used in combination.

- Open-label studies and double-blinded studies have demonstrated the efficacy of botulinum toxin injections in treating limb, head, vocal, palatal, and other tremors.[12,13]

- Gabapentin has also been shown to improve ET in two studies, with a dosage range of 1,800 to 2,400 mg divided 3 times per day.

- Topiramate, clonazepam, and clozapine have also improved tremors in ET in multiple reports.[14] Patients experiencing worsening of tremors associated with anxiety may benefit from anxiolytics.

- As in PD, for patients who continue to have disabling tremors despite optimal medical therapy and an adequate medication trial or who cannot tolerate therapy as a result of side effects, thalamic lesioning or deep brain stimulation is an effective alternative.[15]

CEREBELLAR TREMOR. No medication has been consistently successful in the treatment of cerebellar tremors. Medications that can be tried include clonazepam, propranolol, trihexyphenidyl, levodopa, physostigmine, and topiramate.[17] Thalamic stimulation for disabling tremor may be an option, and referral to an experienced functional surgical center may be helpful.[18]

DYSTONIC TREMOR. Head, arm, and voice tremors resulting from dystonia have been shown to improve with botulinum toxin injections. Other medications that can be tried include anticholinergic agents, levodopa, propranolol, and clonazepam.[19]

ORTHOSTATIC TREMOR. The treatment of choice for orthostatic tremor is low-dose clonazepam. Phenobarbital, primidone, propranolol, levodopa, pramipexole, and gabapentin may also be tried when clonazepam fails or is not tolerated.

ENHANCED PHYSIOLOGIC TREMOR. The most important step in the treatment of enhanced physiologic tremor (EPT) is to find its cause. If a metabolic etiology is found during workup (eg, thyroid, glucose), it should be treated accordingly. In the anxious patient, treatment of the anxiety may improve tremors. If the tremors are drug-induced, decrease the dose or stop the suspected offending drug.

NEUROPATHIC TREMORS. To date, there no successful pharmacologic treatment has been reported for the treatment of neuropathic tremors. Medications such as clonazepam, primidone, and propranolol have been tried with inconsistent benefit. A patient with disabling neuropathic tremor has been reported to have benefited from thalamic deep brain stimulation.[20]

PALATAL TREMORS. Fortunately, palatal tremors are usually not disabling. Patients who are bothered by the ear click associated with essential palatal tremor may benefit from pharmacologic treatment with trihexyphenidyl, valproate, or flunarizine. Injection of botulinum toxin in the tensor veli palatini has also been reported to be beneficial.[21]

DRUG-INDUCED TREMORS. The treatment for drug-induced tremors usually consists of discontinuation or reduction of the dose of the offending agent.

WILSON'S DISEASE. Patients should adhere to a diet low in copper and avoid foods with a high copper content. These include shellfish, liver, pork, duck, lamb, avocados, dried beans, dried fruits, raisins, dates, prunes, bran, mushrooms, wheat germ, chocolate, and nuts. Consider agents that deplete copper: penicillamine (1–2 g/d) with pyridoxine (50 mg/d), trientine (500 mg 2 times daily), tetrathiomolybdate (80–120 mg daily in 3 to 4 divided doses), and zinc (50 mg/d without food). Thalamotomy has been reported to improve medication-resistant tremors.

REFERENCES

1. Deuschl G, Krack P, Lauk M, Timmer J. Clinical neurophysiology of tremor. *J Clin Neurophysiol.* 1996; 13:110–121.
2. Elble RJ. Central mechanisms of tremor. *J Clin Neurophysiol.* 1996; 13:133–144.
3. Wills AJ, Jenkins IH, Thompson PD. Red nuclear and cerebellar but no olivary activation associated with essential tremor: a positron emission tomographic study. *Ann Neurol.* 1994; 36:636–642.
4. Puschmann A, Wszolek ZK. Diagnosis and treatment of common forms of tremor. *Semin Neurol.* 2011; 31(1):65–77.
5. Bain PG, Britton TC, Jenkins IH, et al. Tremor associated with benign IgM paraproteinaemic neuropathy. *Brain.* 1996; 119(pt 3):789–799.
6. Karas BJ, Wilder BJ, Hammond EJ, Bauman AW. Valproate tremors. *Neurology.* 1982; 32(4):428–432.
7. LeDoux MS, McGill LJ, Pulsinelli WA, et al. Severe bilateral tremor in a liver transplant recipient taking cyclosporine. *Mov Disord.* 1998; 13(3):589–596.
8. Tarsy D, Indorf G. Tardive tremor due to metoclopramide. *Mov Disord.* 2002; 17(3):620–621.
9. Deuschl G, Schade-Brittinger C, Krack P, et al. A randomized trial of deep-brain stimulation for Parkinson's disease. *N Engl J Med.* 2006; 355(9):896–908.
10. Pahwa R, Factor SA, Lyons KE, et al. Practice parameter: treatment of Parkinson's disease with motor fluctuations and dyskinesia (an evidence-based review): report of the Quality Standards Subcommittee of the American Academy of Neurology. *Neurology.* 2006; 66(7):983–995.
11. Suchowersky O, Reich S, Perlmutter J, et al. Practice parameter: diagnosis and prognosis of new onset Parkinson's disease (an evidence-based review): report of the

Quality Standards Subcommittee of the American Academy of Neurology. *Neurology.* 2006; 66(7):968–975.

12. Jankovic J, Schwartz K, Clemence W, et al. A randomized, double-blind, placebo-controlled study to evaluate botulinum toxin type A in essential hand tremor. *Mov Disord.* 1996; 11(3):250–256.

13. Wissel J, Masuhr F, Schelosky L. Quantitative assessment of botulinum toxin treatment in 43 patients with head tremor. *Mov Disord.* 1997; 12:722–726.

14. Zesiewicz TA, Elble R, Louis ED, et al. Practice parameter: therapies for essential tremor: report of the Quality Standards Subcommittee of the American Academy of Neurology. *Neurology.* 2005; 64(12):2008–2020.

15. Hubble JP, Busenbark KL, Wilkinson S, et al. Deep brain stimulation for essential tremor. *Neurology.* 1996; 46(4):1150–1153.

16. Ondo WG. Essential tremor: treatment options. *Curr Treat Options Neurol.* 2006; 8(3):256–267.

17. Sechi G, Agnetti V, Sulas FM, et al. Effects of topiramate in patients with cerebellar tremor. *Prog Neuropsychopharmacol Biol Psychiatry.* 2003; 27(6):1023–1027.

18. Foote KD, Okun MS. Ventralis intermedius plus ventralis oralis anterior and posterior deep brain stimulation for posttraumatic Holmes tremor: two leads may be better than one: technical note. *Neurosurgery.* 2005; 56(2 suppl):E445, discussion E.

19. Singer C, Papapetropoulos S, Spielholz NI. Primary writing tremor: report of a case successfully treated with botulinum toxin A injections and discussion of underlying mechanism. *Mov Disord.* 2005; 20(10):1387–1388.

20. Ruzicka E, Jech R, Zarubova K, et al. VIM thalamic stimulation for tremor in a patient with IgM paraproteinaemic demyelinating neuropathy. *Mov Disord.* 2003; 18(10):1192–1195.

21. Penney SE, Bruce IA, Saeed SR. Botulinum toxin is effective and safe for palatal tremor: a report of five cases and a review of the literature. *J Neurol.* 2006; 253(7):857–860.

3

PARKINSONISM

The cardinal tetrad of parkinsonism includes *tremor*, *rigidity*, *akinesia/bradykinesia*, and *postural instability*.[1] The most common cause of parkinsonism is Parkinson's disease (PD), which is discussed in Chapters 2 and 4. Other neurodegenerative causes of parkinsonism include progressive supranuclear palsy, dementia with Lewy bodies, multiple system atrophy, and corticobasal degeneration.

TREMORS

- Tremors are the presenting symptom of PD in 40% to 70% of cases, and between 68% and 100% of patients with PD will have resting tremor at some point during the course of their illness.[2] However, 10% to 20% of patients with PD do not have tremor.

- The tremor in PD is typically *resting*, although postural tremor and action tremor may be present.

- The typical resting tremor in PD is 4 to 6 Hz in frequency and most prominent in the distal extremity (also called pill-rolling tremor because the tremor has a rotatory component).[3]

- Reemergent tremor (with a *latency* of a few seconds before the tremor reemerges during postural holding) occurs in PD.[4]

- Distraction may help "bring out" a resting tremor, especially if the patient is anxious (eg, if the patient is asked to count backward). Certain provocations, such as naming the months of the year backward, may exacerbate the tremor.

- Tremor usually starts in one hand and arm, then progresses to the ipsilateral leg. It later spreads contralaterally.

○ Lips, chin, and jaw tremors are common in PD, but head tremors are rare in PD, although they are common in essential tremor.

○ Head tremor, seen as nodding ("yes–yes" tremor) or shaking ("no–no" tremor), is a feature of essential tremor rather than PD but can rarely occur in PD.[5]

○ Head tremor can also occur in patients with cervical dystonia.

■ Tremors are often the most unpredictable symptom to treat. About half of patients will notice a treatment response, with improvement in tremor, but tremor is seldom completely abolished.

■ Patients can be troubled by the persistence of tremor despite therapy, and they may report that the treatment is not working because tremor remains, even though bradykinesia has improved.

■ Table 3.1 lists the differences between PD tremor and essential tremor.[6]

Table 3.1
Comparison of Parkinson's Disease Tremor and Essential Tremor

Characteristics	Parkinson's Disease Tremor	Essential Tremor
Tremor	At rest ± reemergent tremor	Postural tremor
Frequency	4–6 Hz	5–12 Hz
Distribution	Asymmetric	Mostly symmetric
Body parts affected	Hands ± legs	Hands, head, voice
Writing	Small (micrographia)	Large and tremulous
Course	Progressive	Stable or slowly progressive
Family history	Uncommon (1%)	Common (>30%)
Extrapyramidal signs (bradykinesia, rigidity, and loss of postural reflex)	Present	Absent
Relieving factors	Levodopa, dopamine agonists, anticholinergics	Alcohol, propranolol, primidone, topiramate, gabapentin, clonazepam
Usual site for surgical treatment with deep brain stimulation	Subthalamic nucleus or globus pallidus interna	Ventral intermediate thalamus

Source: Adapted from Ref. 6: Bhidayasiri R. Differential diagnosis of common tremor syndromes. *Postgrad Med J.* 2005; 81:756–762.

RIGIDITY

- Rigidity is an involuntary increase in muscle tone and can affect all muscle groups.

- Typically, cogwheel rigidity, especially when associated with tremor;[7] may result in flexed neck and trunk posture.

- Rigidity is present throughout the range of movement. The term *"lead pipe" rigidity* can be used to describe movement that feels smooth. The term *"cogwheel" rigidity* is used when movement feels ratcheted. Although there may be a subjective coexisting tremor that gives a feeling of cogwheeling, true cogwheeling is a form of rigidity independent of tremor.

- Rigidity is tested by passively moving the limb.

- Mild rigidity may require "activation," such as by asking the patient to open and close the contralateral hand, before it can be appreciated by the examiner.[8]

- Patients describe rigidity as muscle stiffness or sometimes pain. Not uncommonly, patients with PD experiencing significant rigidity initially present to an orthopedist with a "frozen shoulder."[9, 10] Pain in PD may also be caused by dystonia.

BRADYKINESIA/AKINESIA

- *Bradykinesia* is a slowness of initiating voluntary movement and sustaining repetitive movements, with progressive reduction in speed and amplitude.[7]

- *Hypokinesia* is paucity of movement.

- Patient symptoms and functional limitations that reflect bradykinesia and hypokinesia include the following:[7]

  ○ Loss of arm swing

  ○ Difficulty walking, with a tendency to drag a leg in early disease

  ○ Increasingly small handwriting (micrographia)

  ○ Difficulty with fine hand movements—manipulating buttons and zippers and cutting food

  ○ Difficulty turning in bed

  ○ Loss of facial expression, often described as a masklike face (hypomimia)

  ○ Hypophonia (reduced voice volume and modulation)

- Bradykinesia causes significant disability affecting the quality of life of patients with PD and almost always responds to antiparkinsonian therapy.

POSTURAL INSTABILITY

- Patients report poor balance, unsteadiness, and falls.[11]

- Postural instability is examined with the *pull test*.[12]

  ○ The examiner stands behind the patient and pulls back sharply on the patient's shoulders (the feet should be slightly apart, unlike their position in a Romberg test).

  ○ Patients typically correct themselves easily in the early stages. They develop some retropulsion later on, in which they may take two to three steps back but can still correct themselves. Finally, in advanced stages, they may fall if unsupported.

GAIT DYSFUNCTION

- *Shuffling gait* is usually seen in akinetic–rigid syndromes like PD.

- It may be the initial complaint in patients with non–tremor-predominant PD (often termed the *akinetic–rigid* variant or *postural instability–gait dysfunction* variant of PD).

- Other conditions that may present with a shuffling gait include multiple system atrophy (MSA), progressive supranuclear palsy (PSP), corticobasoganglionic degeneration (CBGD), dementia with Lewy bodies (DLB), normal-pressure hydrocephalus (NPH), some dementing processes, and frontal lobe syndromes, among others.

- The patient with a characteristic shuffling gait adopts a stooped posture, with flexion of the neck and shoulders.

  ○ Steps are short. The trunk is flexed and rigid, and the knees tend to be flexed.

  ○ However, the patient with PSP often adopts a more erect truncal posture, whereas truncal flexion can be accentuated in MSA.

  ○ A *cock gait* has been described in parkinsonism resulting from manganese toxicity, with an exaggerated lumbar lordosis and leg movements resembling those of a cock walking. A *magnetic gait* is classically attributed to NPH and is described as slightly wide-based, unsteady, and associated with some difficulty lifting the foot, "as if a magnet underneath is preventing the normal heel–toe stride." However, NPH can also present with a typical shuffling, parkinsonian gait, or the *marche à petit pas* ("walk with small steps") seen in vascular parkinsonism.

  ○ The patient with PD (and also the patient with CBGD) usually has an asymmetric arm swing compared with patients who have other parkinsonian disorders.

- *Festination,*[13] defined as a tendency to increase velocity but with shorter steps, may also be seen in the shuffling patient and is a characteristic, but not specific, finding in PD.

- The symptoms accompanying parkinsonism usually are the ones that give a clue to the diagnosis. For example:

  - When a shuffling gait is associated with urinary incontinence and cognitive impairment, NPH should be considered.[14]

  - When a shuffling gait is associated with early falls and vertical ophthalmoplegia, PSP should be considered.[15]

  - When cognitive impairment occurs early, DLB, CBGD, and PSP should be considered.

  - Prominent autonomic dysfunction suggests MSA.[16]

  - Likewise, marked disequilibrium early in the disease is more suggestive of PSP, DLB, or MSA.

- Other gait abnormalities that may also present with shuffling are the following:

  - *Isolated gait ignition failure.*[17] The patient often presents with difficulty initiating gait and frequent freezing during ambulation, aggravated by turning. The patient usually has normal postural responses but may have mild parkinsonian symptoms.

  - *Frontal gait disorder.*[18] The patient gives the appearance of having the feet "glued" or "magnetized" to the floor. It is very difficult to initiate gait, and when gait is initiated, it may be shuffling in nature. Special maneuvers, like turning, may exacerbate the symptoms. This syndrome can result from extensive, bilateral ischemic white matter disease (atherosclerotic/vascular parkinsonism), hydrocephalus, or other frontal lobe disorders. It has also been called gait apraxia.

EXAMINATION OF THE PATIENT WITH SHUFFLING

- Once a comprehensive history is obtained, a careful evaluation of gait should be performed (Table 3.2).[19]

- Observe trunk posture while the patient is walking. The patient's pace, stance, stride, initiation, and performance in special maneuvers (eg, turning) should be noted.

- With the patient initially seated, ask him or her to stand up without pushing on the arm rests. Although failure to stand without assistance can result from proximal muscle weakness of the lower extremities (eg, a myopathic condition), the same problem is often appreciated in moderate and severe stages of parkinsonism.

■ Ask the patient to initiate walking. It should be an easy, free-flowing process.

○ Hesitation in starting gait is suggestive of an akinetic–rigid syndrome.

■ Once gait is initiated, stride, stance, and velocity should be noted.

○ Shuffling steps are suggestive of an akinetic–rigid syndrome, and the shuffling may range in severity from very short steps to complete inability to ambulate ("magnetic feet").

○ A wide-based gait or difficulty in heel-to-toe walking suggests a concomitant cerebellar disorder such as olivopontocerebellar (OPCA) type of MSA or truncal ataxia.

■ The patient should be observed in special maneuvers, such as when asked to turn in a corner or suddenly change direction. This may cause the patient to "freeze" or may worsen the shuffling.

■ The examiner should pay attention to symptom asymmetry or the development of tremors, which are features suggestive of PD.

■ The postural reflexes should then be examined, and the clinician usually performs this examination by standing behind the patient and giving him or her a good tug on the shoulders.

■ Examine for rigidity, bradykinesia, and tremors.

■ Look for associated features, such as apraxia, ataxia, sensory abnormalities, aphasia, cognitive impairment, and hyperreflexia.

Table 3.2
Important Aspects of Gait Evaluation

Gait Aspect	Characteristics
Posture	Stooped versus upright
Stance	Narrow versus wide-based
Speed	Slow versus normal, with or without festination
Stride	Short, normal, or long
Gait initiation	Is there hesitation? Is it "magnetic"?
Freezing	Is there freezing during gait ignition or during turning?
Symptom asymmetry	Is the parkinsonism symmetric or asymmetric?
Heel–toe walking	Look for truncal ataxia, cerebellar features
Postural reflexes	Early versus late onset
Falls	Backward or forward, early versus late onset

DIFFERENTIAL DIAGNOSIS OF PATIENTS PRESENTING WITH PARKINSONISM

- Patients presenting with parkinsonism as the main feature can be broadly classified as having *primary parkinsonism*, *secondary parkinsonism*, or a *Parkinson-plus syndrome*, as defined in Chapter 1 (Table 3.3).[20]

Parkinson-Plus Syndromes

- Dementia with Lewy bodies (DLB)[21-25]

  - DLB is characterized by progressive dementia with prominent attention and visual defects fluctuation in cognition and attention, visual hallucinations, and parkinsonism.

  - It may be difficult to differentiate from PD dementia because patients with either condition can exhibit fluctuations in sensorium/alertness, frequent falls, hallucinations, and sensitivity to PD medications (Table 3.4).

  - Recurrent visual hallucinations and delusions (may be unrelated to medications).

  - Symmetric akinetic–rigid parkinsonism (bradykinesia and rigidity > tremor).

  - Gait abnormalities and falls occur early.

  - REM sleep behavior disorder is common.

  - There is a partial response to levodopa.

  - Dementia occurs before or within 1 year after onset of parkinsonism in DLB.

Table 3.3
Classification of Disorders With Parkinsonism as the Main Feature

Primary Parkinsonism	Parkinson-Plus Syndromes	Secondary Parkinsonism
Parkinson's disease	Progressive supranuclear palsy (PSP)	Drugs
Juvenile parkinsonism	Multiple system atrophy (MSA)	Metabolic causes
	Corticobasal syndrome (CBS)	Toxins
	Dementia with Lewy bodies (DLB)	Trauma
	Parkinsonism–dementia–amyotrophic lateral sclerosis complex	Postencephalitic parkinsonism
		Prion disorders
		Brain tumor
		Vascular causes

Source: Adapted from Ref. 20: Fahn S, Jankovic J, Hallet M. *Principles and Practice of Movement Disorders.* 2nd ed. Philadelphia, PA: Saunders Elsevier; 2011.

Table 3.4
Comparison of Clinical Presentations of Parkinson's Disease Dementia and Dementia With Lewy Bodies

Parkinson's Disease Dementia	Dementia With Lewy bodies
Cognitive impairment occurs at least 12 months after motor manifestations of the disease (usually 4 to 5 years at least).	Cognitive impairment usually occurs within 12 months of motor manifestations of disease.
Hallucinations occur later and after Parkinson's disease medication use.	Hallucinations occur earlier and sometimes prior to Parkinson's disease medication use.
Tremor is common.	Tremor is less common.
Predominantly unilateral motor symptoms are common.	Bilateral motor symptoms are more common.
Axial symptoms and gait difficulty are less common.	Axial symptoms and gait difficulty are more common.

* Progressive supranuclear palsy[15, 26–31]

  ○ PSP is also known as Steele-Richardson-Olszewski syndrome.

  ○ PSP can have a wide clinical spectrum, with different clinical "variants" described.

    * *Classic PSP/Steele-Richardson variant* is characterized by supranuclear gaze palsy (predominantly vertical gaze), parkinsonism, pseudobulbar affect, prominent frontal lobe syndrome, axial symptoms (neck and trunk) with early falls in the first year after onset, and symmetric symptoms. Resting tremor is uncommon. Gait is broad-based and unsteady, unlike the typical small-stepped shuffling gait in PD, with the typical "surprised" facies, spastic dysarthria, and retrocollis.

    * *Parkinsonian variant* has parkinsonian features very similar to those seen in PD or MSA, but without much response to levodopa and a predominance of postural instability and gait dysfunction.

    * *Gait ignition failure/primary progressive freezing of gait–like variant* may present with minimal parkinsonian features, at least initially, and mainly with gait freezing.

    * *Corticobasoganglionic–like variant:* autosopy-proven PSP has been described in patients who present with limb dystonia, limb apraxia, and alien limb syndrome with or without ophthalmoplegia.

  ○ Some eye findings include choppy pursuits and saccades and "square-wave jerks" (subtle, intermittent, quick movements of the eyes when the patient is asked to fix the gaze on an object). These can be appreciated before vertical ophthalmoplegia, characteristic of PSP, becomes evident.

- Multiple system atrophy[16,32–36]

  ○ Cerebellar dysfunction, parkinsonism, and autonomic dysfunction. MSA is mainly divided into the parkinsonian type (MSA-P, formerly known as *striatonigral degeneration*) and the cerebellar type (MSA-C, formerly known as *olivopontocerebellar atrophy*) (Figure 3.1). MSA-P is between two and four times more common than MSA-C.

  ○ Rapid course, *nocturnal stridor* (typically elicited from a bed partner), early disability and falls, stimulus-sensitive myoclonus, pyramidal tract signs, severe dysarthria and transient response to levodopa, "cold hands," minipolymyoclonus (jerky and irregular, affecting individual fingers without a particular pattern), and profound autonomic dysfunction are some of the features of MSA.

  ○ The mean age at onset is 54 years (younger than in idiopathic PD), and there are no known pathologically proven cases in which symptoms developed before the age of 30 years.

  ○ Resting tremor can be seen initially, as well as asymmetry; facial dyskinesias after levodopa use can also be seen.

  ○ Anterocollis is common, including an exaggerated truncal flexion.

  ○ REM sleep behavior disorder is seen in almost all patients.

  ○ Depression can occur; dementia is less common.

  ○ Although choppy saccades and pursuits are also seen in MSA, just as in other neurodegenerative parkinsonian conditions, the presence of gaze-evoked nystagmus and positioning downbeat nystagmus (ie, nystagmus seen during the Dix-Hallpike maneuver) is more suggestive of MSA.

  ○ Although they are not specific, some imaging clues can be appreciated in MSA (Figures 3.2 and 3.3).

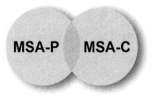

Figure 3.1
The clinical presentations of multiple system atrophy, parkinsonian type, and multiple system atrophy, cerebellar type, can overlap.

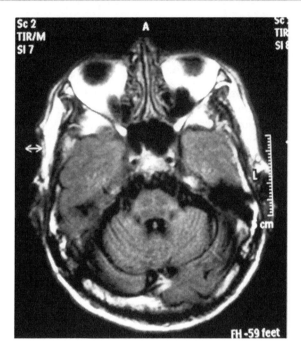

Figure 3.2

Axial FLAIR (fluid attenuation inversion recovery) MRI showing the "hot cross bun sign" in a patient with multiple system atrophy, cerebellar type.

▪ Corticobasal syndrome[37–43]

  ○ Unilateral parkinsonism, myoclonus, limb kinetic apraxia, and early limb dystonia occur.

  ○ Dementia with cortical and subcortical features is common and occurs early.

  ○ Alien limb phenomenon is seen in 50% of patients.

  ○ MSA usually presents in the sixth decade.

  ○ Pharmacotherapy may include antidepressants and a trial of dopaminergic therapy. Clonazepam may help myoclonus, and baclofen can be used for muscle spasm. Botulinum toxin injections may alleviate limb dystonia.

▪ Table 3.5 summarizes the clinical features that may suggest atypical parkinsonism, especially Parkinson-plus syndromes.[44]

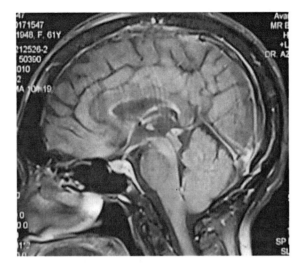

Figure 3.3
Sagittal T1-weighted MRI showing midbrain atrophy ("humming bird sign")
in a patient with progressive supranuclear palsy.

Table 3.5
Clinical Features of Atypical Parkinsonian Disorders

Motor	Oculomotor	Cognitive and Behavioral	Autonomic
• Early instability and falls • Rapid disease progression • Absent, poor, or unsustained response to levodopa • Pyramidal signs • Cerebellar signs • Early dysarthria and/or dysphagia	• Supranuclear gaze palsy • Slowing of saccades • Difficulty initiating saccades (oculomotor apraxia)	• Early dementia • Visual hallucinations, not treatment-induced • Ideomotor apraxia • Sensory or visual neglect/cortical disturbances	• Early autonomic failure unrelated to treatment (orthostatic hypotension, impotence, or urinary disturbances)

Source: Adapted from Ref. 44: Litvan I. Parkinsonian features: when are they Parkinson disease? *JAMA.* 1998; 280:1654–1655.

Secondary Parkinsonism

■ Vascular parkinsonism[45–47]

○ Vascular parkinsonism is also known as *lower body parkinsonism.*

○ The pattern typically involves the lower body (whereas in idiopathic PD, the arms and upper body are more often initially affected). However, the upper body can be involved in vascular parkinsonism.

○ Patients with vascular parkinsonism are more likely to be older and to have postural instability, a history of falling, dementia, corticospinal findings, and incontinence.

○ The original description by Critchley in the 1920s was predominantly one of a gait disorder (*marche à petit pas*, "walk with short steps") with additional features of dementia and pyramidal signs. Classically, the presentation was described as having an acute onset, symmetric and without tremor, but with postural instability and a poor response to dopamine replacement therapy. However, the onset is more commonly insidious. In one series, only about a quarter of cases of vascular parkinsonism were considered to have an acute onset with a new ischemic stroke event, but even here, the new event may have unmasked an insidious process.

○ There are three pathologic patterns of vascular parkinsonism:

• Multiple lacunar infarcts are clinically associated with a gait disorder, pyramidal deficits, cognitive impairment, and pseudobulbar palsy.

• Subcortical arteriosclerotic encephalopathy (Binswanger disease) is clinically associated with a progressive gait disorder and dementia.

• Basal ganglia infarct (usually lacunar) is a rare type.

○ Patients exhibit a wide-based, small-stepped gait and freezing.

○ There is a gradual onset with stepwise progression.

○ Addressing vascular risk (control of hypertension, diabetes, and hypercholesterolemia; consideration of antiplatelet therapy) and advising smoking cessation seem sensible, although these therapeutic strategies have not been studied in vascular parkinsonism.

○ Typically, there is a poor therapeutic response to levodopa in vascular parkinsonism, but some evidence of a levodopa response in patients with pathologic confirmation of vascular parkinsonism was noted in a case review (12 of 17 patients had a good or excellent response documented).

• In clinical practice, it is appropriate to try levodopa, often up to the maximum tolerated dose, and to continue treatment if there is clinical benefit but discontinue it if there is no response, or if adverse effects outweigh any benefit.

○ The results of functional imaging with single photon emission computed tomography (SPECT) or positron emission tomography (PET) to check the integrity of presynaptic neurons are abnormal in idiopathic PD but normal in vascular parkinsonism (unless there is widespread basal ganglia infarction).

■ Drug-induced parkinsonism[48–50]

○ This is the second most common cause of parkinsonism after PD (and may be the most common cause in certain countries).

○ Usually caused by antiemetics (eg, metoclopramide, promethazine, and prochlorperazine) and antipsychotics (eg, chlorpromazine, haloperidol, and risperidone) that possess strong dopamine D2 receptor–blocking properties.

○ Occasionally associated with other tardive syndromes: oral–buccal-lingual dyskinesias, retrocollis (dystonia), and akathisia.

○ Although drug-induced parkinsonism is typically symmetric with predominant rigidity, and with much less tremor and postural instability, it may be difficult to differentiate from PD as it can also have an asymmetric presentation with resting tremor.

○ It may require 6 months or longer for parkinsonian symptoms to resolve after discontinuation of the offending agent; persistence of parkinsonian symptoms persist can be a sign of "conversion" to idiopathic PD.

○ Table 3.6 summarizes the differences between drug-induced parkinsonism and PD.

Table 3.6
Comparison of Characteristics of Drug-Induced Parkinsonism and Parkinson's Disease

Characteristics	Drug-Induced Parkinsonism	Parkinson's Disease
Tremor	Rare	Common
Distribution	Commonly symmetric	Asymmetric
Concurrent choreathetoid dyskinesias	More common (representing tardive dyskinesia)	Uncommon (except when associated with levodopa-induced dyskinesia)
Treatment	Withdrawal of offending medication, anticholinergic agents, amantadine	Levodopa, dopamine agonist, monoamine oxidase B inhibitors, anticholinergics, amantadine

- Normal-pressure hydrocephalus[14,51–53]

  - NPH is a rather rare condition in which parkinsonism is associated with "normal-pressure" hydrocephalus and primary empty sella.

  - In addition to parkinsonism, there are symptoms are of urinary incontinence, gait disturbance, and dementia.

  - NPH is distinguished from PD by the following:

    - Rigidity, tremor, and bradykinesia tend to be less common in NPH than in PD.

    - There is a limited, if any, response to levodopa.

    - Incontinence is usually urinary but may also be bowel incontinence.

  - Dementia may progress less rapidly than in Alzheimer disease or in PD dementia.

  - Structural neuroimaging aids the diagnosis (Figure 3.4).

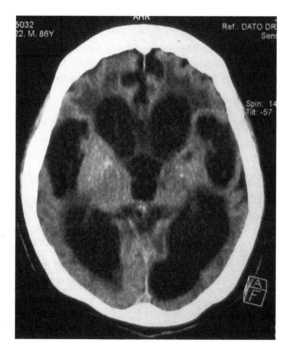

Figure 3.4
CT scan of the brain of a patient with normal-pressure hydrocephalus.

○ Surgical shunting should be considered. However, the risks of surgery may outweigh the potential benefit, particularly when poor prognostic features, including dementia, long-standing symptoms, and cortical atrophy, are present.[54]

○ NPH may be confused with PD or vascular dementia. Many experts feel that NPH is overdiagnosed, and caution should be exercised before high-risk surgical procedures, such as shunting, are considered.

Other Neurodegenerative Disorders Presenting With Parkinsonism

■ Wilson's disease[55–58]

○ Wilson's disease is an autosomal recessive genetic disorder of copper metabolism.

○ It is characterized by hepatic, ophthalmologic, neurological, and psychiatric manifestations (Table 3.7).

○ Movement disorders are protean and can include parkinsonism, tremors (classically described as "wing beating"), dystonia (limb and trunk, and also facial dystonia, termed *risus sardonicus*), and less commonly ataxia, myoclonus, or chorea.

○ The gene responsible is *ATP7B* on chromosome 13.

○ Laboratory findings for Wilson's disease include the following:

  • Serum ceruloplasmin less than 0.2 g/L (normal, 0.2–0.5 g/L)

  • Twenty-four-hour urinary copper greater than 100 mcg per 24 hours (>1.6 mcmol/24 h)

  • Hepatic copper less than 250 mcg/g dry weight

■ Spinocerebellar ataxias[59–61]

○ Some autosomal dominant spinocerebellar ataxias (SCAs) have parkinsonism as part of their clinical presentation.

○ These include SCAs 1, 2, 3, 12, 21, and 27.

○ Dentatorubropallidoluysian atrophy (DRPLA), although not part of the SCAs, can present with ataxia, parkinsonism, myoclonus, and dystonia along with dementia and also follows an autosomal dominant pattern.

Table 3.7
Summary of Clinical Characteristics of Wilson's Disease

System involvement	Clinical features

Neurological manifestations	Tremor
	  May be resting, postural, or kinetic
	    "Wing-beating" appearance suggests proximal
	    upper extremity tremor
	  Head titubation may appear
	Dysarthria
	  Extrapyramidal or cerebellar character
	Dystonia
	  Risus sardonicus (frozen facial expression)
	  Drooling
	  Whispering dysphonia
	Choreiform movements
	Painless variant of painful legs and moving toes
	  syndrome
	Seizures
	Peripheral sensorimotor polyneuropathy
	Olfactory impairment
	Pseudobulbar emotional lability
	Hypersomnia
	Priapism
	Muscle cramps

Psychiatric manifestations	Personality changes (antisocial or criminal
	  behavior)
	Mood disorder, especially depression
	Psychosis unusual
	Sexual preoccupation and disinhibition
	Cognitive impairment
	  Fronto-executive behavior
	  Visuospatial processing
	  Memory impairment

Ophthalmologic manifestations	Kayser-Fleischer rings (deposition of copper within
	  Descemet membrane); virtually always present
	  in persons with neurological or psychiatric
	  manifestations in Wilson's disease
	"Sunflower cataract"

Hepatic manifestations	Asymptomatic enlargement of liver and spleen Hepatitis Elevated unconjugated (indirect) bilirubin Liver cirrhosis

continued

Table 3.7 (cont.)
Summary of Clinical Characteristics of Wilson's Disease

System involvement	Clinical features

Other manifestations	Osteoporosis (may cause spontaneous fractures)
	Joint involvement
	Hemolytic anemia
	Renal tubular dysfunction
	Hyperpigmentation of skin at anterior lower legs
	Gynecologic abnormalities
	   Menstrual irregularities
	   Delayed puberty
	   Gynecomastia
	Cardiovascular abnormalities
	   Congestive cardiac failure
	   Cardiac arrhythmia
	Glucose intolerance
	Parathyroid insufficiency

Table 3.8
Diagnostic Workup of Common Parkinsonian Syndromes

Is there a history of exposure to dopamine receptor blockers?	If yes, consider drug-induced parkinsonism.	Symptoms are usually symmetric.
Is there history of cerebrovascular disease?	Consider vascular parkinsonism, especially if symptoms are symmetric.	Lower-body parkinsonism is usually a presentation of vascular parkinsonism.
Is the patient younger than 50 years old?	Evaluate for Wilson's disease.	Serum ceruloplasmin, 24-hour urinary copper excretion; slit-lamp evaluation; liver biopsy if needed
Abnormal MRI of brain	Consider the following: Vascular parkinsonism	Basal ganglia or periventricular ischemic gliotic changes
	Normal-pressure hydrocephalus	Ventriculomegaly
	Toxic/metabolic cause (hypoxic–anoxic injury, manganese intoxication, iron deposition)	Increased signal in basal ganglia

continued

Table 3.8 (cont.)
Diagnostic Workup of Common Parkinsonian Syndromes

"Normal" MRI of brain	Parkinson's disease	Slowly progressive, levodopa-responsive, asymmetric resting tremors
	Multiple system atrophy	Autonomic disturbances, poor levodopa response; MRI may show atrophic pons.
	Progressive supranuclear palsy	Early falls, dysphagia, poor levodopa response, vertical gaze paresis; MRI may show small midbrain.
	Corticobasoganglionic degeneration	Asymmetric, dystonia, alien hand, poor levodopa response, dystonia; MRI/SPECT may show cortical asymmetry, especially in the temporal lobes.
	Dementia with Lewy bodies	Early hallucinations, poor levodopa response, memory disturbances, fluctuations in mental status

Abbreviation: SPECT, single photon emission tomography.

Table 3.9
Laboratory Clues to Type of Parkinsonism

Investigations	Findings	Diagnosis to Consider
Peripheral blood film	Acanthocytes	Neuroacanthocytosis
Creatine kinase	Elevated	Neuroacanthocytosis
CT of brain	Multifocal infarcts	Vascular parkinsonism
	Enlarged ventricles (hydrocephalus)	Normal-pressure hydrocephalus
MRI of brain	Multifocal infarcts	Vascular parkinsonism
	Midbrain atrophy with "hummingbird sign"	Progressive supranuclear palsy
	Pontine atrophy on sagittal view "Hot cross bun sign" on axial view Hyperintensity of middle cerebral peduncle	Multiple system atrophy, cerebellar type (MSA-C)

continued

Table 3.9 (cont.)
Laboratory Clues to Type of Parkinsonism

Investigations	Findings	Diagnosis to Consider
	Other etiologies with hyperintensity of the middle cerebral peduncle	Spinocerebellar ataxias Fragile X–ataxia syndrome
	Hypodensity of the posterolateral aspect of the putamen on gradient echo Putaminal atrophy Hyperintense putaminal rim on axial T2-weighted sequences	Multiple system atrophy, parkinsonian type (MSA-P)
	Enlarged ventricles (hydrocephalus)	Normal-pressure hydrocephalus
	Increase signal in basal ganglia on T2	Pantothenate kinase–associated neurodegeneration (PKAN; "eye of the tiger" sign) Wilson's disease ("giant panda" sign) Manganese toxicity (mainly putamen) Carbon monoxide poisoning (mainly globus pallidus) Hypoxic–anoxic injury

DIAGNOSTIC WORKUP OF PARKINSONIAN SYNDROMES

- The diagnostic workup of parkinsonian syndromes is summarized in Table 3.8.
- Laboratory features can provide clues to the type of parkinsonism (Table 3.9).
- The treatment of parkinsonism is discussed in Chapter 4.

REFERENCES

1. Fahn S, Jankovic J. *Principles and Practice of Movement Disorders*. Philadelphia, PA: Elsevier; 2007.
2. Pal PK, Samii A, Calne DB. Cardinal features of early Parkinson's disease. In: Factor SA, Weiner WJ, eds. *Parkinson's Disease Diagnosis and Clinical Management*. New York, NY: Demos; 2002:41–56.
3. Sethi KD. Clinical aspects of Parkinson disease. *Curr Opin Neurol*. 2002; 15:457–460.

4. Jankovic J, Schwarts KS, Ondo W. Re-emergent tremor of Parkinson's disease. *J Neurol Neurosurg Psychiatry.* 1999; 67:646–650.

5. Hsu YD, Chang MK, Sung SC, et al. Essential tremor: clinical, electromyographical and pharmacological studies in 146 Chinese patients. *Zhonghua Yi Xue Za Zhi (Taipei).* 1990; 45:93–99.

6. Bhidayasiri R. Differential diagnosis of common tremor syndromes. *Postgrad Med J.* 2005; 81:756–762.

7. Jankovic J. Parkinson's disease: clinical features and diagnosis. *J Neurol Neurosurg Psychiatry.* 2008; 79:368–376.

8. Broussolle E, Krack P, Thobois S, et al. Contribution of Jules Froment to the study of parkinsonian rigidity. *Mov Disord.* 2007; 22:909–914.

9. Riley D, Lang AE, Blair RD, et al. Frozen shoulder and other shoulder disturbances in Parkinson's disease. *J Neurol Neurosurg Psychiatry.* 1989; 52:63–66.

10. Stamey WP, Jankovic K. Shoulder pain in Parkinson's disease. *Mov Disord.* 2007; 22:S247–S248.

11. Williams DR, Watt HC, Lees AJ. Predictors of falls and fractures in bradykinetic rigid syndrome: a retrospective study. *J Neurol Neurosurg Psychiatry.* 2006; 77:468–473.

12. Munhoz RP, Li JY, Kurtinecz M, et al. Evaluation of the pull test technique in assessing postural instability in Parkinson's disease. *Neurology.* 2004; 62:125–127.

13. Alexander N. Gait disorders. In: Pompei P, Murphy JB, eds. *Geriatric Review Syllabus: A Core Curriculum in Geriatric Medicine.* 6th ed. New York, NY: American Geriatrics Society; 2006.

14. Tsakanikas D, Relkin N. Normal pressure hydrocephalus. *Semin Neurol.* 2007; 27(1):58–65.

15. Pearce JMS. Progressive supranuclear palsy (Steele-Richardson-Olszewski syndrome). *Neurologist.* 2007; 13(5):302–304.

16. Osaki Y, Ben-Shlomo Y, Wenning GK, et al. Do published criteria improve clinical diagnostic accuracy in multiple system atrophy? *Neurology.* 2002; 59:1486–1491.

17. Paisset M. Freezing of gait in Parkinson's disease. *Neurol Clin.* 2004; 22:S53–S62.

18. Rubino FA. Gait disorders. *Neurologist.* 2002; 8(4):254–262.

19. Van Garpen JA. Office assessment of gait and station. *Semin Neurol.* 2011; 31(1):78–84.

20. Fahn S, Jankovic J, Hallet M. *Principles and Practice of Movement Disorders.* 2nd ed. Philadelphia, PA: Saunders Elsevier; 2011.

21. Weisman D, McKeith I. Dementia with Lewy bodies. *Semin Neurol.* 2007; 27(1):42–47.

22. Lippa CF, McKeith I. Dementia with Lewy bodies. *Neurology.* 2003; 60:1571–1572.

23. Leverenz JB, McKeith IG. Dementia with Lewy bodies. *Med Clin N Am* 2002; 86: 519–535.

24. McKeith I, Mintzer J, Aarsland D, et al. Dementia with Lewy bodies. *Lancet.* 2004; 3:19–28.

25. Galvin JE. Dementia with Lewy bodies. *Arch Neurol.* 2003; 60:1332–1335.

26. Jankovic J. Parkinsonism-plus syndromes. *Mov Disord.* 1989; 4(suppl 1):S95–S119.

27. Williams DR, Lees AJ. Progressive supranuclear palsy: clinicopathological concepts and diagnostic challenges. *Lancet Neurol.* 2009; 8:270–279.

28. Warren NM, Burn DJ. Progressive supranuclear palsy. *Pract Neurol.* 2007; 7:16–23.

29. Lubarsky M, Juncos JL. Progressive supranuclear palsy: a current review. *Neurologist.* 2008; 14(2):79–88.

30. Burn DJ, Lees AJ. Progressive supranuclear palsy: where are we now? *Lancet Neurol.* 2002; 1:359–369.

31. Pastor P, Tolosa E. Progressive supranuclear palsy: clinical and genetic aspects. *Curr Opin Neurol.* 2002; 15:429–437.
32. Gilman S, Low PA, Quinn N, et al. Consensus statement on the diagnosis of multiple system atrophy. *J Neurol Sci.* 1999; 163:94–98.
33. Papp MI, Kahn JE, Lantos PL. Glial cytoplasmic inclusions in the CNS of patients with multiple system atrophy (striatonigral degeneration, olivopontocerebellar atrophy and Shy-Drager syndrome). *J Neurol Sci.* 1989; 94:79–100.
34. Quinn N. Multiple system atrophy-the nature of the beast. *J Neurol Neurosurg Psychiatry.* 1989; 52(special suppl):78–89.
35. Wenning GK, Ben Shlomo Y, Magalhaes M, Daniel SE, Quinn NP. Clinical features and natural history of multiple system atrophy. An analysis of 100 cases. *Brain.* 1994; 117(pt 4):835–845.
36. Stefanova N, Bucke P, Duerr S, Karl Wenning G. Multiple system atrophy: an update. *Lancet Neurol.* 2009; 8:1172–1178.
37. Bergeron C, Davis A, Lang AE. Corticobasal ganglionic degeneration and progressive supranuclear palsy presenting with cognitive decline. *Brain Pathol.* 1998; 8:355–365.
38. Fratalli CM, Grafman J, Patronas N, Makhlouf F, Litvan I. Language disturbances in corticobasal degeneration. *Neurology.* 2000; 54:990–992.
39. Fratalli CM, Sonies BC. Speech and swallowing disturbances in corticobasal degeneration. *Adv Neurol.* 2000; 82:153–160.
40. Gibb WRC, Lurthert PJ, Marsden CD. Clinical and pathological features of corticobasal degeneration. *Adv Neurol.* 1990; 53:51–54.
41. Grimes DA, Lang AE, Bergeron C. Dementia is the most common presentation of cortical-basal ganglionic degeneration. *Neurology.* 1999; 53:1969–1974.
42. Kertesz A. Corticobasal degeneration. *J Neurol Neurosurg Psychiatry.* 2000; 68:275–276.
43. Rinne JO, Lee MS, Thompson PD, Marsden CD. Corticobasal degeneration. A clinical study of 36 cases. *Brain.* 1994; 117:1183–1196.
44. Litvan I. Parkinsonian features: when are they Parkinson disease? *JAMA.* 1998; 280:1654–1655.
45. Tuite PJ, Krawczewski K. Parkinsonism: a review-of-systems approach to diagnosis. *Semin Neurol.* 2007; 27(2):113–122.
46. Demirkiran M, Bozdemir H, Sarica Y. Vascular parkinsonism: a distinct, heterogeneous clinical entity. *Acta Neurol Scand.* 2001; 104:63–67.
47. Kashmere J, Camicioli R, Martin W. Parkinsonian syndromes and differential diagnosis. *Curr Opin Neurol.* 2002; 15:461–466.
48. Van Garpen JA. Drug-induced parkinsonism. *Neurologist.* 2002; 8(6):363–370.
49. Thanvi B, Treadwell S. Drug-induced parkinsonism: a common cause of parkinsonism in older people. *Postgrad Med J.* 2009; 85:322–326.
50. Lim TT, Ahmed A, Itin I, et al. Is 6 months of neuroleptic withdrawal sufficient to distinguish drug-induced parkinsonism from Parkinson's disease? *Int J Neurosci.* 2013; 123(3):170–174.
51. Graff-Radford NR. Normal pressure hydrocephalus. *Neurol Clin.* 2007; 25:808–832.
52. Malm J, Eklund A. Idiopathic normal pressure hydrocephalus. *Pract Neurol.* 2006; 6:14–27.
53. Wilson RK, Williams MA. Normal pressure hydrocephalus. *Clin Geriatr Med.* 2006; 22:935–951.

54. Marmarou A, Young HF, Aygok GA et al. Diagnosis and management of idiopathic normal-pressure hydrocephalus: a prospective study in 151 patients. *J Neurosurg.* 2005; 102(6); 987–997.

55. Ala A, Walker AP, Ashkan K, Dooley JS, Schilsky ML. Wilson's disease. *Lancet.* 2007; 369:397–408.

56. Pfeiffer RF. Wilson's disease. *Semin Neurol.* 2007; 27(2):123–132.

57. Brewer GJ. Wilson's disease. *Curr Treat Options Neurol.* 2000; 2(3):193–203.

58. Van Wassenaer-van Hall HN, Van den Heuvel AG, Jansen GH, et al. Cranial MR in Wilson disease: abnormal white matter in extrapyramidal and pyramidal tracts. *AJNR Am J Neuroradiol.* 1995; 16:2021–2027.

59. Soong BW, Paulson HL. Spinocerebellar ataxias: an update. *Curr Opin Neurol.* 2007; 20:438–446.

60. Worth PF. Sorting out ataxia in adults. *Pract Neurol.* 2004; 4:130–141.

61. Schols L, Bauer P, Schmidt T, et al. Autosomal dominant cerebellar ataxias: clinical features, genetics, and pathogenesis. *Lancet Neurol.* 2004; 3:291–304.

4

PARKINSON'S DISEASE

OVERVIEW OF PARKINSON'S DISEASE

James Parkinson wrote and published "An Essay on the Shaking Palsy" in 1817.[1] However, in India, paralysis agitans was described under the name *Kampavata* in the Ayurevedic literature as far back as 4500 bc. *Mucuna pruriens* (a tropical legume), which they called Atmagupta, was used to treat Kampavata. The seeds of *Mucuna pruriens* are a natural source of therapeutic quantities of levodopa.[2]

- Parkinson's disease (PD) is a neurodegenerative disease characterized by slowly progressive symptoms of resting tremor, rigidity, akinesia/bradykinesia, and postural instability.

- PD is the second most common neurodegenerative disease after Alzheimer disease.

- PD affects about 2% of the population over 60 years.

- Incidence rates of PD are 8 to 18 per 100,000 person-years.[3] In 3% to 5% of patients with parkinsonism, the onset is before the age of 40 years.[4] Figure 4.1 compares young-onset PD with juvenile parkinsonism.[5,6]

- Age is the single most consistent risk factor. Figure 4.2 outlines factors that have been reported to increase and decrease the risk for developing PD.[3,7–24]

- Although the majority of cases of PD are sporadic, there are known and increasingly reported genetic and familiar forms of PD (Figure 4.3; Tables 4.1 and 4.2).[25–35]

- **Most inherited forms of PD present at a younger age.**

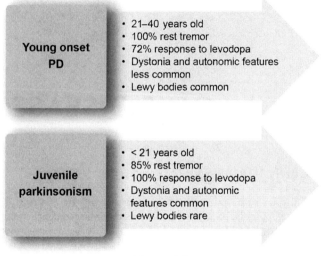

Figure 4.1

Differences between young-onset Parkinson's disease and juvenile-onset parkinsonism.

From Refs. 5, 6.

Mitochondrial Inheritance

- So far, data fail to demonstrate a bias toward maternal inheritance in familial PD.[36]

- There is no association of common haplogroup-defining mitochondrial DNA variants or of the 10398G variant with the risk for PD.

- However, it still remains possible that other inherited mitochondrial DNA variants, or somatic mitochondrial DNA mutations, contribute to the risk for familial PD.

PATHOLOGY

- The traditional view is that the main pathologic process in PD is the degeneration of dopaminergic neurons in the substantia nigra.

- Braak and colleagues have challenged this idea and introduced a six-stage pathologic process (Figure 4.4).[37]

  ○ In this staging system, degeneration of dopaminergic neurons in the substantia nigra occurs in stage 3 (see Figure 4.4; Figure 4.5).

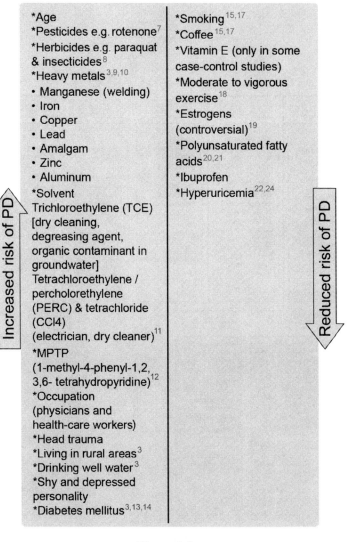

Increased risk of PD

*Age
*Pesticides e.g. rotenone[7]
*Herbicides e.g. paraquat
& insecticides[8]
*Heavy metals[3,9,10]
• Manganese (welding)
• Iron
• Copper
• Lead
• Amalgam
• Zinc
• Aluminum
*Solvent
Trichloroethylene (TCE)
[dry cleaning,
degreasing agent,
organic contaminant in
groundwater]
Tetrachloroethylene /
percholorethylene
(PERC) & tetrachloride
(CCl4)
(electrician, dry cleaner)[11]
*MPTP
(1-methyl-4-phenyl-1,2,
3,6- tetrahydropyridine)[12]
*Occupation
(physicians and
health-care workers)
*Head trauma
*Living in rural areas[3]
*Drinking well water[3]
*Shy and depressed
personality
*Diabetes mellitus[3,13,14]

Reduced risk of PD

*Smoking[15,17]
*Coffee[15,17]
*Vitamin E (only in some
case-control studies)
*Moderate to vigorous
exercise[18]
*Estrogens
(controversial)[19]
*Polyunsaturated fatty
acids[20,21]
*Ibuprofen
*Hyperuricemia[22,24]

Figure 4.2
Known environmental risk and protective factors for Parkinson's disease
genetics and familial forms of Parkinson's disease.

■ The mechanism responsible for neuronal degeneration is probably multifactorial and based on a combination of genetic and environmental factors
(Figure 4.6).[38]

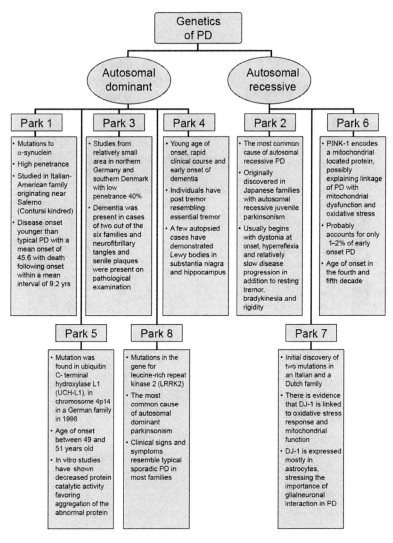

Figure 4.3

Summary of autosomal dominant and autosomal recessive Parkinson's disease.

From Refs. 25–35.

Table 4.1
Autosomal Dominant Parkinson's Disease

Locus	Gene	Chromosomal Location	Clinical Features
PARK 1	Alpha-synuclein	4q21-q23	• Early and late onset • Parkinsonism, dementia, and visual hallucinations of variable severity • Less tremor • Faster clinical deterioration • Concomitant myoclonus • Hyperventilation
PARK 3	Unknown	2p13	• Late onset • Dementia may be present (two of six families studied) • Typical response to dopaminergic agents • Penetrance < 40%
PARK 4	Alpha-synuclein triplication	4q21-q23	• Early onset • Rapid progression • Postural tremor • Asymmetric limb "heaviness" and rigidity • Atypical features (eg, autonomic dysfunction, dementia, weight loss in early stages, myoclonus, and seizures have been described) • Late dementia
PARK 5	*UCHL1*	4p14	• Late onset
PARK 8	*LRRK2*	12p11.2-q13.1	• Late onset • Resembles typical sporadic Parkinson's disease • Response to levodopa good
NA	Syphilin 1	5q23.1-q23.3	• Late onset
NA	*NR4A2*	2q22-q23	• Late onset without atypical features

Table 4.2
Autosomal Recessive Parkinson's Disease

Locus	Gene	Chromosomal Location	Clinical Features
PARK 2	Parkin	6q25.2-q27	• Juvenile onset • Slow progression • High incidence of focal dystonia • Good response to dopaminergic therapy • Symmetric presentation • Levodopa-induced dyskinesias and motor fluctuations common • Hyperreflexia may be present

continued

Table 4.2 (cont.)
Autosomal Recessive Parkinson's Disease

Locus	Gene	Chromosomal Location	Clinical Features
PARK 6	*PINK1*	1p35-p36	• Early onset • Slow progression • Response to levodopa good and long-lasting
PARK 7	*DJ1*	1p36	• Early onset • Slow progression • Variable clinical severity • Sustained response to levodopa • Comorbidity showing psychiatric symptoms

PARK 9
(Kufor-Rakeb
syndrome)
		1p36	• Atypical features such as spasticity,
			  dementia, and progressive supranuclear
			  palsy may be present
			• May produce facial and finger
			  minimyoclonus
			• Response to levodopa good

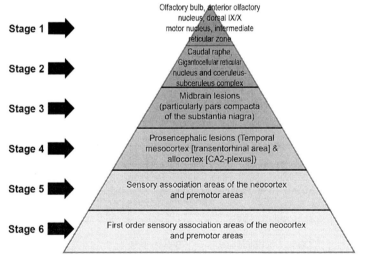

Figure 4.4

Stages of Parkinson's disease–related pathology according to Braak and colleagues.

From Ref. 37: Braak H, Tredici KD, Riib U, et al. Staging of brain pathology related to sporadic Parkinson's disease. Neurobiol Aging. 2003; 24:197–211.

■   There are three basal ganglia pathways:

   ○   Direct pathway (cortex—striatum—GPi—thalamus—cortex)

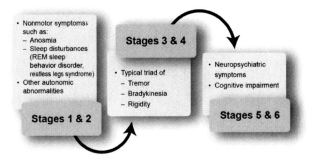

Figure 4.5

Clinical features prevalent within the stages of Parkinson's disease described by Braak and colleagues.

From Ref. 37: Braak H, Tredici KD, Riib U, et al. Staging of brain pathology related to sporadic Parkinson's disease. Neurobiol Aging. 2003; 24:197–211.

- D1 receptors
- Cortical glutaminergic input to the striatal cells
- GABAergic neurons projecting to the globus pallidus internus (GPi)
- GABAergic neurons of the GPi projecting to the ventral anterior/ventrolateral nuclei of the thalamus

○ Indirect pathway (cortex—striatum—GPe—STN—GPi—thalamus—cortex)

- D2 receptors
- Cortical glutaminergic input to the striatal cells
- GABAergic neurons projecting to the globus pallidus externus (GPe)
- GABAergic neurons of the GPe projecting to the subthalamic nucleus (STN)
- STN glutaminergic projection to the GPi
- GPi to thalamus to cortex (similar to the direct pathway)

○ Hyperdirect pathway (cortex—STN)

- Cortex directly to the STN

■ Alteration in the direct pathway leading to PD (Figures 4.7 and 4.8)

○ In **normal subjects,** dopaminergic neurons in the substantia nigra, pars compacta (SNc) act to excite inhibitory neurons in the direct pathway (see Figure 4.7).

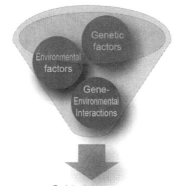

Oxidative stress
(Antioxidants eg vitamin E, C, iron chelators
MAO-B Inhibitors, eg Selegiline, Rasagiline)

Mitochondrial dysfunction
(Bioenergetic agents eg Coenzyme Q_{10})

Excitotoxicity
(Antiglutaminergic agents eg NMDA antagonists
Calcium channel blockers)

Inflammation
(Anti-inflammatory agents eg COX2 inhibitors)

Protein handling dysfunction with Lewy body formation
(Proteosomal enhancers, Heat shock proteins)

Neuronal dysfunction
(Trophic factors eg GDNF, Nurturin)

Apoptosis
(Antiapoptotic agents eg Dopamine agonists,
caspase inhibitors, propargylamines)

Figure 4.6

Etiopathogenesis of Parkinson's disease and possible neuroprotective approaches.

*From Ref. 38: Schapira AHV, Olanow CW. Neuroprotection in
Parkinson disease. JAMA. 2004; 291:358–364.*

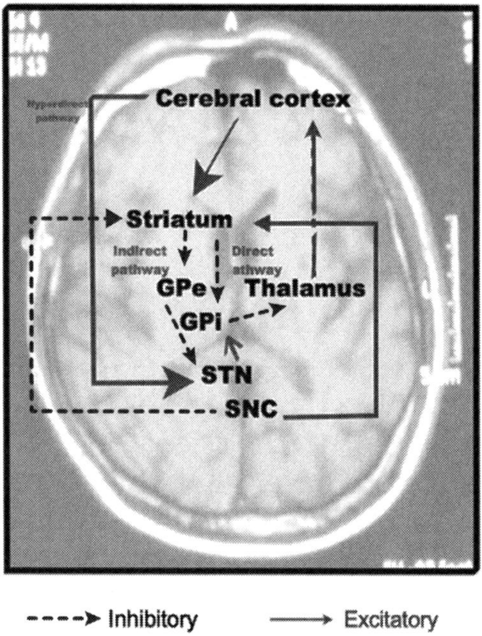

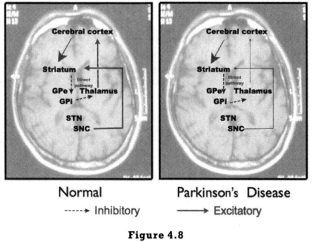

----→ Inhibitory   ——→ Excitatory

Figure 4.7
Normal basal ganglia pathway.

Normal   Parkinson's Disease
-----→ Inhibitory   ——→ Excitatory

Figure 4.8
Direct pathway of the basal ganglia circuit in normal subjects and
subjects with Parkinson's disease.

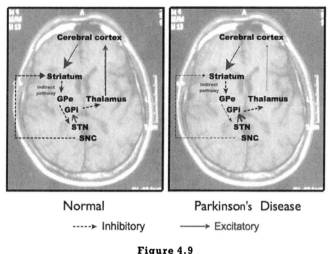

Normal   Parkinson's Disease

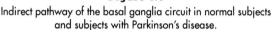

Figure 4.9
Indirect pathway of the basal ganglia circuit in normal subjects
and subjects with Parkinson's disease.

○ In **PD**, dopaminergic cell loss in the SNc results in reduced striatal inhibition of the GPi and substantia nigra, pars reticulata (SNr). The overactivity of the GPi and SNr results in excess inhibition of the thalamus. The final pathway would be a reduced activation of the motor cortex.

■ Alteration in the indirect pathway leading to PD (Figure 4.9)

○ In **normal subjects**, dopaminergic neurons in the SNc act to inhibit excitatory neurons in the indirect pathway.

○ In **PD**, there is dopaminergic cell loss in the SNc, resulting in increased striatal inhibition of the GPe. The reduced inhibition of the STN results in increased excitation of the GPi, which in turn results in excess inhibition of the thalamus. The final pathway would be a reduced activation of the motor cortex.

NEUROPROTECTION TRIALS

■ Although several agents have been tested to evaluate their neuroprotective effect in PD, none has been definitively shown to slow disease progression (Table 4.3).[39–62]

■ Currently, the clinical data for neuroprotective agents for patients with early PD are conflicting and inconclusive.

■ Clinical endpoints available are readily confounded by agents that also carry symptomatic effects.

Table 4.3
Neuroprotective Trials in Parkinson's Disease to Date

Agents	Trial	N	Primary Outcome	Conclusion
Antioxidants (monoamine oxidase B inhibitors and inosine)				
Selegiline (deprenyl) and tocopherol[39]	DATATOP	800	Need for levodopa	Selegiline delayed the need for levodopa therapy; however, this may be due to its symptomatic effect. There is no beneficial effect of vitamin E.
Selegiline (deprenyl)[40]	Tetrud and Langston	54	Need for levodopa	Early selegiline therapy delays the requirement for antiparkinsonian medications, possibly by slowing progression of the disease.
Selegiline (deprenyl)[41]	SINDEPAR	101	UPDRS	Selegiline attenuates deterioration in UPDRS score in patients with early PD. These findings are not readily explained by the drug's symptomatic effects and are consistent with the hypothesis that deprenyl has a neuroprotective effect.
Selegiline[42]	Swedish Selegiline	157	Need for levodopa	Selegiline delayed significantly the need to start levodopa in early PD. After a 2-month washout period (before the start of levodopa therapy), no significant symptomatic effect of selegiline was seen in comparison with the placebo group, supporting the concept of neuroprotective properties of the drug.
Selegiline[43]	Norwegian-Danish	163	UPDRS change	Patients treated with the combination of selegiline and levodopa developed markedly less severe parkinsonism and required lower doses of levodopa during the 5-year study period than did patients treated with levodopa and placebo.

continued

Table 4.3 (cont.)
Neuroprotective Trials in Parkinson's Disease to Date

Agents	Trial	N	Primary Outcome	Conclusion
Rasagiline[44]	TEMPO	404	UPDRS change	Subjects treated with rasagiline, 2 and 1 mg/d, for 12 months showed less functional decline than subjects whose treatment was delayed for 6 months.
Rasagiline[45]	ADAGIO	1,176	UPDRS change	Early treatment with rasagiline at a dose of 1 mg/d provided benefits that suggested a possible disease-modifying effect, but early treatment with rasagiline 2 mg/d did not.
Inosine: phase 2 trial[46]	SURE-PD	90	Tolerability, validity (urate elevation), dosage, and symptomatic efficacy will be assessed after 12 weeks of treatment.	The phase 2 study showed that inosine is safe and well tolerated in PD. Plans are currently under way for a phase 3 trial, as a potential neuroprotectant in PD is warranted.
Agents that enhance mitochondrial function				
Coenzyme Q10[47]	QE2	80	UPDRS change	Coenzyme Q10 was safe and well tolerated at dosages of up to 1,200 mg/d. Less disability developed in subjects assigned to coenzyme Q10 than in those assigned to placebo, and the benefit was greatest in subjects receiving the highest dose.
Coenzyme Q10[48]	QE3	600	UPDRS change	The study was prematurely terminated. It was futile to complete the study because it was very unlikely to demonstrate a statistically significant benefit of active treatment over placebo.

continued

Table 4.3 (cont.)
Neuroprotective Trials in Parkinson's Disease to Date

Agents	Trial	N	Primary Outcome	Conclusion
Isradipine	STEADY-PD	99	Tolerability	The tolerability of isradipine was dose-dependent. No difference in change in UPDRS was noted among doses. A phase 3 trial is under way to assess the efficacy of 10 mg of isradipine in slowing PD progression.
Antiexcitotoxic and antiglutaminergic agents				
Amantadine[49]	Amantadine (retrospective, unblinded study)	836	Better survival (higher 10-year expected survival, absence of dementia, type of parkinsonism=PD and low Hoehn and Yahr Scale stage 1 or 2)	The association of improved survival with amantadine use may stem from symptomatic benefit or may reflect a "neuroprotective" effect.
Riluzole[50]	Jankovic and Hunter	20	UPDRS change	No evidence of symptomatic effect of riluzole was observed. Riluzole was well tolerated.
Riluzole[51]	Riluzole	1,084	Need for symptomatic treatment	Riluzole did not show superiority over placebo in slowing PD progression.
Antiapoptotic agents				
CEP-1347 (potent inhibitor of kinase 3)[52]	PRECEPT	800	UPDRS change	CEP-1347 was ineffective as a disease-modifying treatment in early PD.
TCH346[53]		301	UPDRS change	TCH346 did not show any difference in time to disability requiring dopaminergic therapy or change in UPDRS or quality of life.

continued

Table 4.3 (cont.)
Neuroprotective Trials in Parkinson's Disease to Date

Agents	Trial	N	Primary Outcome	Conclusion
Dopamine agonists and levodopa				
Ropinirole vs levodopa[54]	REAL-PET	186	Fluorodopa PET	Ropinirole is associated with a slower progression of PD than levodopa as assessed by ^{18}F-dopa. PET.
Pramipexole vs levodopa[55]	CALM-PD-CIT	82	Beta-CIT change	Patients initially treated with pramipexole demonstrated a loss of striatal [^{123}I]beta-CIT uptake vs those treated with levodopa during a 46-month period.
Pramipexole[56]	PROUD	535	UPDRS change	Results do not support a disease-modifying effect of pramipexole but confirm its efficacy and tolerability as monotherapy in early PD.
Levodopa[57]	ELLDOPA	360	UPDRS change [^{123}I]beta-CIT change	Levodopa in a dose response pattern significantly reduced the worsening of symptoms of PD. After the washout period, high-dose levodopa (600 mg daily) had better UPDRS scores but more adverse events of dyskinesia, nausea, headache, infection, and hypertonia and showed a greater decline in [^{123}I] beta-CIT uptake.
Anti-inflammatory effects and enhancement of mitochondrial function				
Minocycline and creatine[58]	NINDS NET-PD FS-1	200	UPDRS change	Both creatine and minocycline should be considered for definitive phase 3 trials to determine if they alter the long-term progression of PD.
GDNF[59]	Liatermin	34	UPDRS change	Liatermin did not confer the predetermined level of clinical benefit to patients with PD despite increased ^{18}F-dopa uptake.
Ibuprofen[60]	Harvard epidemiological study	291	Meta-analysis	Ibuprofen is potentially neuroprotective against PD, not shared by other NSAIDs or acetaminophen.

continued

Table 4.3 (cont.)
Neuroprotective Trials in Parkinson's Disease to Date

Agents	Trial	N	Primary Outcome	Conclusion
Agents that enhance mitochondrial function and neuro-immunophilin				
Coenzyme Q10 and GP-1485[61]	NINDS NET-PD FS-Too	213	UPDRS change	Coenzyme Q10 and GPI-1485 may warrant further study in PD, although the data are inconsistent. Additional factors (cost, availability of other agents, more recent data on placebo outcomes, other ongoing trials) should also be considered in the selection of agents for phase 3 studies.
Agents that increase brain-derived neurotrophic factor (BDNF) and glial cell line–derived neurotrophic factor (GDNF)				
Exercise (indirect evidence)[62]	Osaka epide-miology study	438	Epidemiology study	The exercising group showed a reduced mortality.

Abbreviations: ADAGIO, Attenuation of Disease Progression With Azilect Given Once Daily; CALM-PD, Comparison of the Agonist Pramipexole With Levodopa on Motor Complications of PD; DATA-TOP, Deprenyl and Tocopherol Antioxidative Therapy of Parkinsonism; ELLDOPA, Earlier Versus Later Levodopa Therapy in PD; NINDS, National Institute of Neurological Disease and Stroke; NET-PD FS-1, Neuroprotective Exploratory Trials in PD, Futility Study 1; PET, positron emission tomography; PRECEPT, A Randomized Double-Blind Placebo-Controlled Dose-Finding Study to Assess the Efficacy and Safety of CEP 1347 in Patients With Early PD; PROUD, Pramipexole on Underlying Disease; QE2, Coenzyme Q10 Evaluation-2; REAL-PET, Requip as Early Therapy Versus L-dopa PET; SINDEPAR, Sinemet-Deprenyl-Parlodel; STEADY PD, Safety, Tolerability, and Efficacy Assessment of Dynacirc CR for PD; SURE-PD, Safety of Urate Elevation in PD; TEMPO, TVP-1012 in Early Monotherapy for PD Outpatients; UPDRS, Unified Parkinson's Disease Rating Scale.

DIAGNOSIS

■ The diagnosis of PD remains clinical to this day (Figure 4.10). The UK Parkinson's Disease Society Brain Bank Clinical Diagnostic Criteria have been used as a gold standard diagnostic tool in PD research (Table 4.4).[63]

■ At present, there is no biological marker that unequivocally confirms the diagnosis of PD.

  ○ Imaging and other ancillary tests have been utilized (clinically or in PD research) to help confirm the diagnosis of PD (Table 4.5).

  ○ Recently, DaTscan has been approved by the US Food and Drug Administration (FDA) to differentiate neurodegenerative parkinsonism (eg, PD) from nonneurodegenerative parkinsonism (eg, essential tremor, vascular parkinsonism, drug-induced parkinsonism) (Figure 4.11). However, DaTscan is unable to differentiate PD from other Parkinson-plus syndromes (eg, progressive supranuclear palsy, multiple system atrophy, dementia with Lewy bodies).

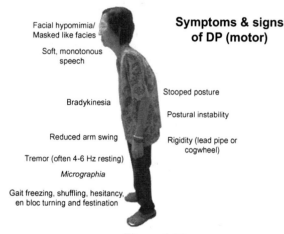

Facial hypomimia/
Masked like facies

Soft, monotonous
speech

**Symptoms & signs
of DP (motor)**

Bradykinesia

Stooped posture

Postural instability

Reduced arm swing

Rigidity (lead pipe or
cogwheel)

Tremor (often 4-6 Hz resting)

Micrographia

Gait freezing, shuffling, hesitancy,
en bloc turning and festination

Figure 4.10
Motor features of Parkinson's disease.

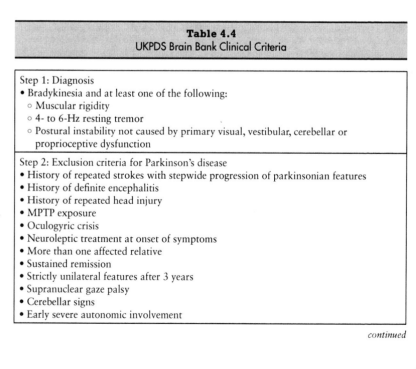

Table 4.4
UKPDS Brain Bank Clinical Criteria

Step 1: Diagnosis
- Bradykinesia and at least one of the following:
  - Muscular rigidity
  - 4- to 6-Hz resting tremor
  - Postural instability not caused by primary visual, vestibular, cerebellar or proprioceptive dysfunction

Step 2: Exclusion criteria for Parkinson's disease
- History of repeated strokes with stepwide progression of parkinsonian features
- History of definite encephalitis
- History of repeated head injury
- MPTP exposure
- Oculogyric crisis
- Neuroleptic treatment at onset of symptoms
- More than one affected relative
- Sustained remission
- Strictly unilateral features after 3 years
- Supranuclear gaze palsy
- Cerebellar signs
- Early severe autonomic involvement

continued

Table 4.4 (cont.)
UKPDS Brain Bank Clinical Criteria

- Early severe dementia with disturbances of memory, language, and praxis
- Babinski sign
- Presence of cerebral tumor or communicating hydrocephalus on CT scan
- Negative response to large doses of levodopa (if malabsorption excluded)

Step 3: Supportive criteria for Parkinson's disease (three or more required for diagnosis of definite Parkinson's disease)
- Unilateral onset
- Resting tremor
- Progressive disorder
- Persistent asymmetry with side of onset affected to greater degree
- Excellent response (70%–100%) to levodopa
- Severe levodopa-induced chorea
- Levodopa response for 5 years or more
- Clinical course of 10 years or more

Abbreviation: UKPDS, UK Parkinson's Disease Society Brain Bank Clinical Diagnostic Criteria.

Source: Adapted from Ref. 63: Gibb WR, Lees AJ. The relevance of the Lewy body to the pathogenesis of idiopathic Parkinson's disease. *J Neurol Neurosurg Psychiatry.* 1988;51:745–752.

Table 4.5
Imaging and Ancillary Tests for Parkinson's Disease

Test	Interpretation	Advantage	Disadvantages
Positron emission tomography (PET) (commonly ^{18}F-dopa used as PET marker for dopamine synthesis)	Reduction of ^{18}F-dopa uptake, particularly in the putamen	Differentiates PD from multiple system atrophy (MSA), progressive supranuclear palsy (PSP), and other types of degenerative parkinsonism	Expensive and not widely available
Single photon emission tomography (SPECT) ([^{123}I]FP-CIT [DaTscan], [^{123}I] beta-CIT, TRO-DAT commonly used as isotope-labeled dopamine transporters)	Reduced presynaptic dopamine activity in PD and other types of neurodegenerative parkinsonism	Differentiates neurodegenerative parkinsonism from other differential diagnoses (eg, essential tremor, drug-induced parkinsonism, vascular parkinsonism)	Unable to differentiate PD from other types of neurodegenerative parkinsonism (eg, PSP, MSA) Expensive

continued

Table 4.5 (cont.)
Imaging and Ancillary Tests for Parkinson's Disease

Test	Interpretation	Advantage	Disadvantages
Diffusion tensor imaging	Fractional anisotropy (FA) in substantia nigra (SN) reduced in PD	Indirect measure of dopaminergic degeneration within SN Cheaper than PET or SPECT and MRI more widely available Differentiates PD from atypical parkinsonism (abnormal FA in putamen) Potentially a noninvasive early biomarker of PD 100% sensitivity and specificity for distinguishing subjects with PD from healthy subjects	Lack of experience in interpretation Not widely performed No correlation between FA and Unified Parkinson's Disease Rating Scale (UPDRS) scores
Proton density–weighted spin-echo (SE) and fast short T1 inversion recovery (STIR) images	Iron deposition in lateral substantia nigra, pars compacta (SNc)	Correlation with progression of motor symptoms Potential biomarker for disease progression	No difference in size of SN between PD and normal subjects
Magnetic resonance spectroscopy (MRS)	Normal or reduced N-acetylaspartate (NAA) and increased lactate Significant increase in lactate/NAA ratio in PD with dementia	Noninvasive technique	Nonspecific False negatives Not able to differentiate PD from atypical parkinsonism
Transcranial ultrasound	Hyperechogenicity from SN in PD	May identify early disease when combined with other noninvasive tests (eg, olfactory testing)	Difficult to perform and time-consuming Nonspecific

continued

Table 4.5 (cont.)
Imaging and Ancillary Tests for Parkinson's Disease

Test	Interpretation	Advantage	Disadvantages
Cardiac sympathetic nerve imaging (ligand includes meta-iodobenzylguanidine [MIBG])	Decreased in PD (dopamine transporter loss) Normal in MSA and other types of neurodegenerative parkinsonism	Sensitive Helps to differentiate PD from MSA	Nonspecific
Olfactory testing (eg, University of Pennsylvania Smell Identification Test [UPSIT])	Impaired olfaction correlates with functional neuroimaging abnormalities	Can identify early PD, even before motor symptoms of PD	Nonspecific
Dopaminergic challenge test	Positive response in PD is a reduction in motor score of 20% (60 min after levodopa or 20 min after apomorphine)	Easy to perform Good predictor of response to treatment	False negatives (some patients may show response to longer-term oral therapy) Difficult to determine if baseline motor score < 10
Sweat test *Axon reflex test:* iontophoresis of 10% acetylcholine in five sites with 2 mA of direct current for 5 minutes; sweat output recorded for this time and for additional 5 min *Thermoregulatory sweat test:* environment of 50% humidity and 50°C (skin at 40°C) for 30 min or core temperature increased by more than 1.5°C; sweat output quantified	Impaired sweat axon reflex in PD and MSA	Studies autonomic function	Unable to definitively differentiate PD from MSA

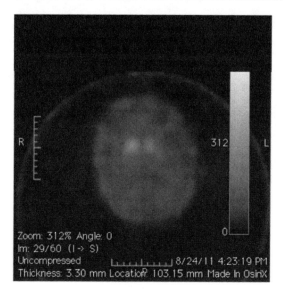

Figure 4.11

Single photon emission computed tomographic scan of a patient with Parkinson's disease showing decreased tracer uptake in the bilateral putamen, suggestive of loss of dopaminergic neuronal terminal density in the striatum.

- The PD motor presentation can be divided into two phenotypes (Figure 4.12).

  - Akinetic–rigid syndrome or postural instability gait dysfunction subtype (PIGD)

  - Tremor-predominant subtype

- Certain clinical features, such as resting tremor, asymmetry of parkinsonian motor symptoms, and good response to levodopa, strongly suggest PD rather than a Parkinson-plus syndrome (Figure 4.13).

- The akinetic–rigid syndrome or PIGD subtype is more challenging to differentiate from other Parkinson-plus syndromes.

Clinical Rating Scale for Parkinson's Disease

- There is currently no biomarker to assess the severity of PD.

- The severity of PD is based mainly on the clinical features.

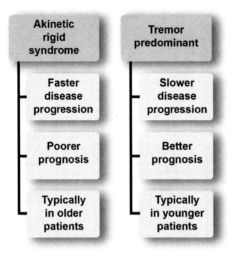

Figure 4.12
Clinical phenotype of Parkinson's disease.

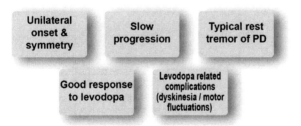

Figure 4.13
Features suggestive of Parkinson's disease compared with other causes of parkinsonism.

■ The Unified Parkinson's Disease Rating Scale (UPDRS) is the most widely used scale to assess PD severity and symptomatic motor improvement in treatment trials and in clinical practice (Table 4.6).[64–67]

Nonmotor Symptoms of Parkinson's Disease

■ Almost all PD patients will develop nonmotor complications (Table 4.7).

○ **Always ask patients (or their caregivers) about these nonmotor symptoms!**

Table 4.6
Comparison of Scales in Parkinson's Disease

Scale	Advantages	Disadvantages
Unified Parkinson's Disease Rating Scale (UPDRS)[64]	• Most widely used "gold standard"	• Length of scale (about 17 min required for experienced users) • Less emphasis on neuropsychiatric symptoms and other nonmotor symptoms
Movement Disorder Society–sponsored revision of Unified Parkinson's Disease Rating Scale (MDS-UPDRS)[65]	• Comprehensive and better instructions and scoring anchor descriptions • Good emphasis on neuropsychiatric symptoms and other nonmotor symptoms • Validated in several languages; ongoing validation in additional languages	• Length of scale • New and therefore not sufficiently tested in clinical trials
Short Parkinson's Evaluation Scale/Scale for Outcomes in Parkinson's Disease (SPES/SCOPA)[66]	• Short and practical • High reproducibility	• Lack of assessment of nonmotor symptoms of PD • Not widely used
Hoehn and Yahr[67]	• Short and easy to administer • Correlates well with disease progression • Correlates well with pathology of PD	• Emphasizes only motor component of PD • Lacking detail and not comprehensive

Source: Adapted from Refs. 64–67.

   ○   If present, determine if they fluctuate, as many of these nonmotor features worsen in the "off" state. In this case, lessening/improving the wearing-off state through dopaminergic medication adjustments may also improve the nonmotor features.

   ○   If these nonmotor features are pervasive and persist regardless of motor state, then a more targeted, symptom-specific approach and treatment are warranted.

■   The nonmotor symptoms of PD decrease quality of life (often more so than the motor features of the disorder) and impose significant caregiver stress and an economic burden on society.

- Some nonmotor symptoms occur very early and even predate the onset of motor symptoms (eg, anosmia, constipation, depression, REM sleep behavior disorder).

- Other nonmotor symptoms, such as behavioral and cognitive dysfunction, are the major contributors of disability in advanced disease states, especially dementia and psychosis (which are typically drug-induced). However, anxiety, apathy, depression, fatigue, and urinary, speech, swallow, and sleep disturbances are also fairly common.

- The dopaminergic treatment seems to be unhelpful for most of the nonmotor symptoms unless these are linked to motor fluctuations.[68]

- Table 4.8 summarize the nonmotor features of PD, along with their possible etiologies and treatment.[69]

Table 4.7
Overview of Nonmotor Symptoms of Parkinson's Disease

Behavioral and cognitive • Depression • Anxiety and panic attacks • Dementia or mild cognitive impairment • Apathy • Impulse control disorders (dopamine dysregulation syndrome: punding, pathologic gambling, compulsive shopping, binge eating, hypersexuality) • Hallucinations • Delusions
Sleep • REM sleep behavior disorder • Restless legs syndrome • Insomnia • Sleep fragmentation
Autonomic dysfunction • Blood pressure control (orthostatic hypotension, supine hypertension) • Gastrointestinal problems (constipation, dysphagia, nausea, drooling of saliva, nausea, reflux, vomiting, gastroparesis) • Bladder dysfunction (hyperactive and disinhibited bladder) • Sexual dysfunction (impotence, decreased libido) • Dry mouth • Hypo/hyperhidrosis
Fatigue
Pain
Weight loss
Skin • Seborrheic dermatitis

Table 4.8
Nonmotor Symptoms of Parkinson's Disease With Possible Etiology and Treatment

Nonmotor Symptoms (Prevalence)	Possible Etiopathophysiology	Treatment
Behavioral and cognitive symptoms		
Depression (up to 72% of patients with PD)	• Involvement of serotoninergic and noradrenergic system in the orbitofrontal–subcortical connections	• Pramipexole[A] • Selective serotonin receptor inhibitors (SSRIs) (eg, sertraline[E], escitalopram, citalopram[E], paroxetine[E], fluoxetine[E]) • Tricyclic antidepressants (TCAs) (eg, nortriptyline[B], desipramine[B], amitriptyline[E]) • Mirtazapine (noradrenergic and serotoninergic antidepressant) • Bupropion (norepinephrine reuptake inhibitor) • Duloxetine and venlafaxine (serotonin and noradrenaline reuptake inhibitors: SNRIs) • Nefazodone[E] (serotonin antagonist and reuptake inhibitor: SARI) • Atomoxetine[E] (SNRI) • Cognitive behavioral therapy • Transcranial magnetic stimulation (rTMS)[E] • Electroconvulsive therapy (ECT)[E] in severe depression
Anxiety and panic attacks (about 40% of PD patients)	• Changes in dopaminergic, noradrenergic, and serotoninergic pathways in the striatal motor system, nucleus accumbens, amygdala, locus ceruleus, and limbic structures • Sensory or behavior "offs" can accompany motor "offs"	• Psychotherapy • Benzodiazepine (eg, lorazepam, clonazepam, or alprazolam)

continued

Table 4.8 (cont.)
Nonmotor Symptoms of Parkinson's Disease With Possible Etiology and Treatment

Nonmotor Symptoms (Prevalence)	Possible Etiopathophysiology	Treatment
Dementia or mild cognitive impairment (40% in cross-sectional studies, 80% in longitudinal studies)	• Alpha-synuclein, beta-amyloid plaque, Lewy body inclusions and deficits in cholinergic output of pedunculopontine nucleus (PPN) • More common in postural instability gait disorder (PIGD) category than tremor-dominant category, older age, greater severity and longer duration of PD, and male gender • Montreal Cognitive Assessment (MOCA) better than Mini-Mental State Examination (MMSE) as screening tool • Predicts nursing home placement	• Provide environmental stability and safety • Manage sleep and mood disorders • Keep PD drugs for motor control at a minimum • Withdraw anticholinergics • Cholinesterase inhibitors (eg, rivastigmine[A], donepezil[E], and galantamine[E]) • N-methyl-d-aspartate receptor antagonist (ie, memantine[E]) • Only rivastigmine is FDA-approved for PD dementia in the United States
Apathy (38%–51% patients with PD)	• Involvement of dopaminergic pathways in the mesial frontal–anterior cingulate cortex connections • Risk factors include older age, male sex, higher depression scores, worsening of speech and motor skills with axial involvement, higher scores on the motor Unified Parkinson's Disease Rating Scale (UPDRS), dementia	• Responds slightly to dopaminergic drugs
Impulse control disorders, dopamine dysregulation syndrome: punding (1.4%–14%), pathologic gambling (3.4%–8% of PD patients), compulsive shopping, binge eating, hypersexuality (4.3% of PD patients)	• Dopaminergic activity in the ventral and dorsal striatum, nucleus accumbens, and mesolimbic network	• Decrease PD medications, especially dopamine agonists

continued

Table 4.8 (cont.)
Nonmotor Symptoms of Parkinson's Disease With Possible Etiology and Treatment

Nonmotor Symptoms (Prevalence)	Possible Etiopathophysiology	Treatment
Punding: repetitive, stereotypic, pointless motor behaviors	• Associated with dopaminergic medication, but not exclusively • More prevalent in male patients and patients with early onset of disease, right-sided onset of motor manifestations, past history of depression or bipolar disorder, disinhibition, irritability, and appetite disorders	• SSRI • Atypical antipsychotics (controversial, reports showing that quetiapine may worsen punding in patients with PD) • Amantadine[E] for pathologic gambling
Hallucinations (30%–40% of PD patients)	• Often visual hallucinations consisting of people or animals; occur in dim lighting; last only seconds to minutes	• Decrease or eliminate anti-PD medications in the following order: Anticholinergics ⬇ Amantadine ⬇ Monoamine oxidase B (MAO-B) inhibitors ⬇ Dopamine agonists ⬇ Catechol O-methyltransferase (COMT) inhibitors ⬇ Levodopa • Atypical antipsychotics with "milder" dopamine blocker (ie, clozapine[A] or quetiapine[E]); avoid olanzapine[C] • Mild cases may benefit from cholinesterase inhibitors or memantine
Delusions (8% of PD patients)	• Commonly paranoid, typically beliefs of abandonment or spousal infidelity	
Psychosis (lifetime prevalence in PD 25% to nearly 50%)	• Risk factors include older age, longer duration of illness, severe motor impairment, presence of depression and RBD, significant autonomic impairment, and visual acuity	
Sleep (60%–98% of PD patients)		
REM sleep behavior disorder (25%–50% of PD patients)	• Degeneration of lower brainstem nuclei involving laterodorsal tegmentum, pedunculopontine nucleus (PPN), perilocus ceruleus, medial medulla, and ventrolateral reticulospinal tracts (Braak stages 1 and 2)	• Low-dose clonazepam • Melatonin

continued

Table 4.8 (cont.)
Nonmotor Symptoms of Parkinson's Disease With Possible Etiology and Treatment

Nonmotor Symptoms (Prevalence)	Possible Etiopathophysiology	Treatment
Excessive daytime sleepiness (up to 50% of PD patients)	• Strongly associated with dopamine agonists • Risk for motor vehicle accidents	• Reduce dose of PD medications, particularly dopamine agonists • Reduce sedating medications, such as benzodiazepines, sedative antidepressants • Stimulants such as modafinil[E], sodium oxybate, methylphenidate, and anti-H3 drugs • Patients report feeling more alert with pedunculopontine deep brain stimulation
Restless legs syndrome (7.9%–50% of PD patients) and periodic limb movements during sleep (30%–80% of PD patients)	• Involvement of dopaminergic pathways other than nigrostriatal dopaminergic pathways	• Iron supplementation • Dopamine agonist (ie, pramipexole, ropinirole, or rotigotine patch) • Anticonvulsants, opioids, or benzodiazepines
Insomnia	• Degeneration of lower brainstem nuclei involving laterodorsal tegmentum, PPN, perilocus ceruleus, medial medulla, and ventrolateral reticulospinal tracts (Braak stages 1 and 2) • Most commonly caused by undertreated nocturnal parkinsonism, which is very responsive to levodopa therapy	• Benzodiazepines (eg, alprazolam) • Hypnotics (eg, eszopiclone[E]) • Melatonin[E] • Controlled-release formulation of levodopa/carbidopa[E]
Sleep fragmentation		• Benzodiazepines (eg, alprazolam, clonazepam) • Controlled-release formulation of levodopa/carbidopa
Autonomic dysfunction		
Orthostatic hypotension (35%–58% of PD patients)		• Increase intake of fluids, salt, and caffeine • Elevation of head of bed • Use abdominal ring binder or compression stockings • Advise patient to shift position from supine to sitting or standing slowly

continued

Table 4.8 (cont.)
Nonmotor Symptoms of Parkinson's Disease With Possible Etiology and Treatment

Nonmotor Symptoms (Prevalence)	Possible Etiopathophysiology	Treatment
		• Medications (fludrocortisone[E], midodrine[E], pyridostigmine, droxidopa)
Constipation	• Immobility • Drugs (eg, anticholinergics • Reduced fluid and food intake • Parasympathetic involvement (Lewy bodies in dorsal nucleus of vagus) prolonging colonic transit	• Physical exercise • Stop anticholinergics • Adequate intake of fluid, fruits, vegetables, fiber • Laxatives: lactulose (10–20 g/d), polyethylene glycol (macrogol[B]) • Apomorphine and duodopa
Gastroparesis		• Use of domperidone[B] • Botulinum toxin in the pyloric sphincter, electric stimulation, or surgery • Exercise, diet with high intake of liquid and dietary fiber, symbiotic yogurt, and medications such as macrogol
Urinary symptoms, such as urge incontinence (37%–70% of PD patients)	• Overactivity of the detrusor muscle attributed to loss of inhibition of D1 receptors in the micturition center in the pons	• Anticholinergic agents (eg, oxybutynin, solifenacin, tolterodine) • Darifenacin (selective M2–M3 muscarinic receptor)
Erectile dysfunction (42% of PD patients)	• Correlated with higher UPDRS, left-sided prominence of motor symptoms, lower educational level, cognitive impairment, fatigue, apathy, and low testosterone levels	• Sildenafil[E] or other phosphodiesterase inhibitors • Apomorphine
Sweating (45%–75% of PD patients)	• Decreased dopaminergic activity in the hypothalamus	• Use of cool, comfortable clothing

continued

Table 4.8 (cont.)
Nonmotor Symptoms of Parkinson's Disease With Possible Etiology and Treatment

Nonmotor Symptoms (Prevalence)	Possible Etiopathophysiology	Treatment
		• Maintaining low room temperature • Increasing intake of fluids • Control of motor fluctuations and avoidance of "wearing off"
Nausea	• More frequently related to medications	• Avoid use of metoclopramide as it potentially causes extrapyramidal side effects • Slow upward titration of PD medications • Add Lodosyn (pure carbidopa) • Antiemetics without extrapyramidal side effects (eg, trimethobenzamide, ondansetron, domperidone)
Drooling, sialorrhea, dysphagia (up to 75% of PD patients)	• Involvement of the dorsal motor nucleus of the vagus and the peripheral autonomic nervous system (myenteric plexus)	• Botulinum toxin A[A] and B[A] for treatment of sialorrhea • Anticholinergics (eg, glycopyrrolate[A]) for sialorrhea • Gum chewing for drooling and dysphagia
Hyposmia (40% of PD patients) and rhinorrhea	• Lewy bodies and Lewy neuritis in the olfactory nucleus and tract and amygdala	• No pharmacologic treatment for anosmia
Fatigue (about 44% of PD patients)	• Probable causes include mood disorders, changes in neurotransmitters, hormonal imbalance (eg, testosterone deficiency), changes in expression of cytokines and other inflammatory factors, changes in life patterns, sleep disturbances, apathy, and dysautonomia	• Medications (eg, amantadine, methylphenidate[E], modafinil[E], duodopa, selegiline, sodium oxybate, and levodopa)

continued

Table 4.8 (cont.)
Nonmotor Symptoms of Parkinson's Disease With Possible Etiology and Treatment

Nonmotor Symptoms (Prevalence)	Possible Etiopathophysiology	Treatment
Weight loss (65% of PD patients)	• Imbalance between food intake and consumption of energy • Associated with loss of appetite, taste, olfaction, and motility of bowels; low levels of leptins; dysphagia; drooling; gastroesophageal reflux; nausea; vomiting; constipation; depression; side effects of medications; loss of income; muscle wasting; rigidity; excess of movement (dyskinesia)	• Behavior therapies • Consider supplements • Mirtazapine
Pain (40% of PD patients)[69]	• May be associated with motor fluctuations, early morning dystonia, or musculoskeletal pain	

- Tables 4.9 through 4.15 summarize the levels of efficacy of described treatments for nonmotor complications of PD as follows:[70]

  ○ **Efficacious.** Evidence shows that the intervention has a positive effect on studied outcomes; supported by data from at least one high-quality (score ≥ 75%) randomized controlled trial without conflicting level 1 data.[A]

  ○ **Likely efficacious.** Evidence suggests, but is not sufficient to show, that the intervention has a positive effect on studied outcomes; supported by data from any level 1 trial without conflicting level 1 data.[B]

  ○ **Unlikely efficacious.** Evidence suggests that the intervention does not have a positive effect on studied outcomes; supported by data from any level 1 trial without conflicting level 1 data.[C]

  ○ **Nonefficacious.** Evidence shows that the intervention does not have a positive side effect on studied outcomes; supported by data from at least one high-quality (score ≥ 75%) randomized controlled trial without conflicting level 1 data.[D]

  ○ **Insufficient evidence.** There is not enough evidence either for or against efficacy of the intervention in the treatment of PD; all the circumstances not covered by the previous statement.[E]

Table 4.9
Evidence on Drugs Used for Depression in Parkinson's Disease

Drugs	Efficacy	Safety	Practice implications
Dopamine agonists			
Pramipexole	Efficacious	Acceptable risk without specialized monitoring	Clinically useful
Pergolide	Insufficient evidence	Acceptable risk with specialized monitoring	Not useful
Tricyclic antidepressants (TCAs)			
Nortriptyline	Likely efficacious	Acceptable risk without specialized monitoring	Possibly useful
Desipramine	Likely efficacious	Acceptable risk without specialized monitoring	Possibly useful
Amitriptyline	Insufficient evidence	Acceptable risk without specialized monitoring	Investigational
Selective serotonin receptor inhibitors (SSRIs)			
Citalopram	Insufficient evidence	Acceptable risk without specialized monitoring	Investigational
Sertraline	Insufficient evidence	Acceptable risk without specialized monitoring	Investigational
Paroxetine	Insufficient evidence	Acceptable risk without specialized monitoring	Investigational
Fluoxetine	Insufficient evidence	Acceptable risk without specialized monitoring	Investigational
Monoamine oxidase inhibitors			
Moclobemide	Insufficient evidence	Insufficient evidence (combined treatment with TCAs and SSRIs carries an unacceptable risk)	Investigational

continued

Table 4.9 (cont.)
Evidence on Drugs Used for Depression in Parkinson's Disease

Drugs	Efficacy	Safety	Practice implications
Selegiline	Insufficient evidence	Acceptable risk without specialized monitoring	Investigational
Newer antidepressants			
Atomoxetine	Insufficient evidence	Acceptable risk without specialized monitoring	Investigational
Nefazodone	Insufficient evidence	Unacceptable risk	Not useful
Alternative therapies			
Omega-3 fatty acids	Insufficient evidence	Acceptable risk without specialized monitoring	Investigational
Nonpharmacologic interventions			
Transcranial magnetic stimulation (rTMS)	Insufficient evidence	Acceptable risk without specialized monitoring	Investigational
Electroconvulsive therapy (ECT)	Insufficient evidence	Insufficient evidence	Investigational

Source: Adapted from Ref. 70: Seppi K, Weintraub D, Coelho M, et al. The Movement Disorder Society Evidence-Based Medicine Review Update: Treatments for the non-motor symptoms of Parkinson's disease. *Mov Disord.* 2011; 26(suppl 3):S42–S80.

Table 4.10
Evidence on Drugs Used for Fatigue in Parkinson's Disease

Drugs	Efficacy	Safety	Practice Implications
Methylphenidate	Insufficient evidence	Insufficient evidence	Investigational
Modafinil	Insufficient evidence	Insufficient evidence	Investigational

Source: Adapted from Ref. 70: Seppi K, Weintraub D, Coelho M, et al. The Movement Disorder Society Evidence-Based Medicine Review Update: Treatments for the non-motor symptoms of Parkinson's disease. *Mov Disord.* 2011; 26(suppl 3):S42–S80.

Table 4.11
Evidence on Drug Used for Pathologic Gambling in Parkinson's Disease

Drug	Efficacy	Safety	Practice Implications
Amantadine	Insufficient evidence	Acceptable risk without specialized monitoring	Investigational

Source: Adapted from Ref. 70: Seppi K, Weintraub D, Coelho M, et al. The Movement Disorder Society Evidence-Based Medicine Review Update: Treatments for the non-motor symptoms of Parkinson's disease. *Mov Disord.* 2011; 26(suppl 3):S42–S80.

Table 4.12
Evidence on Drugs Used for Dementia in Parkinson's Disease

	Efficacy	Safety	Practice Implications
Acetylcholinesterase inhibitors			
Donepezil	Insufficient evidence	Acceptable risk without specialized monitoring	Investigational
Rivastigmine	Efficacious	Acceptable risk without specialized monitoring	Clinically useful
Galantamine	Insufficient evidence	Acceptable risk without specialized monitoring	Investigational
N-methyl-D-aspartate (NMDA) receptor antagonist			
Memantine	Insufficient evidence	Acceptable risk without specialized monitoring	Investigational

Source: Adapted from Ref. 70: Seppi K, Weintraub D, Coelho M, et al. The Movement Disorder Society Evidence-Based Medicine Review Update: Treatments for the non-motor symptoms of Parkinson's disease. *Mov Disord.* 2011; 26(suppl 3):S42–S80.

Motor Fluctuations

■ About 40% of patients treated with levodopa develop motor fluctuations and/or dyskinesias within 4 to 6 years of initiating therapy.[71]

■ The pathogenesis of motor fluctuations remains unclear but appears to be associated with two major factors:[72]

  ○ Progression of PD

Table 4.13
Evidence on Drugs Used for Psychosis in Parkinson's Disease

Drugs	Efficacy	Safety	Practice Implications
Clozapine	Efficacious	Acceptable risk with specialized monitoring	Clinically useful
Olanzapine	Unlikely efficacious	Unacceptable risk	Not useful
Quetiapine	Insufficient evidence	Acceptable risk without specialized monitoring	Investigational

Note: Recent randomized controlled trials have shown the efficacy of pimavanserin, a serotonin (5-HT) receptor 2A antagonist, in alleviating Parkinson's disease psychosis without worsening parkinsonism.

Source: Adapted from Ref. 70: Seppi K, Weintraub D, Coelho M, et al. The Movement Disorder Society Evidence-Based Medicine Review Update: Treatments for the non-motor symptoms of Parkinson's disease. *Mov Disord.* 2011; 26(suppl 3):S42–S80.

Table 4.14
Evidence on Drugs Used for Autonomic Dysfunction in Parkinson's Disease

Drugs	Efficacy	Safety	Practice Implications
Orthostatic hypotension[a]			
Fludrocortisone	Insufficient evidence	Insufficient evidence	Investigational
Domperidone	Insufficient evidence	Insufficient evidence	Investigational
Midodrine	Insufficient evidence	Insufficient evidence	Investigational
Dihydroergotamine	Insufficient evidence	Insufficient evidence	Investigational
Etilefrine hydrochloride	Insufficient evidence	Insufficient evidence	Investigational
Indomethacin	Insufficient evidence	Insufficient evidence	Investigational
Yohimbine	Insufficient evidence	Insufficient evidence	Investigational
Threo-3-(3,4)-dihydroxyphenyl-L-serine	Insufficient evidence	Insufficient evidence	Investigational
Sexual dysfunction			
Sildenafil	Insufficient evidence	Insufficient evidence	Investigational
Gastrointestinal motility problems (constipation)			
Macrogol	Likely efficacious	Acceptable risk without specialized monitoring	Possibly useful

continued

Table 4.14 (cont.)
Evidence on Drugs Used for Autonomic Dysfunction in Parkinson's Disease

Drugs	Efficacy	Safety	Practice Implications
Gastrointestinal motility problems (anorexia, nausea, and vomiting associated with levodopa and/or dopamine agonist treatment)			
Domperidone	Likely efficacious	Acceptable risk without specialized monitoring	Possibly useful
Metoclopramide	Insufficient evidence	Unacceptable risk	Not useful
Sialorrhea			
Ipratropium bromide spray	Insufficient evidence	Insufficient evidence	Investigational
Glycopyrrolate	Efficacious	Insufficient evidence	Possibly useful
Botulinum toxin B	Efficacious	Acceptable risk with specialized monitoring	Clinically useful
Botulinum toxin A	Efficacious	Acceptable risk with specialized monitoring	Clinically useful
Urinary frequency, urinary urgency, and/or urge incontinence			
Oxybutynin	Insufficient evidence	Insufficient evidence	Investigational
Tolterodine	Insufficient evidence	Insufficient evidence	Investigational
Flavoxate	Insufficient evidence	Insufficient evidence	Investigational
Propiverine	Insufficient evidence	Insufficient evidence	Investigational
Prazosin	Insufficient evidence	Insufficient evidence	Investigational
Desmopressin	Insufficient evidence	Insufficient evidence	Investigational

[a]Droxidopa, a prodrug of norepinephrine and epinephrine capable of crossing the blood–brain barrier, has recently been shown in randomized controlled trials to mitigate orthostatic hypotension in primary autonomic disorders, such as Parkinson's disease and multiple systems atrophy.

Source: Adapted from Ref. 70: Seppi K, Weintraub D, Coelho M, et al. The Movement Disorder Society Evidence-Based Medicine Review Update: Treatments for the non-motor symptoms of Parkinson's disease. *Mov Disord.* 2011; 26(suppl 3):S42–S80.

○ Molecular and functional alterations of basal ganglia structures as a consequence of the *pulsatile dopaminergic stimulation* caused by the repeated oral administration of levodopa

■ Motor fluctuations are more likely to occur as the disease progresses (Figure 4.14).[73]

Table 4.15
Evidence on Drugs Used for Disorders of Sleep and Wakefulness in Parkinson's Disease

Drugs	Efficacy	Safety	Practice Implications
Insomnia			
Controlled-release formulation of levodopa/ carbidopa	Insufficient evidence	Acceptable risk without specialized monitoring	Investigational
Pergolide	Insufficient evidence	Acceptable risk with specialized monitoring	Not useful
Eszopiclone	Insufficient evidence	Acceptable risk without specialized monitoring	Investigational
Melatonin 3–5 mg	Insufficient evidence	Acceptable risk without specialized monitoring	Investigational
Melatonin 50 mg	Insufficient evidence	Insufficient evidence	Investigational
Excessive daytime somnolence and sudden onset of sleep			
Modafinil	Insufficient evidence	Insufficient evidence	Investigational

Source: Adapted from Ref. 70: Seppi K, Weintraub D, Coelho M, et al. The Movement Disorder Society Evidence-Based Medicine Review Update: Treatments for the non-motor symptoms of Parkinson's disease. *Mov Disord.* 2011; 26(suppl 3):S42–S80.

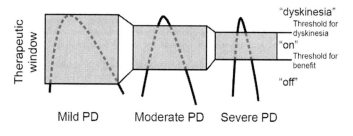

Figure 4.14
Changes in the clinical effect of Parkinson's disease as the disease progresses.
The therapeutic window narrows over time and as PD advances.

From Ref. 73: Dopamine agonists in early Parkinson's disease. Obeso JA et al. In: Olanow CW, Obeso JA, eds. Beyond the Decade of the Brain. Vol 2. Kent, UK: Wells Medical Ltd; 1997:11–35.

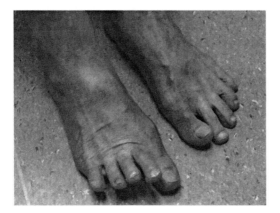

Figure 4.15
Striatal toes. Dystonic posturing of the right second to fifth toes
secondary to levodopa therapy.

- *Mild or early PD* is characterized by a smooth or extended duration of target clinical response; low incidence of dyskinesia.

- *Moderate PD* is generally characterized by diminished duration of target clinical response; increased incidence of dyskinesia.

- *Severe or advanced PD* is often characterized by short duration of target clinical response; "on" time is associated with dyskinesia, either choreic, ballistic, or dystonic in presentation (Figure 4.15). **In addition, this stage can be dominated by nonmotor features (eg, cognitive decline or dementia, psychosis).**

TREATMENT

- Levodopa remains the most effective medication for the treatment of PD.

- The disadvantage of levodopa is its greater likelihood of causing motor fluctuations, especially dyskinesias.

- However, it must be noted that dyskinesias, when they occur, are often less bothersome to the patient than they are to their caregivers. The majority of PD patients would typically prefer to be slightly dyskinetic than to be parkinsonian.

- The other medical therapies for PD consist of dopamine agonists, monoamine oxidase B (MAO-B) inhibitors, amantadine, anticholinergic agents, and catechol O-methyltransferase (COMT) inhibitors (Figure 4.16; Table 4.16).[74,75] In some countries, such as Japan, adenosine A2A antagonists are included among approved drug classes for PD.

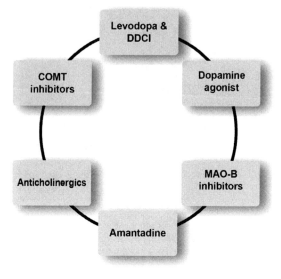

Figure 4.16
Current medical therapy for Parkinson's disease.

■ Figure 4.17 summarizes their mechanisms of action.

■ None of the medications has been shown to alter the progressive course of PD.

■ Delaying the use of levodopa early in the course of treatment delays the development of dyskinesia and motor fluctuations (Table 4.17).[76,77]

■ While the treatment for PD should be individualized to the patient, a general guideline/algorithm can be used based mainly on the patient's age and severity of motor symptoms (Figure 4.18).

  ○ Older patients are less likely to develop levodopa-induced dyskinesias and therefore are generally best initiated on levodopa, regardless of disease severity.

  ○ Younger patients are more likely to develop levodopa-induced dyskinesias, and therefore careful consideration before dopamine agonists or other adjunctive medications are initiated may be in order if their benefits outweigh the risks.

  ○ The superiority of levodopa over all other anti-PD oral medications, with regard to motor improvement, is clear; therefore, when functional disability is significant, it is best to use levodopa regardless of age or other factors.

Table 4.16
Medical Therapy for Parkinson's Disease

Medication Group[a]	Medications	Available Doses	Side Effects	Indications and Precautions
Levodopa	Carbidopa/levodopa (Sinemet)	10/100 mg, 25/100 mg, 50/200 mg	Nausea, vomiting, hypotension, hallucinations, somnolence, dyskinesias	• Most efficacious treatment for PD ("gold standard") • Greater likelihood for development of motor complications, dyskinesias • Better tolerated (compared with dopamine agonists), especially in the elderly
	Carbidopa/levodopa controlled release (Sinemet CR)	50/200 mg	Nausea, vomiting, hypotension, hallucination, somnolence, dyskinesias	
	Carbidopa/ levodopa/ entacapone (Stalevo)	12.5/50/200 mg, 25/100/200 mg, 37.5/150/200 mg	Nausea, vomiting, hypotension, hallucination, dyskinesias, somnolence, diarrhea, orange urine	
Dopamine agonist (ergot)	Bromocriptine	2.5 mg, 5 mg	Nausea, vomiting, leg edema, somnolence, valvular fibrosis	• Less efficacious than levodopa/ carbidopa • Pramipexole has been shown to be effective in tremor (75) and has possible antidepressant effect • Less tolerated than levodopa (more sedation, hallucinations, edema) • Watch for idiosyncratic class side effects: pedal edema, impulse control disorder, "sleep attacks" (ie, suddenly falling asleep without warning), weight gain
Dopamine agonists (nonergot)	Pramipexole (Mirapex)	0.125 mg, 0.25 mg, 0.5 mg, 1 mg, 1.5 mg	Nausea, vomiting, leg edema, somnolence, impulse control disorder, weight gain	
	Ropinirole (Requip)	0.25 mg, 0.5 mg, 1 mg, 2 mg, 3 mg, 4 mg, 5 mg	Nausea, vomiting, leg edema, somnolence, impulse control disorder, weight gain	
	Piribedil (Trivastal)	50 mg	Nausea, vomiting, leg edema, somnolence, impulse control disorder, weight gain	

continued

105

Table 4.16 (cont.)
Medical Therapy for Parkinson's Disease

Medication Group[a]	Medications	Available Doses	Side Effects	Indications and Precautions
	Pramipexole extended release (Mirapex ER)	0.375 mg, 0.75 mg, 1.5 mg, 2.25 mg, 3 mg, 3.75 mg, and 4.5 mg	Nausea, vomiting, leg edema, somnolence, impulse control disorder, weight gain	
	Ropinirole extended release (Requip ER)	2 mg, 4 mg, 8 mg, 12 mg	Nausea, vomiting, leg edema, somnolence, impulse control disorder, weight gain	
	Rotigotine transdermal patch (Neupro)	2 mg, 4 mg, 6 mg	Rash, nausea, vomiting, somnolence	
	Apomorphine (Apokyn)	0.02 mL, 0.06 mL	Nausea, vomiting, dizziness, somnolence, skin changes	• Dopamine agonist with strong D1 and D2 receptor–stimulating properties • Lipophilic, therefore diffuses directly across blood–brain barrier, bypassing the active transport mechanism needed for levodopa absorption • Onset within 10 minutes of injection • Short half-life, lasting about 60–90 minutes • Useful as a rescue agent for "off" states

Drug class	Drug	Dosage	Side effects	Notes
Monoamine oxidase B (MAO-B) inhibitors	Selegiline (Eldepryl)	5 mg	Insomnia, hallucinations, confusion	• Indicated for monotherapy in early PD as well as adjunctive therapy with levodopa • Very well tolerated • "Debatable" neuroprotective effect • Reactions with tyramine-rich foods and selective serotonin reuptake inhibitors (SSRIs) no longer significant concerns
	Rasagiline (Azilect)	0.5 mg, 1 mg	Insomnia, hallucinations, confusion, possible serotonin syndrome (when mixed with serotonin and noradrenaline reuptake inhibitor [SNRI], tricyclic antidepressant [TCA])	
Catechol O-methyltransferase (COMT) inhibitors	Entacapone (Comtan)	200 mg	Orange urine, diarrhea, dyskinesia	• Effective to treat end-of-dose wearing-off effect • Must be used with levodopa/carbidopa • Uncommonly causes diarrhea
	Tolcapone (Tasmar)	100 mg, 200 mg	Orange urine, nausea, vomiting, abnormal liver function	
Anticholinergic agents	Trihexyphenidyl (benzhexol, Artane)	1 mg, 2 mg	Dry mouth, urinary retention, blurred vision, cognitive impairment, hallucination	• Useful for tremor • Limited effect on other parkinsonian motor symptoms • Not advisable in elderly in view of side effects of cognitive impairment and psychosis
	Benztropine (Cogentin)	0.5 mg	Dry mouth, urinary retention, blurred vision, cognitive impairment, hallucinations	
N-methyl-D-aspartate (NMDA) antagonist	Amantadine	100 mg	Dizziness, dry mouth, livedo reticularis, leg edema, hallucinations, tachyphylaxis	• Useful for dyskinesia • Useful for mild, early PD

[a]Istradefylline, the first adenosine A 2A antagonist, is now approved in some countries as an adjunctive treatment with levodopa to improve wearing-off symptoms.

Source: Adapted from Ref. 74: Bhidayasiri R, Brenden N. 10 commonly asked questions about Parkinson disease. Neurologist. 2011; 17:57–62.

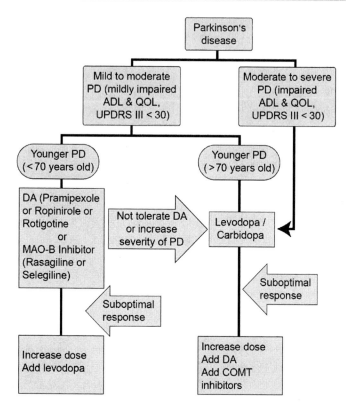

Figure 4.17

Mode of action of dopa-decarboxylase inhibitors, catechol O-methyltransferase (COMT) inhibitors, and monoamine oxidase B (MAO-B) inhibitors.

Table 4.17
Levodopa Versus Dopamine Agonist

Levodopa Advantages	Dopamine Agonist Advantages
• More efficacious with better symptomatic control than dopamine agonist • Easier administration • Quicker titration • Fewer side effects (eg, somnolence, pedal edema, impulse control disorder, weight gain) • Less costly	• Less likely to cause motor fluctuations, especially dyskinesias • Generic equivalents now available at lower cost • Brand name formulations may be taken once daily

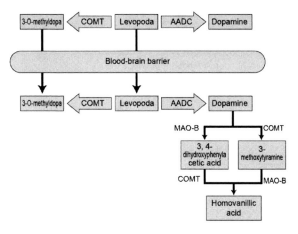

Figure 4.18
Treatment algorithm for the pharmacologic management of Parkinson's disease.

○ Similarly, given the superiority of levodopa in providing motor improvement and its better tolerability profile (compared with dopamine agonists), it is best to use levodopa when the exact diagnosis of the parkinsonian disorder is in question (eg, when a Parkinson-plus syndrome is a consideration).

■ Table 4.18[78–80] outlines the treatment options for motor fluctuations in PD, and Tables 4.19 through 4.23[81] summarize the levels of efficacy of described treatments for motor complications of PD according to the same criteria presented above (for nonmotor complications of PD).

■ *Advanced therapies in PD* are typically referred to as nonoral therapies and are generally reserved for patients who have significant motor fluctuations despite "optimized" pharmacologic adjustments and titrations with available oral symptomatic agents (Table 4.24). The three most commonly used advanced therapies in PD are the following:

○ *Deep brain stimulation surgery* (see also Chapter 16).

  • Several targets are currently approved in PD: STN, GPi, and ventral intermediate nucleus (VIM) of the thalamus.

○ *Levodopa/carbidopa intestinal gel infusion*

  • Delivery of levodopa in liquid gel form through an ambulatory pump via a percutaneous endoscopic gastrostomy tube that ends in the jejunum

  • Approved in most European countries and undergoing FDA evaluation in the United States

Table 4.18
Treatment for Motor Complications

Motor Fluctuations[a]	Treatment
Delayed "on" response	• Take additional doses of short-acting levodopa • Liquid levodopa • Apomorphine injection
Early morning akinesia	• Controlled-release levodopa at bedtime • Dispersible levodopa in the early morning • Apomorphine injection
End-of-dose wearing off[b]	• Increase dosage frequency • Add long-acting levodopa • Add COMT inhibitors, dopamine agonists, or MAO-B inhibitors • Convert to carbidopa/levodopa/entacapone (Stalevo) • DBS
Unpredictable "on–off" effects	• Liquid levodopa • Apomorphine injection
Episodes of freezing	• Physical therapy or occupational therapy
Dyskinesias	• **Treatment**
Peak-dose dyskinesia	• Reduce previous dose of levodopa • Discontinue COMT inhibitors and MAO-B inhibitors • Add amantadine • Avoid controlled-release levodopa • Add or increase dopamine agonist • DBS
"Off dystonia"	• Increase levodopa dose • Botulinum toxin • Baclofen (79) • Lithium (80)
Diphasic dyskinesia	• Increase levodopa dose • DBS

Abbreviations: COMT, catechol O-methyltransferase; DBS, deep brain stimulation; MAO-B, monoamine oxidase B.

[a]Recent reports of intrajejunal levodopa/carbidopa intestinal gel in a double-blinded, double-dummy randomized clinical trial and a large, long-term, multicenter, prospective, open-label study have shown improvement of up to 4 hours in wearing off, without worsening of dyskinesias.

[b]Istradefylline, the first adenosine A 2A antagonist, is now approved in some countries as an adjunctive treatment with levodopa to improve wearing-off symptoms; zonisamide has also been shown to improve wearing-off states in a randomized controlled trial.

Source: Adapted from Ref. 78: Adler CH. Relevance of motor complications in Parkinson's disease. *Neurology.* 2002; 58(suppl 1):S51–S56.

Table 4.19

Evidence on Dopamine Agonists in Parkinson's Disease

Dopamine Agonists		Prevention/ Delay of Clinical Progression	Symptomatic Monotherapy	Symptomatic Adjunct to Levodopa	Prevention/ Delay of Motor Complications[a]	Treatment of Motor Complications[a]
Nonergot dopamine agonists						
Piribedil	Efficacy	Insufficient evidence	Efficacious	Efficacious	Insufficient evidence	Insufficient evidence (E, D)
	Safety	Acceptable risk without specialized monitoring				
	Practice implications	Investigational	Clinically useful	Clinically useful	Investigational (F, D)	Investigational (F, D)
Pramipexole	Efficacy	Insufficient evidence	Efficacious	Efficacious	Efficacious (E, D)	Efficacious (F) Insufficient evidence (D)
	Safety	Acceptable risk without specialized monitoring				
	Practice implications	Investigational	Clinically useful	Clinically useful	Clinically useful (F, D)	Clinically useful (F)
Pramipexole ER	Efficacy	Insufficient evidence	Efficacious	Insufficient evidence	Insufficient evidence (E, D)	Insufficient evidence (E, D)
	Safety	Acceptable risk without specialized monitoring				
	Practice implications	Investigational	Clinically useful	Investigational	Investigational (F, D)	Investigational (F, D)
Ropinirole	Efficacy	Insufficient evidence	Efficacious	Efficacious	Insufficient evidence (F) Efficacious (D)	Efficacious (F) Insufficient evidence (D)
	Safety	Acceptable risk without specialized monitoring				
	Practice implications	Investigational	Clinically useful	Clinically useful	Investigational (F) Clinically useful (D)	Clinically useful (F) Investigational(D)

continued

Table 4.19 (cont.)
Evidence on Dopamine Agonists in Parkinson's Disease

Dopamine Agonists		Prevention/ Delay of Clinical Progression	Symptomatic Monotherapy	Symptomatic Adjuvant to Levodopa	Prevention/ Delay of Motor Complications[a]	Treatment of Motor Complications[a]
Ropinirole XL	Efficacy	Insufficient evidence	Likely efficacious	Efficacious	Insufficient evidence (F) / Efficacious (D)	Efficacious (F) / Insufficient evidence (D)
	Safety	Acceptable risk without specialized monitoring				
	Practice implications	Investigational	Possibly useful	Clinically useful	Investigational (F) / Clinically useful (D)	Clinically useful (F) / Investigational (D)
Rotigotine patch	Efficacy	Insufficient evidence	Efficacious	Efficacious	Insufficient evidence (F, D)	Efficacious (F) / Insufficient evidence (D)
	Safety	Acceptable risk without specialized monitoring				
	Practice implications	Investigational	Clinically useful	Clinically useful	Investigational (F, D)	Clinically useful (F) / Investigational (D)
Apomorphine	Efficacy	Insufficient evidence	Insufficient evidence	Efficacious	Insufficient evidence (F, D)	Efficacious (F) / Insufficient evidence (D)
	Safety	Acceptable risk without specialized monitoring when used as parenteral therapy				
	Practice implications	Investigational	Investigational	Clinically useful	Investigational (F, D)	Clinically useful (F) / Investigational (D)
Ergot dopamine agonists						
Bromocriptine	Efficacy	Insufficient evidence	Likely efficacious	Efficacious	Insufficient evidence (F) / Likely efficacious (D)	Likely efficacious (F) / Insufficient evidence (D)
	Safety	Acceptable risk with specialized monitoring				
	Practice implications	Investigational	Possibly useful	Clinically useful	Investigational (F) / Possibly useful (D)	Possibly useful (F) / Investigational (D)

Cabergoline	Efficacy	Insufficient evidence	Efficacious	Efficacious	Efficacious (F, D)	Likely efficacious (F) Insufficient evidence (D)
	Safety	Acceptable risk with specialized monitoring				
	Practice implications	Investigational	Clinically useful	Clinically useful	Clinically useful (F, D)	Possibly useful (F) Investigational (D)
Dihydroergo-cryptine	Efficacy	Insufficient evidence	Efficacious	Insufficient evidence	Insufficient evidence (E, D)	Insufficient evidence (F, D)
	Safety	Acceptable risk with specialized monitoring				
	Practice implications	Investigational	Clinically useful	Investigational	Investigational (F, D)	Investigational (F, D)
Lisuride	Efficacy	Insufficient evidence	Likely efficacious	Likely efficacious	Insufficient evidence (F, D)	Insufficient evidence (F, D)
	Safety	Acceptable risk with specialized monitoring				
	Practice implications	Investigational	Possibly useful	Possibly useful	Investigational (F, D)	Investigational (E, D)
Pergolide	Efficacy	Unlikely efficacious	Efficacious	Efficacious	Insufficient evidence (F) Likely efficacious (D)	Efficacious (F) Insufficient evidence (D)
	Safety	Acceptable risk with specialized monitoring				
	Practice implications	Unlikely useful	Clinically useful	Clinically useful	Investigationally useful (F) Possibly useful (D)	Clinically useful (F) Investigational (D)

[a] D, dyskinesia; F, motor fluctuations.

Source: Adapted from Ref. 81: Fox SH, Katzenschlager R, Lim SY, et al. The Movement Disorder Society Evidence-Based Medicine Review Update: Treatments for the motor symptoms of Parkinson's disease. Mov Disord. 2011; 26(suppl 3):S2–S41.

Table 4.20

Evidence on Levodopa in Parkinson's Disease

Levodopa		Prevention/Delay of Clinical Progression	Symptomatic Monotherapy	Symptomatic Adjuvant to Levodopa	Prevention/Delay of Motor Complications[a]	Treatment of Motor Complications[a]
Standard formulation	Efficacy	Insufficient evidence	Efficacious	Not applicable	Non-efficacious (F, D)	Efficacious (F) Insufficient evidence (D)
	Safety	Acceptable risk without specialized monitoring				
	Practice implications	Investigational	Clinically useful	Not applicable	Not useful (F, D)	Clinically useful (F) Investigational (D)
Controlled-release formulation	Efficacy	Insufficient evidence	Efficacious	Not applicable	Non-efficacious (F, D)	Insufficient evidence (F, D)
	Safety	Acceptable risk without specialized monitoring				
	Practice implications	Investigational	Clinically useful	Not applicable	Not useful	Investigational (F, D)
Rapid-onset oral formulation	Efficacy	Insufficient evidence	Insufficient evidence	Insufficient evidence	Insufficient evidence (F, D)	Insufficient evidence (F, D)
	Safety	Acceptable risk without specialized monitoring				
	Practice implications	Investigational	Investigational	Investigational	Investigational (F, D)	Investigational (F, D)
Infusion formulations	Efficacy	Insufficient evidence	Insufficient evidence	Insufficient evidence	Insufficient evidence (F, D)	Likely efficacious (F, D)
	Safety	Acceptable risk without specialized monitoring				
	Practice implications	Investigational	Investigational	Investigational	Investigational (F, D)	Investigational (F, D)

[a]D, dyskinesia; F, motor fluctuations.

Source: Adapted from Ref. 81: Fox SH, Katzenschlager R, Lim SY, et al. The Movement Disorder Society Evidence-Based Medicine Review Update: Treatments for the motor symptoms of Parkinson's disease. *Mov Disord.* 2011; 26(suppl 3)S2–S41.

Table 4.21
Evidence on COMT Inhibitors in Parkinson's Disease

COMT Inhibitors		Prevention/Delay of Clinical Progression	Symptomatic Monotherapy	Symptomatic Adjuvant to Levodopa	Prevention/Delay of Motor Complications[a]	Treatment of Motor Complications[a]
Entacapone	Efficacy	Insufficient evidence	Not applicable	Efficacious (for subjects with motor complications) Non-efficacious (for nonfluctuating subjects)	Non-efficacious (F, D)	Efficacious (F) Insufficient evidence (D)
	Safety	Acceptable risk without specialized monitoring				
	Practice implications	Investigational	Not applicable	Clinically useful (for subjects with motor complications) Not useful (for nonfluctuating subjects)	Not useful (F, D)	Clinically useful (F) Investigational (D)
Tolcapone	Efficacy	Insufficient evidence	Not applicable	Efficacious	Insufficient evidence (E, D)	Efficacious (F) Insufficient evidence (D)
	Safety	Acceptable risk with specialized monitoring				
	Practice implications	Investigational	Not applicable	Possibly useful	Investigational (E, D)	Possibly useful (F) Investigational (D)

Abbreviation: COMT, catechol O-methyltransferase.

[a]D, dyskinesia; F, motor fluctuations.

Source: Adapted from Ref. 81: Fox SH, Katzenschlager R, Lim SY, et al. The Movement Disorder Society Evidence-Based Medicine Review Update: Treatments for the motor symptoms of Parkinson's disease. *Mov Disord.* 2011; 26(suppl 3):S2–S41.

115

Table 4.22
Evidence on MAO-B Inhibitors in Parkinson's Disease

MAO-B Inhibitors		Prevention/Delay of Clinical Progression	Symptomatic Monotherapy	Symptomatic Adjuvant to Levodopa	Prevention/Delay of Motor Complications[a]	Treatment of Motor Complications[a]
Selegiline	Efficacy	Insufficient evidence	Efficacious	Insufficient evidence	Insufficient evidence (F) Non-efficacious (D)	Insufficient evidence (F, D)
	Safety	Acceptable risk without specialized monitoring				
	Practice implications	Investigational	Clinically useful	Investigational	Investigational (F) Not useful(D)	Investigational (F, D)
Orally disintegrating selegiline	Efficacy	Insufficient evidence	Insufficient evidence	Insufficient evidence	Insufficient evidence (F, D)	Insufficient evidence (F, D)
	Safety	Acceptable risk without specialized monitoring				
	Practice implications	Investigational	Investigational	Investigational	Investigational (F, D)	Investigational (F, D)
Rasagiline	Efficacy	Insufficient evidence	Efficacious	Efficacious	Insufficient evidence (F, D)	Efficacious (F) Insufficient evidence (D)
	Safety	Acceptable risk without specialized monitoring				
	Practice implications	Investigational	Clinically useful	Clinically useful	Investigational (F, D)	Clinically useful (F) Investigational (D)

Abbreviation: MAO-B, monoamine oxidase B.

[a]D, dyskinesia; F, motor fluctuations.

Source: Adapted from Ref. 81: Fox SH, Katzenschlager R, Lim SY, et al. The Movement Disorder Society Evidence-Based Medicine Review Update: Treatments for the motor symptoms of Parkinson's disease. *Mov Disord.* 2011; 26(suppl 3):S2–S41.

Table 4.23
Evidence on Anticholinergics, Amantadine, Clozapine, and Zonisamide in Parkinson's Disease

Drugs		Prevention/Delay of Clinical Progression	Symptomatic Monotherapy	Symptomatic Adjuvant to Levodopa	Prevention/Delay of Motor Complications[a]	Treatment of Motor Complications[a]
Anticholinergics	Efficacy	Insufficient evidence	Likely efficacious	Likely efficacious	Insufficient evidence (F, D)	Insufficient evidence (F, D)
	Safety	Acceptable risk without specialized monitoring				
	Practice implications	Investigational	Clinically useful	Clinically useful	Investigational (F, D)	Investigational (F, D)
Amantadine	Efficacy	Insufficient evidence	Likely efficacious	Likely efficacious	Insufficient evidence (F, D)	Insufficient evidence (F) Efficacious (D)
	Safety	Acceptable risk without specialized monitoring				
	Practice implications	Investigational	Possibly useful	Possibly useful	Investigational (F, D)	Investigational (F) Clinically useful (D)
Clozapine	Efficacy	Insufficient evidence	Insufficient evidence	Insufficient evidence	Insufficient evidence (F, D)	Insufficient evidence (F) Efficacious (D)
	Safety	Acceptable risk with specialized monitoring				
	Practice implications	Investigational	Investigational	Investigational	Investigational (F, D)	Investigational (F) Possibly useful (D)
Zonisamide	Efficacy	Insufficient evidence	Insufficient evidence	Efficacious	Insufficient evidence (F, D)	Insufficient evidence (F, D)
	Safety	Acceptable risk without specialized monitoring				
	Practice implications	Investigational	Investigational	Clinically useful	Investigational (F, D)	Investigational (F, D)

[a]D, dyskinesia; F, motor fluctuations.

Source: Adapted from Ref. 81: Fox SH, Katzenschlager R, Lim SY, et al. The Movement Disorder Society Evidence-Based Medicine Review Update: Treatments for the motor symptoms of Parkinson's disease. *Mov Disord.* 2011; 26(suppl 3):S2–S41.

Table 4.24
Advanced Therapies in Parkinson's Disease

Therapy	Advantages	Disadvantages
DBS surgery	• Proven longevity of efficacy of > 10 years in patients with advanced PD • Several targets (STN, GPi, VIM) depending on symptomatology and patient profile • Generally maintenance-free once device implanted • Current "gold standard" against which all other advanced therapies are compared, with the most impressive improvement in motor fluctuations • Most effective among patients with dyskinesia and medication-resistant tremors	• Patients must be cognitively intact, emotionally stable, and physically healthy (with the fewest comorbidities) • Most invasive (ie, brain surgery) of the advanced therapies in PD • Side effects potentially irreversible • May "disqualify" patient from future brain surgical interventions (eg, gene therapy, stem cells)
Levodopa/ carbidopa intestinal gel infusion	• Less invasive than DBS • May be considered for patients who have mild to moderate cognitive impairment • May still be suitable for older, less physically robust patients with PD • Ability to convert to levodopa monotherapy	• Patient hooked to an external pump, which can interfere less with independence • Pump size and weight can be a disadvantage to some patients • More maintenance and social support needed • Gastrointestinal complications can occur with varying frequency
Subcutaneous apomor- phine infusion	• Least invasive of all advanced therapies • Minimal maintenance • Device small, patients can be relatively independent • May also improve depression and anxiety	• Fewest randomized clinical trials or comparison studies with other advanced therapies • Some maintenance and social support needed • Less longevity of use in comparison with other advanced therapies

Abbreviations: DBS, deep brain surgery; GPi, globus pallidus internus; STN, subthalamic nucleus; VIM, ventral intermediate nucleus.

○ *Subcutaneous apomorphine infusion*

   •   Continuous subcutaneous apomorphine infusion (similar to an insulin pump for diabetics)

   •   Approved in most European countries and about to undergo regulatory clinical trials in the United States

REFERENCES

1. Parkinson J. An essay on the shaking palsy. London, UK: Sherwood, Neely and Jones; 1817. Reprinted in: Neuropsychiatric classics. *J Neuropsychiatry Clin Neurosci.* 2002; 14:223–236.
2. Manyam Vala B. Paralysis agitans and levodopa in "Ayurveda": ancient Indian medical treatise. *Mov Disord.* 1990; 5(1):47–48.
3. De Lau LML, Breteler MMB. Epidemiology of Parkinson's disease. *Lancet Neurol.* 2006; 5:525–535.
4. Schrag A, Schott JM. Epidemiological, clinical, and genetic characteristics of early-onset parkinsonism. *Lancet Neurol.* 2006; 5:355–363.
5. Schrag A, Ben-Schlomo Y, Brown R, et al. Young-onset Parkinson's disease revisited—clinical features, natural history, and mortality. *Mov Disord.* 1998; 13:885–894.
6. Bhidayasiri R, Brenden N. 10 commonly asked questions about Parkinson disease. *Neurologist.* 2011; 17:57–62.
7. Gorell JM, Johnson CC, Rybicki BA, et al. The risk of Parkinson's disease with exposure to pesticides, farming, well water, and rural living. *Neurology.* 1998; 50:1346–1350.
8. Semchuk KM, Love EJ, Lee RG. Parkinson's disease and exposure to agricultural work and pesticide chemicals. *Neurology.* 1992; 42:1328–1335.
9. Dexter DT, Wells FR, Lees AJ, et al. Increased nigral iron content and alterations in other metal ions occurring in brain in Parkinson's disease. *J Neurochem.* 1989; 52:1830–1836.
10. Gorell JM, Johnson CC, Rybicki BA, et al. Occupational exposure to metals as risk factors for Parkinson's disease. *Neurology.* 1997; 48:650–658.
11. Goldman SM, Quinlan PJ, Webster Ross G, et al. Solvent exposures and Parkinson's disease risk in twins. *Ann Neurol.* 2011; 71(6):776–784.
12. Langston JW, Ballard P, Tetrud JW, Irwin I. Chronic Parkinsonism in humans due to a product of meperidine-analog synthesis. *Science.* 1983; 219:979–980.
13. Xu Q, Park Y, Huang X, et al. Diabetes and risk of Parkinson's disease. *Diabetes Care.* 2011; 34:910–915.
14. Tanner CM, Goldman SM, Aston DA, et al. Smoking and Parkinson's disease in twins. *Neurology.* 2001; 58:581–588.
15. Ross GW, Abbott RD, Petrovitch H, et al. Association of coffee and caffeine intake with the risk of Parkinson disease. *JAMA.* 2000; 283:2674–2679.
16. Ascherio A, Zhang SM, Hernan MA, et al. Prospective study of caffeine consumption and risk of Parkinson's disease in men and women. *Ann Neurol.* 2001; 50:56–63.
17. Fink JS, Bains La, Beiser A, et al. Caffeine intake and the risk of incident Parkinson's disease: the Framingham Study. *Mov Disord.* 2001; 16:984.
18. Xu Q, Park Y, Huang X, et al. Physical activities and future risk of Parkinson disease. *Neurology.* 2010; 75:341–348.
19. Saunders-Pullman R. Estrogens and Parkinson disease: neuroprotective, symptomatic, neither, or both? *Endocrine.* 2003; 21:81–87.
20. Abbott RD, Ross GW, White LR, et al. Environmental, life-style, and physical precursors of clinical Parkinson's disease: recent findings from the Honolulu-Asia Aging Study. *J Neurol.* 2003; 250(suppl 3):III30–III39.
21. De Lau LM, Bornebroek M, Witteman JC, et al. Dietary fatty acids and the risk of Parkinson disease: the Rotterdam study. *Neurology.* 2005; 64:2040–2045.

22. Davis JW, Grandinetti A, Waslien CI, et al. Observations on serum uric acid levels and the risk of idiopathic Parkinson's disease. *Am J Epidemiol.* 1996; 144:480–484.

23. de Lau LML, Koudstaal PJ, Hofman A, Breteler MMB. Serum uric acid levels and the risk of Parkinson disease. *Ann Neurol.* 2005; 58:797–800.

24. Weisskopf MG, O'Reilly E, Chen H, et al. Plasma urate and risk of Parkinson's disease. *Am J Epidemiol.* 2007; 166:561–567.

25. Kitada T, Asakawa S, Hattori N, et al. Mutations in the parkin gene cause autosomal recessive juvenile parkinsonism. *Nature.* 1998; 392:605–608.

26. Gasser T. Genetics of Parkinson's disease. *Curr Opin Neurol.* 2005; 18:363–369.

27. Bonifati V, Rizzu P, Van Baren MJ, et al. Mutations in the DJ-1 associated with autosomal recessive early-onset parkinsonism. *Science.* 2002; 299:256–259.

28. Bandopadhyay R, Kingsbury AE, Cookson MR, et al. The expression of DJ-1(PARK7) in normal human CNS and idiopathic Parkinson's disease. *Brain.* 2004; 127:420–430.

29. Golbe LI, Di Iorio G, Bonavita V, et al. A large kindred with autosomal dominant Parkinson's disease. *Ann Neurology.* 1990; 27:276–282.

30. Golbe LI, Di Iorio G, Sanges G, et al. Clinical genetic analysis of Parkinson's disease in the Contursi kindred. *Ann Neurol.* 1996; 40:767–775.

31. Hughes AJ, Daniel SE, Blankson S, Lees AJ. A clinicopathologic study of 100 cases of Parkinson's disease. *Arch Neurol.* 1993; 50:140–148.

32. Gasser T, Mueller-Myhsok B, Wszolek ZK, et al. A susceptibility locus for Parkinson's disease maps to chromosome 2p13. *Nat Genet.* 1998; 18:262–265.

33. Farrer M, Gwinn-Hardy K, Muenter M, et al. A chromosome 4p haplotype segregating with Parkinson's disease and postural tremor. *Hum Mol Genet.* 1999; 8(1):81–85.

34. Muenter MD, Howard FM, Okazaki H, et al. A familial Parkinson-dementia syndrome. *Ann Neurol.* 1998; 43:768–781.

35. Saigoh K, Wang YL, Suh JG, et al. Intragenic deletion in the gene encoding ubiquitin carboxy-terminal hydroxylase in GAD mice. *Nat Genet.* 1999; 23:47–51.

36. Simon DK, Pankratz N, Kissell DK, et al. Maternal inheritance and mitochondrial DNA variants in familial Parkinson's disease. *BMC Med Genet.* 2010; 11(53):1–9.

37. Braak H, Tredici KD, Riib U, et al. Staging of brain pathology related to sporadic Parkinson's disease. *Neurobiol Aging.* 2003; 24:197–211.

38. Schapira AHV, Olanow CW. Neuroprotection in Parkinson disease. *JAMA.* 2004; 291:358–364.

39. Parkinson Study Group. Effect of deprenyl on the progression of disability in early Parkinson's disease. *NEJM.* 1989; 321(20):1364–1371.

40. Tetrud JW, Langston JW. The effect of deprenyl (selegiline) on the natural history of Parkinson's disease. *Science.* 1989; 245:519–522.

41. Olanow CW, Hauser RA, Gauger L, et al. The effect of deprenyl and levodopa on the progression of Parkinson's disease. *Ann Neurol.* 1995; 38:771–777.

42. Palhagen S, Heinonen EH, Hagglund J, et al. Selegiline delays the onset of disability in de novo parkinsonian patients. Swedish Parkinson Study Group. *Neurology.* 1998; 51(2):520–525.

43. Larsen JP, Boas J, Erdal JE. Does selegiline modify the progression of early Parkinson's disease? Results from a five-year study. The Norwegian-Danish Study Group. *Eur J Neurol.* 1999; 6:539–547.

44. Parkinson Study Group. A controlled, randomized, delayed-start study of rasagiline in early Parkinson disease. *Arch Neurol.* 2004; 61:561–566.

45. Olanow CW, Rascol O, Hauser R, et al. A double-blind, delayed-start trial of rasagiline in Parkinson's disease. *NEJM*. 2009; 361:1268–1278.

46. Parkinson Study Group. Safety of urate elevation in Parkinson's disease (SURE-PD). http://www.clinicaltrials.gov/ct2/show/NCT00833690?term=SURE-PD&rank=1

47. Shults CW, Oakes D, Kieburtz K, et al. Effects of coenzyme Q10 in early Parkinson disease: evidence of slowing of the functional decline. *Arch Neurol*. 2002; 59:1541–1550.

48. Parkinson Study Group. MOVE-PD (A Phase II Study to Evaluate the Safety and Efficacy of RM-131 in Patients with Parkinson's Disease & Chronic Constipation). http://www.parkinson-study-group.org/parkinson-research/clinical-trials-in-progess

49. Uitti RJ, Rajput AH, Ahlskog JE, et al. Amantadine treatment is an independent predictor of improved survival in Parkinson's disease. *Neurology*. 1996; 46:1551–1556.

50. Jankovic J, Hunter C. A double-blind, placebo-controlled and longitudinal study of riluzole in early Parkinson's disease. *Parkinsonism Relat Disord*. 2002; 8(4):271–276.

51. Rascol O, Olanow W, Brooks D, et al. A 2-year, multicenter, placebo-controlled, double-blind, parallel-group study of the effect of riluzole on Parkinson's disease progression. *Mov Disord*. 2002; 17(suppl 5):P80.

52. Shoulson I, Parkinson Study Group, PRECEPT Investigators. CEP-1347 treatment fails to favorably modify the progression of Parkinson's disease (PRECEPT) study: S61.003. *Neurology*. 2006; 67:185.

53. Olanow CW, Schapira AH, LeWitt PA, et al. TCH346 as a neuroprotective drug in Parkinson's disease: a double blind, randomized controlled trial. *Lancet Neurol*. 2006; 5:1013–1020.

54. Whone AL, Watts RL, Stoessl AJ, et al. Slower progression of Parkinson's disease with ropinirole versus levodopa: the REAL-PET study. *Ann Neurol*. 2003; 54:93–101.

55. Parkinson Study Group. Dopamine transporter brain imaging to assess the effects of pramipexole vs levodopa on Parkinson disease progression. *JAMA*. 2002; 287:1653–1661.

56. Schapira A, Albrecht S, Barone P, et al. Immediate vs. delayed-start pramipexole in early Parkinson's disease: the PROUD study. *Parkinsonism Relat Disord*. 2009; 15:S2–S81.

57. Parkinson Study Group. Levodopa and the progression of Parkinson's disease. *NEJM*. 2004; 351:2498–2508.

58. NINDS NET-PD Investigators. A randomized, double-blind, futility clinical trial of creatine and minocycline in early Parkinson disease. *Neurology*. 2006; 66:664–671.

59. Lang AE, Gill S, Patel NK, et al. Randomized controlled trial of intraputaminal glial cell line-derived neurotrophic factor infusion in Parkinson disease. *Ann Neurol*. 2006; 59:459–466.

60. Gao X, Chen H, Schwarzschild, Ascherio A. Use of ibuprofen and risk of Parkinson disease. *Neurology*. 2011; 76:863–869.

61. NINDS NET-PD Investigators. A randomized clinical trial of coenzyme Q10 and GPI-1485 in early Parkinson's disease. *Neurology*. 2007; 68:20–28.

62. Kuroda K, Tatara K, Takatorige T, Shinsho F. Effect of physical exercise on mortality in patients with Parkinson's disease. *Acta Neurol Scand*. 1992; 86(1):55–59.

63. Gibb WR, Lees AJ. The relevance of the Lewy body to the pathogenesis of idiopathic Parkinson's disease. *J Neurol Neurosurg Psychiatry*. 1988; 51:745–752.

64. Fahn S, Elton R, Members of the UPDRS Development Committee. Unified Parkinson's disease rating scale. In: Fahn S, Marsden CD, Calne DB, Goldstein M, eds.

Recent Developments in Parkinson's Disease. Vol 2. Florham Park, NJ: Macmillan Health Care Information; 1987:53-63, 293–304.

65. Goetz CG, Tilley BC, Shaftman SR, et al. Movement Disorder Society-sponsored revision of the Unified Parkinson's Disease Rating Scale (MDS-UPDRS): scale presentation and clinimetric testing results. *Mov Disord.* 2008; 23(15):2129–2170.

66. Marinus J, Visser M, Stinggelbout AM, et al. A short scale for the assessment of motor impairments and disabilities in Parkinson's disease: the SPES/SCOPA. *J Neurol Neurosurg Psychiatry.* 2004; 75:388–395.

67. Hoehn MM, Yahr MD. Parkinsonism: onset, progression and mortality. *Neurology.* 1967; 17:427–442.

68. Chaudhuri KR, Healy, DG, Schapira AHV. Non-motor symptoms of Parkinson's disease: diagnosis and management. *Lancet Neurol.* 2006; 5:235–245.

69. Snider SR, Fahn S, Isgreen WP, Cote LJ. Primary sensory symptoms in Parkinson's disease. *Neurology.* 1976; 26:423–429.

70. Seppi K, Weintraub D, Coelho M, et al. The Movement Disorder Society Evidence-Based Medicine Review Update: Treatments for the non-motor symptoms of Parkinson's disease. *Mov Disord.* 2011; 26(suppl 3):S42–S80.

71. Adler CH. Relevance of motor complications in Parkinson's disease. *Neurology.* 2002; 58(suppl 1):S51–S56.

72. Chase TN, Oh JD. Striatal mechanisms and pathogenesis of parkinsonian signs and motor complications. *Ann Neurol.* 2000; 47(suppl 1):S122–S129.

73. Obeso JA et al. In: Olanow CW, Obeso JA, eds. Beyond the Decade of the Brain. Vol 2. Dopamine agonists in early Parkinson's disease. Tunbridge Wells, UK: Wells Medical Ltd;1997:11–35.

74. Bhidayasiri R, Brenden N. 10 commonly asked questions about Parkinson disease. *Neurologist.* 2011; 17:57–62.

75. Pogarell O, Gasser T, van Hilten J. Pramipexole in patients with Parkinson's disease and marked drug resistant tremor: a randomized, double blind, placebo controlled multicenter study. *J Neurol Neurosurg Psychiatry.* 2002; 72:713–720.

76. Rascol O, Brooks DJ, Korczyn AD, et al. A five-year study of the incidence of dyskinesia in patients with early Parkinson's disease who were treated with ropinirole or levodopa. *N Engl J Med.* 2000; 342:1484–1491.

77. Hauser RA, McDermott MP, Messing S. Factors associated with the development of motor fluctuations and dyskinesias in Parkinson disease. *Arch Neurol.* 2006; 63:1756–1760.

78. Adler CH. Relevance of motor complications in Parkinson's disease. *Neurology.* 2002; 58(suppl 1):S51–S56.

79. Nauseida PA, Weiner WJ, Klawans HL. Dystonic foot response of parkinsonism. *Arch Neurol.* 1980; 37:132–136.

80. Quinn N, Marsden CD. Lithium for painful dystonia in Parkinson's disease. *Lancet.* 1986; 1(8494):1377.

81. Fox SH, Katzenschlager R, Lim SY, et al. The Movement Disorder Society Evidence-Based Medicine Review Update: Treatments for the motor symptoms of Parkinson's disease. *Mov Disord.* 2011; 26(suppl 3):S2–S41.

5

DYSTONIA

"*Dystonia* is a neurologic syndrome characterized by involuntary, sustained, patterned, and often repetitive muscle contractions of opposing muscles causing twisting movements or abnormal postures. Partly because of its rich expression and a variable course, dystonia is frequently not recognized or misdiagnosed."[1]

The prevalence of generalized primary torsion dystonia in Rochester, Minnesota, was reported to be 3.4 per 100,000 population, and that of focal dystonia to be 30 per 100,000.[2]

PHENOMENOLOGY OF DYSTONIC MOVEMENTS

- The main features of dystonia include the following:

  - The movements are of relatively long duration, whereas in chorea or myoclonus, the involuntary movements are brief.

  - Both the agonist and antagonist muscles of a body part simultaneously contract to result in twisting of the affected body part.

  - The same muscle groups are generally involved, whereas in chorea, the involuntary movements are random and involve different muscle groups.

- Other features include the following:

  - *Primary dystonia* almost always begins by affecting a single part of the body (focal dystonia) and then gradually generalizes; most often, the spread is to contiguous body parts.

  - The younger the age at onset, the more likely it is for the dystonia to spread (eg, a childhood onset with leg involvement usually eventually leads to generalized dystonia, whereas an adult onset with cranial or cervical involvement usually remains focal).[3,4]

  - Dystonia is almost always worsened by voluntary movement. Dystonic movements may be aggravated during voluntary movement and may be termed *action dystonia*. Abnormal dystonic movements that appear only during certain actions are termed *task-specific dystonia*. An example is writer's cramp.

○ As the dystonia progresses, even nonspecific voluntary action can elicit dystonia; eventually, actions in other parts of the body can induce dystonic movements of the primarily affected body part, termed *overflow dystonia*.

○ Dystonia is usually worsened by fatigue and stress and is suppressed by sleep, hypnosis, or relaxation.

○ A unique and intriguing feature of dystonia is that the movements can be suppressed by a tactile or proprioceptive "sensory trick" (*geste antagoniste*); lightly touching (and sometimes simply the act of touching) the affected body part can often reduce the muscle contractions.

○ Surprisingly, pain is not very common in dystonia except in cervical dystonia, in which up to 75% of patients experienced pain in one study.[5]

○ Dystonia can present with tremor (dystonic tremor) or myoclonus (dystonia–myoclonus). Dystonic tremor resulting from cervical dystonia can be distinguished from essential tremor because the dystonic tremor is usually less regular or rhythmic than essential tremor and is associated with a head tilt and chin deviation.

○ Rarely, children and adolescents with primary or secondary dystonia can develop a sudden and marked increase in the severity of dystonia, termed *dystonic storm*.

CLASSIFICATION OF DYSTONIA

■ By distribution

○ *Focal:* affects a single body part (eg, torticollis, writer's cramp, blepharospasm, foot dystonia, lingual dystonia, spasmodic dysphonia).

○ *Segmental:* affects one or more contiguous body parts (eg, Meige syndrome).

○ *Multifocal:* involves two or more noncontiguous body parts.

○ *Hemidystonia:* involves half of the body; usually associated with a structural lesion (eg, tumor in the contralateral putamen).

○ *Generalized:* the entire body is affected.

■ By clinical features

○ *Continual*

- Primary (or idiopathic) dystonia

    - May be inherited or sporadic.

    - Can have an early onset (younger than 26 years of age) or a late onset 26 years and older.

        □ Dystonias with an early onset tend to become severe and are more likely to spread to involve multiple parts of the body.

        □ Dystonias with a later onset tend to remain focal.

- Secondary dystonia

    - Secondary dystonia may be generalized, segmental, focal or multifocal, and associated with other neurologic disorders.

    - Unilateral dystonia/hemidystonia is often symptomatic and usually results from a stroke, trauma, arteriovenous malformation, or tumor.

○ *Fluctuating*

- Paroxysmal dyskinesias can vary from chorea-ballism to the sustained contractions of dystonia. *Paroxysmal* is the term most commonly used for periodic choreoathetotic and dystonic involuntary movements, while *episodic* is most commonly used for periodic ataxic involuntary movements. Paroxysmal dyskinesias are generally classified into four types (Table 5.1):[6]

    - Paroxysmal kinesigenic dyskinesia (PKD)

        □ Usually lasts for seconds to minutes; precipitated by sudden movement, startle, or hyperventilation; occurs many times a day; patients may experience a sensory "aura" prior to the attack.

        □ The majority of cases are primary (familial with autosomal dominant inheritance or sporadic); causes of secondary PKD include multiple sclerosis, head injury, hypoxia, hypoparathyroidism, and basal ganglia and thalamic strokes.

        □ Affecting PRRT2 (proline-rich transmembrane protein, which seems to manifest in embryonic neural tissue).

        □ PKD may respond to anticonvulsants such as carbamazepine, especially when the paroxysmal attacks are brief; females may respond better than males.

Table 5.1
Summary of Features of Major Causes of Paroxysmal Dyskinesias

CHARACTERISTICS	PKD	PNKD	PED
Male-to-female ratio	4:1	3:2	Unclear
Age at onset	5–15 y (even 1–20 y; limits more lenient if positive family history)	< 5 y	2–20 y
Inheritance	AD, sporadic	AD, sporadic	AD
Duration of attacks	< 5 min, often < 1 min	Several minutes to hours	5–30 min
Frequency	Very frequent: 100/d–1/mo	Occasional: 3/d–2/y	1/d–1/mo
Asymmetry	Common	Less common	
Ability to suppress attacks	Able	Able	
Precipitating factors	Identifiable triggers (eg, sudden movement, startle, hyperventilation, fatigue, stress)	Alcohol, caffeine, exercise, excitement	Prolonged exercise, stress, caffeine, fatigue
Associated features	Dystonia, chorea, epilepsy; no pain or loss of consciousness	Chorea, dystonia, ataxia	Dystonia, chorea
Treatment	Phenytoin, carbamazepine, barbiturates, acetazolamide	Clonazepam, oxazepam	

Abbreviations: AD, autosomal dominant; PED, paroxysmal exertional dyskinesia; PKD, paroxysmal kinesigenic dyskinesia; PNKD, paroxysmal nonkinesigenic dyskinesia.

Source: Adapted from Ref. 6: Bruno MK, Hallett M, Gwinn-Hardy K, et al. Clinical evaluation of idiopathic paroxysmal kinesigenic dyskinesia: new diagnostic criteria. *Neurology.* 2004; 63(12):2280–2287.

- Paroxysmal nonkinesigenic dyskinesia (PNKD)
  - Often consists of any combination of dystonic postures, chorea, athetosis, and ballism; may be unilateral or bilateral; longer duration and smaller frequency of attacks compared with PKD.
  - Precipitated by alcohol, coffee, tea, stress, or fatigue.
  - Cases can be primary (familial with autosomal dominant inheritance or sporadic) or secondary, caused by multiple sclerosis, hypoxia, encephalitis, metabolic causes, psychogenic, and other conditions.

- □ Not sensitive to anticonvulsants.
  - – Paroxysmal exertional dyskinesia
    - □ Attacks are briefer than those in PNKD, lasting 5 to 30 minutes; precipitated by prolonged exercise.
    - □ Most familial cases exhibit autosomal dominant inheritance.
    - □ May respond to anticonvulsant or antimuscarinic agents.
  - – Paroxysmal hypnogenic dyskinesia
    - □ Attacks can be brief or prolonged.
    - □ Several cases may be due to supplementary motor or frontal lobe seizures.
- Diurnal
  - – Aromatic acid decarboxylase deficiency (usually in infancy): axial hypotonia, athetosis, ocular convergence spasm, oculogyric crises, limb rigidity.
  - – GTP (guanosine triphosphate) cyclohydrolase I deficiency (DYT5): first step in tetrahydrobiopterin synthesis, childhood onset, may be diurnal, improves with low-dose levodopa, abnormal phenylalanine loading test.
- Other causes: side effect of levodopa therapy, acute dystonic reaction to neuroleptics, gastroesophageal reflux, oculogyric crisis (sudden, transient conjugate eye deviation).

■ By etiology

○ *Primary (idiopathic) dystonia:* may be familial (Table 5.2)[7–30] or sporadic. In the pure dystonic syndromes, dystonia is the main and only clinical sign (except for dystonic tremor).

- Of the DYTs, types 1, 2, 4, 6, 7, 13, 17, and 21 (shaded in gray in Table 5.2) are primary dystonias.

○ *Dystonia-plus:* "nonneurodegenerative" conditions in which signs and symptoms other than dystonia, such as parkinsonism and myoclonus, are present; these are generally not neurodegenerative disorders and are better classified as neurochemical disorders.

- Among the DYTs, those with dystonia plus parkinsonism include types 3, 5, 12, and 16, and those with dystonia plus myoclonus include types 11 and 15.

- **Dopa-responsive dystonia**

Table 5.2
Genetic Classification of the Dystonias

Type	Chromosome/Gene	Inheritance	Features	Reference
DYT1	9q34 (torsin A); deletion of one pair of GAG triplets	AD, penetrance rate 30%–40%	1 per 2,000 in Ashkenazi Jewish population, commercial testing available, early onset (testing < 26 y/o useful), limbs affected first, pure dystonia, MRI normal	Ozelieus et al, 1997[7]
DYT2		AR	Described in Spanish gypsies	Khan et al, 2003[8]
DYT3	Xq13.1 (TAF1)	X-linked	"Lubag," male Filipinos, dystonia–parkinsonism	Nolte et al, 2003[9]
DYT4	19p13.12-13 (TUBB4A)		"Whispering dysphonia" family	Parker, 1985[10] Hersheson et al, 2013[11]
DYT5	14q22.1 (GCH1)	AD	Dopa-responsive dystonia	Ichinose et al, 1994[12]
DYT6	8p21-q22 (THAP1)	AD	Mixed type, in Mennonite/ Amish populations, childhood and adult onset, site of onset in arm/cranial region > leg/neck, usually remains in upper body	Almasy et al, 1997[13]
DYT7	18p	AD	Adult-onset familial torticollis in a northwestern German family, occasional arm involvement	Leube et al, 1996[14]
DYT8	2q33-q35 (MR1)	AD	Paroxysmal nonkinesigenic dyskinesia	Fouad et al, 1996[15]; Fink et al, 1996[16]
DYT9	1p21	AD	Paroxysmal dyskinesia with spasticity	Auberger et al, 1996[17]
DYT10	16p11.2-q12.1	AD	Paroxysmal kinesigenic dyskinesia	Tomita et al, 1999[18]
DYT11	7q21-q23/ epsilon- sarcoglycan (SGCE)	AD	Myoclonus–dystonia syndrome, alcohol-responsive	Zimprich et al, 2001[19]

continued

Table 5.2 (cont.)
Genetic Classification of the Dystonias

Type	Chromosome/Gene	Inheritance	Features	Reference
DYT12	19q12-13.2 (*ATP1A3*)	AD	Rapid-onset dystonia–parkinsonism	Kramer et al, 1999[20]
DYT13	1p36.13-p36.32	AD	Adult onset, familial, cranial–cervical–brachial predominant, site of onset usually neck, remains segmental	Valente et al, 2001[21]
DYT14	14q14	AD	Dopamine-responsive dystonia	Grotzsch et al, 2002[22]
DYT15	18p11	AD	Myoclonus–dystonia syndrome	Grimes et al, 2002[23]
DYT16	2q31.2 (*PRKRA*)	AR	Dystonia–parkinsonism in early adolescence, possibly with developmental delay, particularly speech	Camargos et al, 2008[24]
DYT17	20p11.2-q13.12	AR	Cervical dystonia in adolescence, progressing to segmental or generalized with dysphonia	Chouery et al, 2008[25]
DYT18	1p35-p31.3 (*SLC2A1*)	AD	Paroxysmal exercise-induced dyskinesia with or without epilepsy or hemolytic anemia	Suls et al, 2008[26]
DYT19	16q13-q22.1		Episodic kinesigenic dyskinesia 2, probably synonymous with DYT10	Valente et al, 2000[27]
DYT20	2q31		Paroxysmal nonkinesigenic dyskinesia 2	Spacey et al, 2006[28]
DYT21	2q14.3-q21.3	AD	Late-onset torsion dystonia	Norgren et al, 2011[29]
DYT22	11p14.2	AD	Craniocervical dystonia with prominent tremor	Charlesworth et al, 2012[30]

Abbreviations: AD, autosomal dominant; AR, autosomal recessive.
Note: Dystonias within areas shaded in gray are "primary dystonias."

Table 5.3
Features Distinguishing Dopa-Responsive Dystonia, Juvenile Parkinson's Disease,
and Childhood Primary Torsion Dystonia

Feature	DRD	Juvenile PD	Childhood PTD
Gender predisposition	Female	Male	None
Dystonia presentation	Dystonia throughout course, occasionally improves with sleep; starts on the foot or leg; with bradykinesia	Dystonia at onset, may be diurnal and improves with sleep; starts on the foot; with parkinsonism	Dystonia throughout course, without diurnal pattern or sleep benefit; no signs of parkinsonism or bradykinesia
Treatment response	Low-dose carbidopa/ levodopa (Sinemet) and anticholinergic drugs	Higher doses of carbidopa/levodopa (Sinemet); all other anti-PD agents, including anticholinergic drugs	Unlikely to respond to carbidopa/ levodopa (Sinemet) but responds to anticholinergic drugs
Course	Plateaus	Progressive	Usually progressive

- GTP cyclohydrolase I deficiency (DYT5): childhood onset (younger than 16 years), females more often affected than males, may be diurnal (worse at night), improves with low-dose levodopa, adult onset with parkinsonism or focal dystonia, abnormal phenylalanine loading test
- Autosomal recessive with mutation of tyrosine hydroxylase gene[31]
- Other biopterin deficiencies[32]
- May be mistaken for juvenile Parkinson's disease or childhood primary torsion dystonia (Table 5.3)

- **Dopamine agonist–responsive dystonia:** aromatic acid decarboxylase deficiency, autosomal recessive mode of inheritance.

- **Rapid-onset dystonia parkinsonism:** autosomal dominant, *ATP1A3* gene mutations on chromosome 19q13, adolescent or adult onset, dystonia generalizing over a few days to weeks with rostrocaudal progression and prominent bulbar features, parkinsonism but minimal or no tremor at onset, generally stabilizing within a few weeks with slow or no progression, little or no response to levodopa or dopamine agonists.[33]

- **Myoclonus–dystonia syndrome:** dystonia (most commonly cervical dystonia and writer's cramp) with myoclonic jerks that responds to alcohol; autosomal dominant with incomplete penetrance and prominent maternal imprinting; mutations in epsilon-sarcoglycan gene (*SGCE*, DYT11) on chromosome 7q21/18p11 in majority of cases but some cases mutation-negative; upper part of body affected; childhood, adolescent, or adult onset; slowly progressive and tending to plateau; may be associated with other psychiatric features, such as substance abuse, anxiety, psychosis.[34]

○ *Secondary dystonia:* due to environmental insult (Table 5.4).[35]

○ *Heredodegenerative dystonias:* due to neurodegenerative diseases, usually inherited, usually not pure dystonia (Table 5.5).

○ A feature of another neurological disease (eg, tics, paroxysmal dyskinesias, Parkinson's disease, progressive supranuclear palsy).

○ *Pseudodystonia*

- Not true dystonia, but sustained abnormal postures are present

- Examples include stiff-person syndrome, Isaacs syndrome, Satoyoshi syndrome, chronic inflammatory myopathy,[36] Sandifer syndrome, bone disease, ligamentous absence, congenital muscular torticollis (commonly associated with a sternomastoid tumor), juvenile rheumatoid arthritis, seizures

- Psychogenic dystonia is suggested by the following:

  – Abrupt onset

  – Changing characteristics over time

  – Movements that do not "fit" with known patterns

  – Accompanied by other types of movements (eg, rhythmic shaking, bizarre gait, astasia–abasia, excessive startle or slowness)

  – Associated with other features (eg, false weakness and sensory complaints, psychiatric disorders, secondary gain, pending litigation, multiple somatizations)

  – Spontaneous remission

  – Improvement with distraction

  – Paroxysmal or intermittent nature

  – Twisting facial movements (especially side-to-side movements of mouth)

Table 5.4
Symptomatic Causes of Dystonia

Perinatal cerebral injury with kernicterus	Athetoid cerebral palsy, delayed-onset dystonia
Infection	Viral encephalitis Encephalitis lethargica Reye syndrome Subacute sclerosing panencephalitis Creutzfeldt-Jakob disease HIV infection
Drugs	Levodopa and dopamine agonists Dopamine receptor blockers Fenfluramine Anticonvulsants Flecainide Ergots Some calcium channel blockers
Toxins	Manganese Carbon monoxide Carbon disulfide Cyanide Methanol Disulfiram 3-Nitrorpropionic acid Wasp sting toxin
Metabolic	Hypoparathyroidism
Brain/brainstem lesions	Paraneoplastic brainstem encephalitis Primary antiphospholipid syndrome Cerebrovascular accident, ischemic injury Central pontine myelinolysis Multiple sclerosis Tumors Arteriovenous malformation Trauma Surgery (thalamotomy)
Spinal cord lesions, syringomyelia	
Peripheral lesions	Lumbar stenosis Trauma Electrical injury

Table 5.5
Heredodegenerative Disorders With Dystonic Manifestations

Inheritance	Disease	Features	Diagnosis
X-linked	Lubag (X-linked dystonia–parkinsonism) (DYT3)	Male Filipinos living on Panay Island; young adult onset; cranial or generalized dystonia; parkinsonism can appear at onset or develop later; progressive, disabling	Clinical; gene test not currently commercially available
X-linked	Deafness–dystonia syndrome (Mohr-Tranebjaerg syndrome)	Early deafness, optic atrophy, and dystonia appearing later in males (X-linked transmission)	Clinical; no commercially available genetic testing
X-linked	Pelizaeus-Merzbacher disease	Deficiency in myelin-specific lipids; partial to total absence of myelination; ataxia, nystagmus, hypotonia starting in early childhood; dystonia occurs later and progresses slowly; may present with spastic paraparesis in adulthood	Leukodystrophy findings on MRI; genetic testing commercially available (*PLP* gene sequencing)
X-linked	Rett syndrome	X-linked dominant (therefore occurs only in girls); characteristically combines psychomotor regression, loss of purposeful use of hands, stereotypy, ataxia, and apraxia of gait with microcephaly; dystonia and oculogyric crises in >50%; patients normal at birth and start exhibiting symptoms after 2 years of age	Clinical; genetic testing commercially available (*MECP2* gene sequencing)
Autosomal dominant	Juvenile parkinsonism	May present with dystonia initially (see Table 5.2)	Clinical and genetic
Autosomal dominant with complete penetrance	Huntington's disease	Usually presents with chorea but dystonia common; usually manifests between ages of 30 and 54 but can present at any age; progressive disorder with varying degrees of cognitive and psychiatric dysfunction	Genetic testing, *IT15* gene CAG expansion

continued

Inheritance	Disease	Features	Diagnosis
Autosomal dominant with incomplete penetrance	Machado-Joseph disease (SCA3)	Mainly affecting families descended from ancestors who lived in the Portuguese Azore Islands (but not exclusively); dystonia in about 20%; type 1, predominantly pyramidal–extrapyramidal signs; type 2, cerebellar plus pyramidal; type 3, cerebellar plus distal amyotrophy	Genetic testing, CAG expansion 14q
Autosomal dominant	Dentatorubro-pallidoluysian atrophy	Degeneration of cerebellar efferent and pallidoluysian systems; dystonia not usually prominent; adult onset: ataxia, choreoathetosis, dementia; juvenile onset: presents like progressive myoclonic epilepsy	Genetic testing, CAG expansion 21p
	Other spinocerebellar ataxias	Because of great phenotypic variability, complete ataxia genetic screening profile recommended	Genetic testing
Autosomal recessive	Wilson's disease	Can also present with tremor, dystonia, parkinsonism, or any other movement disorder, usually before age 50; abnormal metabolism of copper and linked to chromosome 13; damage results in copper accumulation (see Figure 5.2)	Kayser-Fleischer rings, ceruloplasmin gene defects on chromosome 13, liver biopsy
Autosomal recessive	Niemann-Pick type C disease	Dystonic lipidosis; sea-blue histiocytosis; in type C, no specific enzymatic deficit described; sphingomyelinase activity normal in most tissues; patients with later onset present with characteristic supranuclear gaze palsy, mental decline, gait disorder, ataxia, and dystonia	Defective cholesterol sterification/ sphingomyelinase

continued

Table 5.5 (cont.)
Heredodegenerative Disorders With Dystonic Manifestations

Inheritance	Disease	Features	Diagnosis
Mostly autosomal recessive	Juvenile neuronal ceroid lipofuscinosis	Marked by storage of lipopigments; infantile, late infantile, juvenile, and adult forms; juvenile form presents without visual failure and with myoclonic epilepsy, dementia, and behavioral and extrapyramidal signs, especially facial dyskinesias	Pathology (rectal biopsy)
Autosomal recessive	GM1 gangliosidosis	Characterized by visceromegaly, cognitive decline, dysmorphism, and a cherry red spot in macular region; types 1, 2, and 3 in children; type 3 presents at 2 to 27 years of age with variable manifestations, including ataxia, dystonia, and myopathy; in adults, GM1 characterized by dystonia and early-onset parkinsonism with prolonged survival	Beta-D-galactosidase deficiency
Autosomal recessive	GM2 gangliosidosis	Deficiency of lysosomal hexosaminidase; more frequent among Ashkenazi Jews from eastern Europe; infantile GM2 has aggressive course with spastic tetraparesis, seizures, and blindness and with dystonia later in course; in juvenile, chronic, and adult GM2, dystonia may be presenting feature (usually legs)	Hexosaminidase deficiency
Autosomal recessive	Metachromatic leukodystrophy	Deficiency in cerebroside sulfatase leading to sulfatide accumulation; may present with mental decline, behavioral dysfunction, and dystonia	Aryl sulfatase A deficiency

continued

Table 5.5 (cont.)
Heredodegenerative Disorders With Dystonic Manifestations

Inheritance	Disease	Features	Diagnosis
X-linked	Lesch-Nyhan syndrome	May present with generalized dystonia; onset in children with mental retardation, self-mutilation, hyperuricemia	Hypoxanthine guanine phosphoribosyl transferase deficiency
Autosomal recessive	Homocystinuria	May present in children with generalized dystonia, focal deficits, ectopia lentis, skeletal deformities, and mental retardation; neuroimaging may show focal ischemic lesions, sinus thrombosis	Amino acid chromatography
Autosomal recessive	Glutaric acidemia	Along with cerebral palsy, one of the leading causes of dystonia in first year of life; generalized dystonia with mental retardation	Glutaric acid in urine, glutaryl-CoA dehydrogenase deficiency
Autosomal recessive	Methylmalonic aciduria	Generalized dystonia in children with acute encephalopathy	Chromatography of organic acids; methylmalonic CoA mutase
Autosomal recessive	Ataxia-telangiectasia	Generalized dystonia in children with ataxia and neuropathy; cerebellar atrophy on imaging	Clinical; low levels of immunoglobulin A
Autosomal recessive	Neurodegeneration with brain iron accumulation; pantothenate kinase–associated neurodegeneration	Formerly called Hallervorden-Spatz syndrome; characterized by iron deposition in pallidum; dystonia may be associated with tics and other movement disorders	Pathology; imaging showing pallidal T2 hypointensity ("eye of the tiger" sign)
Autosomal dominant and X-linked	Neuroacanthocytosis	Usually starts in third decade with orobuccolingual hyperkinesia, lip smacking, vocalizations, and even orolingual action dystonia leading to lip and tongue automutilation; 50% with seizures; most with polyneuropathy, distal amyotrophy, pes cavus	Acanthocytes in peripheral smear; Kell antigen determination

continued

Table 5.5 (cont.)
Heredodegenerative Disorders With Dystonic Manifestations

Inheritance	Disease	Features	Diagnosis
Mitochondrial	Leigh disease	Generalized dystonia in children with hypotonia, ataxia, optic atrophy	Pyruvic acid and alanine levels, mitochondrial DNA mutations, cytochrome oxidase activity

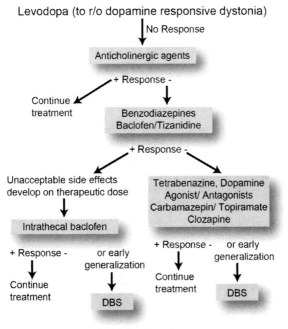

Figure 5.1
Treatment algorithm for generalized dystonia. (This treatment algorithm is not applicable to dystonia caused by treatable metabolic disorders).
Abbreviation: DBS, Deep Brain Stimulation Surgery

TREATMENT

Focus on the etiology. Management can be difficult. Patients do not consistently respond to one type of therapy, and multiple strategies may be needed (Figure 5.1).

■ Oral medications (Table 5.6)

■ Chemodenervation: botulinum toxin, the product of an anaerobic bacterium, *Clostridium botulinum*, is purified and injected into the affected muscles to prevent the release of acetylcholine from nerve terminals to the neuromuscular junctions, thereby preventing muscle contraction.

    ○ Four strains are available: type A (onabotulinumtoxinA/Botox, abobotulinumtoxinA/Dysport, incobotulinumtoxinA/Xeomin) and type B (rimabotulinumtoxinB/Myobloc).

    ○ Injection sites

       ● Blepharospasm

          – Start with very low doses (eg, 2.5 U of type A for each injection site).

          – Inject the upper orbicularis oculi muscle as close to the eyelid margin as possible for maximum efficacy and the fewest side effects.

Table 5.6
Medications Commonly Used for the Symptomatic Treatment of Dystonia

Medication	Typical Starting Dose (mg/d)	Typical Therapeutic Dose (mg/d)	Comments
Carbidopa/ levodopa	25/100	Up to 800	To be given 3 times per day; always try levodopa first, especially if young patient, to rule out dopa-responsive dystonia, which requires only low dose
Trihexyphenidyl	1–2	Up to 120	In divided doses; if increased very slowly, young patients able to tolerate high doses
Benztropine	0.5–1	Up to 8	Watch for anticholinergic side effects
Baclofen	5–10	Up to 120	GABA agonist; do not abruptly discontinue (risk for seizures)
Clonazepam	0.5–1	Up to 5	
Tetrabenazine	25	Up to 75	
Tizanidine	2	24	Unlike baclofen, tizanidine carries minimal risk for seizures with abrupt discontinuation

Abbreviation: GABA, gamma-aminobutyric acid.

- Avoid the middle upper eyelid area (where the levator palpebrae lies) to prevent ptosis.

- Use a 30-gauge, 0.5-in needle.

- Cervical dystonia

  - Sternocleidomastoid muscle: responsible for anterocollis and contralateral chin deviation

  - Splenius capitis: responsible for retrocollis (the most common presentation of tardive dystonia) and ipsilateral chin deviation

  - Trapezius: responsible for ipsilateral shoulder elevation

  - Levator scapulae: responsible for ispsilateral shoulder elevation

  - Scalene complex: responsible for ipsilateral head tilt

  - Submentalis: responsible for anterocollis

- Usual doses (Table 5.7)

  - Inco-, ona-, and abobotulinumtoxinA come in various units/vials of powdered forms to be diluted with preservative-free normal saline.

  - RimabotulinumtoxinB comes in premixed 2,500-/5,000-/10,000-U vials.

  - In cervical dystonia, for which all four toxins are approved, the typical starting doses of each toxin are as follows:

    - OnabotulinumtoxinA (Botox): 120 to 240 U

    - IncobotulinumtoxinA (Xeomin): 120 to 240 U

    - AbobotulinumtoxinA (Dysport): 500 U

    - RimabotulinumtoxinB (Myobloc): 2,500 to 10,000 U

- Botulinum toxin doses may need to be increased or decreased depending on certain factors (Table 5.8):

- Treatment of Wilson's disease (Figure 5.2)

  - Low-copper diet, with avoidance of foods having a high copper content (ie, >0.2 mg): shellfish, liver, pork, duck, lamb, avocados, dried beans, dried fruits, raisins, dates, prunes, bran, mushrooms, wheat germ, chocolate, and nuts.

  - Consider agents that deplete copper: penicillamine (1–2 g/d) with pyridoxine (50 mg/d), trientine (500 mg 2 times daily), tetrathiomolybdate (80–120 mg daily in 3 to 4 divided doses), and zinc (50 mg/d without food).

- Dystonic emergencies

Presentation	Muscle	Average Starting Dose (Botox)	Average Dose (Botox)	Starting Dose Range (Myobloc)
Blepharospasm	Orbicularis oculi	2.5–5 U per site	5–10 U per site	250–1,000 U per side
	Procerus	2.5–5 U per site	2.5–10 U per site	250–500 U
Hemifacial spasm[a]	Orbicularis oris	2.5 U per site	2.5–5 U per site	125–750 U
	Levator anguli oris	2.5–10 U	2.5–10 U	125–250 U
	Depressor anguli oris	2.5–10 U	2.5–10 U	125–250 U
	Mentalis	2.5–5 U	2.5–10 U	125–250 U
	Platysma	2.5–5 U	2.5–15 U	500–2,500 U
	Zygomaticus	2.5–5 U	2.5–10 U	125–500 U
Jaw-closing dystonia	Masseter	40 U per side	20–60 U per side	1,000–3,000 U per side
	Temporalis	20 U per side	20–40 U per side	1,000–3,000 U per side
Jaw-opening dystonia	Pterygoids	5–20 U	5–20 U	1,000–3,000 U per side
	Digastric	5–15 U	5–15 U	250–750 U per side
Cervical dystonia				
• Anterocollis	Sternocleidomastoid	40 U	40–70 U	1,000–3,000 U
• Retrocollis	Splenius capitis	60 U	50–150 U	1,000–5,000 U
	Trapezius	60 U	50–150 U	1,000–5,000 U
• Torticollis (chin deviation)	Ipsilateral splenius capitis	60 U	50–150 U	1,000–5,000 U
	Contralateral sternocleidomastoid	40 U	40–70 U	1,000–3,000 U
• Laterocollis (head tilt)	Scalenes	30 U	15–50 U	1,000–3,000 U
• Shoulder elevation	Levator scapulae	80 U	25–100 U	1,000–4,000 U
	Trapezius	60 U	50–150 U	1,000–5,000 U
Shoulder abduction	Deltoid	50 U	50–150 U	

continued

140

Presentation	Muscle	Average Starting Dose (Botox)	Average Dose (Botox)	Starting Dose Range (Myobloc)
Shoulder adduction	Pectoralis complex	100 U	75–150 U	2,500–5,000 U
	Latissimus dorsi	100 U	50–150 U	2,500–5,000 U
Elbow extension	Triceps	50 U	25–100 U	
Elbow flexion	Biceps	100 U	50–150 U	2,500–5,000 U
	Brachialis	60 U	40–100 U	1,000–3,000 U
	Brachioradialis	60 U	40–100 U	1,000–3,000 U
Wrist flexion	Flexor carpi radialis[b]	50 U	25–100 U	1,000–3,000 U
	Flexor carpi ulnaris[b]	40 U	20–70 U	1,000–3,000 U
Wrist extension	Extensor carpi radialis	20 U	25–100 U	500–1,500 U
	Extensor carpi ulnaris[b]	20 U	20–40 U	500–1,500 U
Wrist pronation	Pronator quadratus[b]	25 U	10–50 U	1,000–2,500 U
	Pronator teres[b]	40 U	25–75 U	1,000–2,500 U
Wrist supination	Supinator	20 U	15–45 U	
Finger flexion	Flexor digitorum profundus[b]	20 U	20–40 U	1,000–3,000 U
	Flexor digitorum superficialis[b]	20 U	20–40 U	1,000–3,000 U
Fisting	Flexor carpi radialis[b]	50 U	25–100 U	1,000–3,000 U
	Flexor carpi ulnaris[b]	40 U	20–70 U	1,000–3,000 U
	Extensor carpi ulnaris	20 U	10–30 U	500–1,500 U
	Extensor carpi radialis	20 U	15–40 U	500–1,500 U
	Flexor digitorum profundus[b]	20 U	20–40 U	1,000–3,000 U
	Flexor digitorum superficialis[b]	20 U	20–40 U	1,000–3,000 U
	Flexor pollicis longus[b]	20 U	10–30 U	1,000–2,500 U
	Opponens pollicis[b]	5 U	2.5–10 U	500–1,500 U
Finger extension	Extensor indicis	5 U	2.5–10 U	500–1,000 U
Thumb extension	Extensor pollicis longus	5 U	2.5–10 U	
Thumb in palm	Flexor pollicis longus[b]	20 U	10–30 U	1,000–2,500 U
	Opponens pollicis[b]	5 U	2.5–10 U	500–1,500 U
	Adductor pollicis[b]			500–2,500 U

continued

141

Presentation	Muscle	Average Starting Dose (Botox)	Average Dose (Botox)	Starting Dose Range (Myobloc)
Thumb protrusion	Extensor pollicis longus	5 U	2.5–10 U	
	Abductor pollicis longus	5 U	5–15 U	
Little finger abduction	Abductor digiti minimi	5 U	2.5–10 U	125–250 U
Hip flexion	Iliopsoas	150 U	50–200 U	3,000–7,500 U
	Rectus femoris	100 U	75–200 U	2,500–5,000 U
Hip adduction	Adductor magnus/ longus/brevis	200 U	75–300 U	5,000–10,000 U
Knee flexion	Semimembranosus	100 U	50–200 U	2,500–7,500 U
	Semitendinosus	100 U	50–200 U	2,500–7,500 U
	Biceps femoris	100 U	50–200 U	2,500–7,500 U
	Gastrocnemius	150 U	50–200 U	3,000–7,500 U
Knee extension	Rectus femoris	100 U	75–200 U	3,000–7,500 U
	Vastus lateralis	100 U	50–200 U	3,000–7,500 U
	Vastus medialis	100 U	50–200 U	3,000–7,500 U
Plantar flexion (equinus)	Gastrocnemius	100 U	50–200 U	3,000–7,500 U
	Soleus	100 U	50–200 U	2,500–5,000 U
Foot inversion	Tibialis posterior	75 U	50–150 U	3,000–7,500 U
Foot dorsiflexion	Tibialis anterior	75 U	50–150 U	2,500–5,000 U
Toe flexion	Flexor digitorum longus	75 U	50–100 U	2,500–5,000 U
	Flexor digitorum brevis	25 U	20–40 U	2,500–5,000 U
	Flexor hallucis longus	50 U	25–75 U	1,500–3,500 U
Striatal toe	Extensor hallucis longus	50 U	20–100 U	2,000–4,000 U

[a]*Hemifacial spasm* is not considered a form of dystonia, even though it can cause blepharospasm and facial spasms. It is consistently unilateral, defined as a neurological disorder manifested by involuntary, recurrent twitches of the eyelids; the perinasal and perioral muscles; and the zygomaticus, platysma, and other muscles of only one side of the face. It is usually due to a compression or irritation of the facial nerve by an aberrant artery or abnormal vasculature around the brainstem. Although microvascular decompression of the facial nerve has a high success rate, it also has risks, such as permanent facial paralysis, stroke, and deafness, so that botulinum toxin injection is the treatment of choice.

[b]Start with lower doses if injecting these muscles for upper limb dystonia; doses provided are recommended for upper limb spasticity.

142

Table 5.8
Dose Modifiers to Consider for the Injection of Botulinum Toxin

Clinical Factor	Starting Dose: Low End of the Range	Starting Dose: High End of the Range
Patient weight	Low	High
Patient age	Elderly	Young
Muscle bulk	Very small	Very large
Number of regions injected	Many	Few
Severity of disease/dystonic spams	Mild	Severe
Concern for weakness	High	Low
Results of previous therapy	Too much weakness	Inadequate denervation
Likely duration of therapy	Chronic	Acute

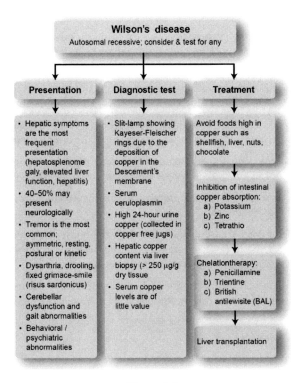

Figure 5.2
The presentation, diagnosis, and treatment of Wilson's disease.

○ Status dystonicus ("dystonic storm," "dystonic crisis") is a rare, potentially life-threatening neurological emergency that can complicate the course of an otherwise slowly progressive or static dystonic condition.

  ● Differentiate from neuroleptic malignant syndrome.

  ● Manage aggressively in an intensive care setting because metabolic disturbances (hyperpyrexia, renal failure from rhabdomyolysis, dehydration), respiratory failure, and aspiration pneumonia from muscle spasms that interfere with bulbar function are common etiologies of morbidity and mortality.

  ● Consider the "Marsden cocktail"—a combination of tetrabenazine (dopamine-depleting drug), haloperidol, or pimozide (D2 receptor antagonist) and trihexyphenidyl (anticholinergic agent).

  ● If needed, intravenous sedation and ventilation, with or without paralytic agents, can be administered.

○ Neuroleptic malignant syndrome occurs with the addition of a neuroleptic drug.

  ● A similar presentation is seen with the abrupt withdrawal of levodopa and other dopamine replacement therapy in Parkinson's disease (eg, the old practice of "levodopa holiday").

  ● The clinical presentation may be slow in onset, with fever, muscle stiffness, fluctuating consciousness, and autonomic instability.

  ● The creatine phosphokinase level is often elevated because of muscle injury (and can be used to monitor the disease course).

  ● Other differential diagnoses include serotonin syndrome, dystonic storm, anticholinergic poisoning, and malignant hyperthermia.

  ● **First, and most importantly, stop the neuroleptic drug or reinstitute levodopa!**

  ● Supportive care includes lowering the body temperature, administering intravenous fluids, preventing deep vein thrombosis, and monitoring blood pressure and electrolytes.

  ● Consider bromocriptine (2.5 mg 3 times daily), dantrolene (1–10 mg/kg intravenously, followed by maintenance at 600 mg/d), benzodiazepines.

■ Surgical therapies

  ○ Peripheral surgical procedures

    ● Rhizotomy

    ● Ramisectomy

- Myotomy
- Intrathecal baclofen
- ○ Central nervous system ablative procedures (please see Chapter 16)
  - Pallidotomy
  - Thalamotomy
- ○ Deep brain stimulation (please see Chapter 16)
  - Globus pallidus internus (GPi) stimulation
  - Ventrolateral thalamic stimulation
- Other therapies
  - ○ Limb immobilization, focal splinting
  - ○ Support groups
  - ○ Physical therapy (gait, transfers, strengthening, stretching)
  - ○ Occupational therapy (assistive devices to regain some independence)

REFERENCES

1. Fahn S. The varied clinical expressions of dystonia. *Neurol Clin.* 1984; 2:541–554.
2. Nutt JG, Muenter MD, Aronson A, Kurlan LT, Melton LJ. Epidemiology of focal and generalized dystonia in Rochester, Minnesota. *Mov Disord.* 1988; 3:188–194.
3. Marsden CD. The focal dystonias. *Clin Neuropharmacol.* 1986; 9(suppl 2):S49–S60.
4. Fahn S. Generalized dystonia: concept and treatment. *Clin Neuropharmacol.* 1986; 9(suppl 2):S37–S48.
5. Chan J, Brin MF, Fahn S. Idiopathic cervical dystonia: clinical characteristics. *Mov Disord.* 1991; 6:119–126.
6. Bruno MK, Hallett M, Gwinn-Hardy K, et al. Clinical evaluation of idiopathic paroxysmal kinesigenic dyskinesia: new diagnostic criteria. *Neurology.* 2004; 63(12): 2280–2287.
7. Ozelius LJ, Hewett JW, Page CE, et al. The early onset torsion dystonia gene (DYT1) encodes at ATP binding protein. *Nat Genet.* 1997; 17:40–48.
8. Khan NL, Wood NW, Bhatia KP. Autosomal recessive DYT2-like primary torsion dystonia: a new family. *Neurology.* 2003; 61:1801–1803.
9. Nolte D, Niemann S, Muller U. Specific sequence changes in multiple transcript system DYT3 are associated with X-linked dystonia parkinsonism. *Proc Natl Acad Sci U S A.* 2003; 100:10347–10352.
10. Parker N. Hereditary whispering dystonia. *J Neurol Neurosurg Psychiatry.* 1985; 45:218–224.
11. Hersheson J, Mencacci N, Davis M. Mutations in the autoregulatory domain of β-tubulin 4a cause hereditary dystonia. *Ann Neurol.* 2013; 73(4):546–553.

12. Ichinose H, Ohye T, Takahashi E, et al. Hereditary progressive dystonia with marked diurnal fluctuation caused by mutations in the GTP cyclohydrolase I gene. *Nat Genet.* 1994; 8:236–242.

13. Almasy L, Bressman SB, Raymond D, et al. Idiopathic torsion dystonia linked to chromosome 8 in two Mennonite families. *Ann Neurol.* 1997; 42:670–673.

14. Leube B, Rudnicki D, Ratzlaff T, Kessler KR, et al. Idiopathic torsion dystonia; assignment of a gene to chromosome 18p in a German family with adult onset, autosomal dominant inheritance and purely focal distribution. *Hum Mol Genet.* 1996; 5:1673–1677.

15. Fouad GT, Servidei S, Durcan S, Bertini E, Ptacek LJ. A gene for familial paroxysmal dyskinesia (FPD1) maps to chromosome 2q. *Am J Hum Genet.* 1996; 59:135–139.

16. Fink JK, Rainier S, Wilkowski J, et al. Paroxysmal dystonic choreoathetosis: tight linkage to chromosome 2q. *Am J Hum Genet.* 1996; 59:140–145.

17. Auburger G, Ratzlaff T, Lunkes A, et al. A gene for autosomal dominant paroxysmal choreoathetosis spasticity maps to the vicinity of a potassium channel gene cluster on chromosome 1p. *Genomics.* 1996; 31:90–94.

18. Tomita H, Nagamitsu S, Wakui K, et al. Paroxysmal kinesigenic choreoathetosis locus maps to chromosome 16p11.2-q12.1. *Am J Hum Genet.* 1999; 65:1688–1697.

19. Zimprich A, Grabowski M, Asmus F, et al. Mutations in the gene encoding epsilon-sarcoglycan cause myoclonus-dystonia syndrome. *Nat Genet.* 2001; 29:66–69.

20. Kramer PL, Mineta M, Klein C, et al. Rapid onset dystonia parkinsonism: linkage to chromosome 19q13. *Ann Neurol.* 1999; 46:176–182.

21. Valente EM, Bentivoglio AR, Cassetta E, et al. DYT13, a novel primary torsion dystonia locus, maps to chromosome 1p36.13-36.32 in an Italian family with cranial-cervical or upper limb onset. *Ann Neurol.* 2001; 49:362–366.

22. Grotzsch H, Pizzolato GP, Ghika J, et al. Neuropathology of a case of dopa-responsive dystonia associated with new genetic locus, DYT14. *Neurology.* 2002; 58:1839–1842.

23. Grimes DA, Han F, Lang AE, et al. A novel locus for inherited myoclonus dystonia on 18p11. *Neurology.* 2002; 59:1183–1186.

24. Camargos S, Scholz S, Simon-Sanchez, et al. DYT16, a novel young-onset dystonia-parkinsonism disorder: identification of a segregating mutation in the stress-response protein PRKRA. *Lancet Neurol.* 2008; 7:207–215.

25. Chouery E, Kfoury J, Delague V, et al. A novel locus for autosomal recessive primary torsion dystonia (DYT17) maps to 20p11.22-q13.12. *Neurogenetics.* 2008; 9:287–293.

26. Suls A, Dedeken P, Goffin K, et al. Paroxysmal exercise-induced dyskinesia and epilepsy is due to mutations in SLC2A1, encoding the glucose transporter GLUT1. *Brain.* 2008; 131:1831–1844.

27. Valente EM, Spacey SD, Wali GM, et al. A second paroxysmal kinesigenic choreoathetosis locus (EKD2) mapping on 16q13-q22.1 indicates a family of genes which give rise to paroxysmal disorders on human chromosome 16. *Brain.* 2000; (123): 2040–2045.

28. Spacey SD, Adams PJ, Lam PCP, et al. Genetic heterogeneity in paroxysmal nonkinesigenic dyskinesia. *Neurology.* 2006; 66:1588–1590.

29. Norgren N, Mattson E, Forsgren L, Holmberg M. A high-penetrance form of late-onset torsion dystonia maps to a novel locus (DYT21) on chromosome 2q14.3-q21.3. *Neurogenetics.* 2011; 12:137–143.

30. Charlesworth G, Plagnol V, Holmstrom KM. Mutations in ANO3 cause dominant craniocervical dystonia: ion channel implicated in pathogenesis. *Am J Hum Genet* 2012; 91:1041–1050.

31. Segawa M. Dopa-responsive dystonia. *Handb Clin Neurol.* 2011; 100:539–557.
32. Friedman J, Roze E, Abdenur JE, et al. Sepiapterin reductase deficiency: a treatable mimic of cerebral palsy. *Ann Neurol.* 2012; 71(4):520–530.
33. Brashear A, Dobyns WB, de Carvalho Aquiar P, et al. The phenotypic spectrum of rapid-onset dystonia-parkinsonism (RDP) and mutations in the ATP1A3 gene. *Brain.* 2007; 130(pt 3):828–835.
34. Nardocci N. Myoclonus-dystonia syndrome. *Handb Clin Neurol.* 2011; 100:563–575.
35. Dressler D. Nonprimary dystonias. *Handb Clin Neurol.* 2011; 100:513–538.
36. Preston DC, Finkleman RS, Munsat TL, Dystonia postures generated from complex repetitive discharges. *Neurology.* 1996; 46:257–258.

6

CHOREA

DEFINITIONS

- Phenomenology: chorea, athetosis, and ballism generally represent a continuum of involuntary, hyperkinetic movement disorders.

- *Chorea* consists of involuntary, continuous, abrupt, rapid, brief, unsustained, irregular movements that flow randomly from one body part to another.

- *Ballism* is a form of chorea characterized by forceful, flinging, high-amplitude, coarse movements; ballism and chorea are often interrelated and may occur in the same patient.

- *Athetosis* is a slow form of chorea and consists of writhing movements resembling dystonia. However, unlike in dystonia, the movements are not sustained, patterned, or painful.

- Other related disorders that can be confused with chorea, athetosis, or ballism are the following:

  - *Akathisia:* a feeling of inner restlessness and anxiety associated with an inability to sit or stand still.

  - *Restless legs syndrome:* a symptom complex of discomfort or unusual sensation in the legs (or arms) that is characteristically relieved by movement of the affected limb(s).

CHOREA

- Clinical features

  - Patients can partially/temporarily volitionally suppress chorea.

  - *Parakinesia* is the act of "camouflaging" some of the choreiform movements by incorporating them into semipurposeful activities.

○   *Motor impersistence* is the inability to maintain voluntary contraction, manifested on examination with "milkmaid grip" (impersistence of grasp) and inability to maintain tongue protrusion.

○   The examiner must differentiate chorea from pseudochoreoathetosis (chorea or athetosis secondary to a defect of proprioception).

○   Chorea may be a manifestation of a primary neurologic disorder (eg, Huntington's disease) or may be secondary to a systemic, toxic, or metabolic disorder.

■   Differential diagnosis: see Figure 6.1[1]

■   Inherited forms of chorea

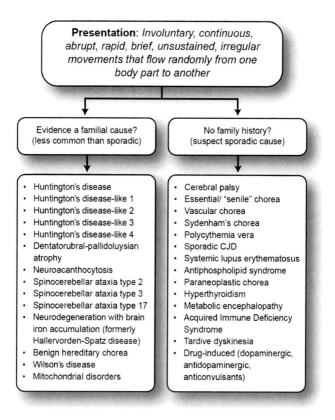

Presentation: *Involuntary, continuous, abrupt, rapid, brief, unsustained, irregular movements that flow randomly from one body part to another*

Evidence a familial cause? (less common than sporadic)

No family history? (suspect sporadic cause)

- Huntington's disease
- Huntington's disease-like 1
- Huntington's disease-like 2
- Huntington's disease-like 3
- Huntington's disease-like 4
- Dentatorubral-pallidoluysian atrophy
- Neuroacanthocytosis
- Spinocerebellar ataxia type 2
- Spinocerebellar ataxia type 3
- Spinocerebellar ataxia type 17
- Neurodegeneration with brain iron accumulation (formerly Hallervorden-Spatz disease)
- Benign hereditary chorea
- Wilson's disease
- Mitochondrial disorders

- Cerebral palsy
- Essential/ "senile" chorea
- Vascular chorea
- Sydenham's chorea
- Polycythemia vera
- Sporadic CJD
- Systemic lupus erythematosus
- Antiphospholipid syndrome
- Paraneoplastic chorea
- Hyperthyroidism
- Metabolic encephalopathy
- Acquired Immune Deficiency Syndrome
- Tardive dyskinesia
- Drug-induced (dopaminergic, antidopaminergic, anticonvulsants)

Figure 6.1
Differential diagnosis of chorea.

○ *Huntington's disease* (HD) is an autosomal dominant neurodegenerative disorder (each child of an affected parent has a 50% chance of developing the disease) caused by an abnormal expansion of the *IT15* gene on chromosome 4, which encodes the protein huntington. This protein is ubiquitously expressed in persons with Huntington's disease, but its function is still poorly understood.[2]

- Most people develop HD between 30 and 54 years of age, but HD can manifest in individuals as young as 4 years or as old as 80 years of age.

- CAG repeats: normal, 10 to 35; indeterminate, 36 to 39; definite, 40 or more.

- There is a triad of motor, cognitive, and psychiatric symptoms.

- Motor symptoms: impairment related to involuntary (chorea) and voluntary movements, reduced manual dexterity, dysarthria, dysphagia, gait instability, and falls are common; parkinsonism and dystonia can be seen in patients with an earlier onset of disease.

  - In the treatment of chorea, nondrug interventions should be considered first as patients are often not bothered by mild chorea and exhibit no functional impairment related to choreiform movements.

  - Pharmacologic treatment for chorea may worsen other aspects of movement, cognition, or mood.

  - Chorea may diminish over time, so that the need for treatment is reduced.

- Cognitive symptoms: initially characterized by loss of speed and flexibility of thinking (executive dysfunction); later, dysfunction becomes more global.

- Psychiatric symptoms: depression (most common), irritability, agitation, impulsivity, mania, obsessive–compulsive disorder, anxiety, apathy, and social withdrawal can all emerge in the same patient.

  - Ask about substance abuse.

  - Always ask about suicidality, particularly given that impulsivity is common.

- Diagnosis: based on the clinical presentation, family history, and genetic testing (genetic counseling required for asymptomatic individuals with a family history before genetic testing).

  - Always disclose the results of genetic testing in person and with a relative, caregiver, or friend of the patient present.

- Prenatal testing (as early as 8–10 weeks) is possible.

- Nonpharmacologic approaches are important in addressing functional difficulties and behavioral dysfunction in HD (Table 6.1).

○ *Huntington-like syndromes* (Table 6.2)[3–10]

○ *Inherited "paroxysmal" disorders that can include choreiform movement* (see Table 6.3 for clinical overview)[11]

Table 6.1
Helpful Tips for Managing Functional and Behavioral Problems
in Patients With Huntington's Disease

Problem	Solution
Dysphagia	The patient should eat slowly and without distractions.
	Foods should be of appropriate size and texture.
	Eating may need to be supervised.
	All caregivers should know the Heimlich maneuver.
Communication	Allow the patient enough time to answer questions.
	Offer cues and prompts to get the patient started.
	Break down tasks or instructions into small steps.
	Use visual cues to demonstrate what you are saying.
	Alphabet boards, yes–no cards, and other devices can be used for patients in more advanced stages.
Executive dysfunction	Rely on routines.
	Make lists that help organize tasks.
	Prompt each activity with external cues.
	Offer limited choices instead of open-ended questions.
	Use short sentences with one or two pieces of information.
Impulsivity	A predictable daily schedule can reduce confusion, fear, and outbursts.
	It is possible that a behavior is a response to something else that needs your attention (eg, pain).
	Let the patient know that yelling is not the best way to get your attention.
	Hurtful and embarrassing statements are generally not intentional. Be sensitive to the patient's efforts to apologize or show remorse afterward.
	Do not badger the person after the fact.

continued

Table 6.1 (cont.)
Helpful Tips for Managing Functional and Behavioral Problems
in Patients With Huntington's Disease

Problem	Solution
Irritability and outbursts	Try to keep the environment as calm as possible.
	Speak in a low, soft voice. Keep your hand gestures quiet.
	Avoid confrontations.
	Redirect the patient away from the source of anger.
	Respond diplomatically, acknowledging the patient's irritability as a symptom of frustration.

Source: Adapted from Ref. 3: Rosenblatt A, Ranen NG, Nance MA, Paulsen JS. *A Physician's Guide to the Management of Huntington's Disease.* 2nd ed. New York, NY: Huntington's Disease Society of America; 1999.

- Sporadic forms of chorea

  - *Essential chorea* is adult-onset, nonprogressive chorea in a patient without a family history or other symptoms suggestive of HD and without evidence of striatal atrophy. "Senile chorea" is essential chorea with onset after age 60 without dementia or psychiatric disturbance.

  - *Infectious chorea* has been described as an acute choreiform manifestation of bacterial meningitis, encephalitis, tuberculous meningitis, aseptic meningitis, HIV encephalitis, or toxoplasmosis.

  - *Postinfectious/autoimmune chorea*[12]

    - **Sydenham disease** (St. Vitus' dance, the eponym sometimes used by patients) is related to infection with group A streptococci, and the chorea may be delayed for 6 months or longer. The distribution is often asymmetric. The chorea can be accompanied by arthritis, carditis, irritability, emotional lability, obsessive–compulsive disorder, or anxiety. Serologic testing reveals elevated titers of anti-streptolysin O (ASO).

    - **Systemic lupus erythematosus** is associated with anti-phospholipid syndrome (characterized by migraine, chorea, and venous and/or arterial thrombosis). The patient tests positive for anti-phospholipid antibodies and anti-cardiolipin antibodies. Other features are spontaneous abortions, arthralgias, Raynaud phenomenon, digital infarctions, transient ischemic attacks, and cardiovascular accidents.

    - **Chorea gravidarum** is often associated with a recurrence of systemic lupus erythematosus or with a prior history of Sydenham chorea but can also be associated with other metabolic or systemic disturbances.

Table 6.2
Summary of Huntington-Like Syndromes

Disease	MOI	Chr	Gene	Triplet Repeat	Protein	Features
Huntington's disease–like 1[4]	AD	20p	HDL1	No		Similar to HD-like 2 but seizures can occur
Huntington's disease–like 2[5]	AD	16q23	HDL2	CTG/CAG	Junctophilin 3	Onset in the fourth decade; chorea, dystonia, parkinsonism, dysarthria, hyperreflexia, gait abnormality, psychiatric symptoms, weight loss, dementia; acanthocytosis common; predominantly African Americans
Huntington's disease–like 3	AR	4p15.3		No		Begins at 3 to 4 years of age; chorea, ataxia, gait disorder, spasticity, seizures, mutism, dementia
Neuroacanthocytosis[6]	AR, some AD or sporadic	9q21-22	CHAC	No	Chorein	After HD, most common hereditary chorea; begins third to fourth decade; lip and tongue biting, orolingual dystonia, motor and phonic tics, generalized chorea, parkinsonism, vertical ophthalmoparesis, seizures, cognitive and personality changes, dysphagia, dysarthria, amyotrophy, areflexia, axonal neuropathy, elevated creatine phosphokinase and acanthocytes on peripheral smear
McLeod syndrome[7]	X-linked recessive	X	XK	No	XK	Form of neuroacanthocytosis; depression, bipolar and personality disorders, chorea, vocalizations, seizures, hemolysis, liver disease, high creatine kinase; usually no lip biting or dysphagia

Disease	MOI	Chr	Gene	Repeat	Protein	Clinical features
Benign hereditary chorea[8]	AD	14q13.1-21.1		No		Nonprogressive chorea with childhood onset; slight motor delay, ataxia; may be self-limiting
SCA2	AD	12q23-24.1	SCA2	CAG	Ataxin 2	Commercially available gene testing
SCA3	AD	14q32.1	SCA3	CAG	Ataxin 3	Machado-Joseph disease; Azorean descent; parkinsonism, dystonia, chorea, neuropathy, ataxia; commercially available testing
SCA17	AD	6q27	SCA17	CAG	TATA-binding protein	Commercially available gene testing
DRPLA[9]	AD	12		CAG	JNK	Japan > Europe, Africa, southern United States (Haw River syndrome); starts in fourth decade; combination of choreoathetosis, dystonia, tremor, parkinsonism, dementia
Neurodegeneration with brain iron accumulation (NBIA) type 1 (formerly Hallervorden-Spatz disease)[10]	AR	20p112.3-13	PANK2	No	Pantothenate kinase	Childhood onset, progressive rigidity, dystonia, choreoathetosis, spasticity, optic nerve atrophy, dementia, acanthocytosis; "eye of the tiger" MRI abnormality
Wilson's disease	AR	13q14.3	ATB7B	No	Cu ATPase	May present with tremor, parkinsonism, dystonia, chorea, usually before age 50. Please see also Chapters 2 and 5.

Abbreviations: AD, autosomal dominant; AR, autosomal recessive; Chr, chromosome; DRPLA, dentatorubropallidoluysian atrophy; HD, Huntington's disease; JNK, c-Jun N-terminal kinase; MOI, mode of inheritance; SCA, spinocerebellar ataxia.

Table 6.3
Summary of Features of Major Causes of Paroxysmal Dyskinesias

	PKD	PNKD	PED
Male-to-female ratio	4:1	3:2	Unclear
Age at onset	5–15 y	< 5 y	2–20 y
Inheritance	AD or sporadic	AD or sporadic	AD
Duration of attacks	< 5 min	Several minutes to hours	5–30 min
Frequency	Very frequent: 100/d–1/mo	Occasional, 3/d–2/y	1/d–1/mo
Asymmetry	Common	Less common	
Ability to suppress attacks	Able	Able	
Precipitating factors	Sudden movement, startle, hyperventilation, fatigue, stress	Alcohol, caffeine, exercise, excitement	Prolonged exercise, stress, caffeine, fatigue
Associated features	Dystonia, chorea, epilepsy	Chorea, dystonia, ataxia	Dystonia, chorea
Treatment	Phenytoin, carbamazepine, barbiturates, acetazolamide	Clonazepam, oxazepam	

Abbreviations: AD, autosomal dominant; PED, paroxysmal exertional dyskinesia; PKD, paroxysmal kinesigenic dyskinesia; PNKD, paroxysmal nonkinesigenic dyskinesia.

○ *Post-pump chorea* is a sequela of cardiac surgery (for congenital heart disease) in children that is associated with a prolonged time on the pump, deep hypothermia, and circulatory arrest. It may respond to dopamine receptor blockers.

○ *Polycythemia vera* is more common in men, but chorea is seen more often in women in association with facial erythrosis or splenomegaly. The onset is usually after 50 years, and the chorea is often bilateral and symmetric. Treatment is reduction of hyperviscosity and administration of antidopaminergic drugs.

○ *Vascular chorea* is described in congophilic angiopathy and other stroke disorders.

○ *Paraneoplastic chorea* is mostly associated with anti-CRMP-5 or anti-CV2 antibodies (commercially testing available).

Table 6.4
Drugs Reported to Cause Tardive Syndromes

Amoxapine (tricyclic antidepressant)
Cinnarizine (calcium channel blocker)
Chlorpromazine
Chlorprothixene
Clebopride
Clozapine (?)
Droperidol
Flunarizine (calcium channel blocker)
Fluphenazine
Haloperidol
Loxapine
Mesoridazine
Metoclopramide
Molindone
Olanzapine
Perazine
Pimozide
Prochlorperazine
Quetiapine (?)
Remoxipride
Risperidone
Sulpiride
Thioridazine
Thiothixene
Tiapride
Trifluoperazine
Triflupromazine
Veralipride

○ *Drug-induced chorea*

  • Most often occurs acutely in association with dopaminergic/anti-
    dopaminergic drugs and anticonvulsants.

  • Tardive chorea is stereotypic oral–buccal–lingual dyskinesia after
    chronic exposure to dopamine receptor blockers (Table 6.4).

○ *Metabolic etiologies:* often asymmetric chorea

  • Hypo- and hypercalcemia

  • Hypo- and hyperglycemia

  • Hyperthyroidism

  • Hypo- and hypernatremia

  • Hypomagnesemia

- Hypo- and hyperparathyroidism

- Liver disease (acquired hepatocerebral degeneration)

○ *Multiple sclerosis:* Although rarely, any movement disorder can be associated with multiple sclerosis. Chorea and/or tremor may be the most common movement disorder presentation. Ballism has also been reported.

■ Workup: see Figure 6.2.

■ Treatment (Table 6.5)[13,14]

○ The first step is always to identify the underlying etiology and correct it if possible (eg, metabolic cause).

○ Dopamine receptor blockers (eg, typical and atypical antipsychotic agents) or dopamine-depleting agents (eg, tetrabenazine or reserpine) can be used if the chorea is disrupting quality of life.[15]

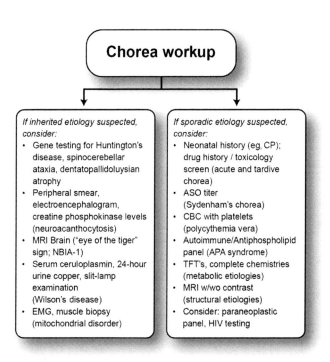

Figure 6.2
Initial workup for a patient presenting with chorea.

Table 6.5
Medications Used to Suppress Chorea

Class	Medication	Starting Dose	Maximum Dose	Adverse Events
Dopamine receptor blockers	Haloperidol	0.5–1 mg/d	6–8 mg/d	Sedation, parkinsonism, dystonia, akathisia, hypotension, constipation, dry mouth, weight gain, confusion
	Fluphenazine	0.5–1 mg/d	6–8 mg/d	Same
	Risperidone	0.5–1 mg/d	6 mg/d	Same
	Thiothixene	1–2 mg/d	6 mg/d	Same
	Thioridazine	10 mg/d	100 mg/d	Same
	Clozapine	12.5 mg/d	600 mg/d	Parkinsonism avoided but rare agranulocytosis; weekly monitoring of white cell count required for first 6 months, then every 2 weeks thereafter
	Quetiapine	25 mg/d	800 mg/d	Less parkinsonism
Benzodiazepines	Clonazepam	0.5 mg/d	4 mg/d	Sedation, ataxia, apathy, withdrawal seizures
	Diazepam	1.25 mg/d	20 mg/d	Same
NMDA receptor antagonist	Amantadine	100 mg/d	400 mg/d	Hallucinations, confusion, leg swelling, livedo reticularis, anticholinergic effects
Dopamine-depleting agents	Reserpine	0.1 mg/d	3 mg/d	Hypotension, sedation, parkinsonism, depression
	Tetrabenazine	25 mg/d	100 mg/d	Hypotension (less), parkinsonism, depression

Abbreviation: NMDA, N-methyl-d-aspartate.

○ Benzodiazepines, valproic acid, amantadine, levetiracetam, and riluzole have also been reported to mitigate chorea.

○ Anticoagulation, immunosuppressants, and plasmapheresis have been used with variable success in autoimmune choreas; consider steroids.

○ Consider stereotactic surgery for severe and disabling cases of chorea or ballism (see Chapter 16 for details).[16]

○ *Tardive dyskinesia*

● The severity of the tardive syndrome and the absolute need for neuroleptic therapy often dictate the treatment approach for this group of disorders.

● Continuing to use drugs known to cause tardive phenomena is not the best approach, and increasing the dose is often a temporary solution at best.

● Because tardive dyskinesia (TD) remits in a majority of patients if they are kept off dopamine receptor blockers, it is best to avoid any antipsychotic drug. When this is not possible, as is often the case, clozapine is best but can be logistically difficult to use (requirement for frequent white blood cell counts).

● To suppress mild TD, low doses of a benzodiazepine or vitamin E, in addition to a switch to clozapine or quetiapine, may be helpful.

● For moderate to severe TD, dopamine-depleting drugs, such as tetrabenazine, may be the most effective agents.

● Only as a last resort, to treat persistent, disabling, and treatment-resistant TD, should neuroleptics be resumed in the absence of active psychosis.

BALLISM

Damage to the subthalamic nucleus and the pallidal–subthalamic pathways is posited to play a critical role; other structures have been implicated/described (thalamus).

■ Etiology

○ When caused by a hemorrhagic or ischemic stroke, ballism is often preceded by hemiparesis.

○ It is also described in anterior parietal stroke.

○ Less common causes are abscess, arteriovenous malformation, cerebral trauma, hyperosmotic hyperglycemia, multiple sclerosis, tumor, basal ganglia strokes or calcification, encephalitis, vasculitis.

- Prognosis and treatment

  - The prognosis for spontaneous remission is often good.

  - Dopamine receptor blockers are most frequently used to treat movements when they are functionally impairing.

  - Dopamine-depleting agents may be considered.

  - Valproic acid and clonazepam have been reported to mitigate ballism.

  - For violent, treatment-refractory ballism, ventrolateral thalamotomy has been described.

ATHETOSIS

Chorea often evolves into athetosis and vice versa, and they can coexist (choreoathetosis).

- Most often accompanies cerebral palsy; can be seen in errors of metabolism, including acidurias, lipidoses, and Lesch-Nyhan syndrome.

- Treatment: usually does not respond to therapy; try levodopa first (to rule out dopa-responsive dystonia, particularly when the patient is less than 40 years old and onset predominantly in lower extremity), then anticholinergic drugs (similar to treatment algorithm for dystonia).

AKATHISIA AND RESTLESS LEGS SYNDROME

- *Akathisia* is characterized by a feeling of inner restlessness and anxiety that is associated with an inability to sit or stand still.

  - Patients subjectively describe feeling fidgety and nervous, which is often objectively manifested by complex stereotyped movements.

  - Subjectively, the most common complaint is the inability to keep the legs still, but patients can also describe a vague inner tension, emotional unease, or anxiety.

  - Objectively, patients are seen rocking from foot to foot, walking in place, shifting weight while sitting, and occasionally grunting, moaning, and/or rocking the trunk.

  - Depending on the timing of its appearance, akathisia may be subclassified as acute or chronic.

    - Chronic akathisia is further subdivided into akathisia occurring early in the course of neuroleptic therapy but persisting (*acute persistent akathisia)* and akathisia associated with long-term therapy (*tardive akathisia).*

- It is often difficult to distinguish between these two subtypes because of imprecise information about the onset of akathisia relative to the initiation of neuroleptic treatment.

○ Tardive akathisia and tardive dystonia are the most distressing and disabling of the tardive syndromes. Therefore, the offending dopamine receptor blocker should be stopped if possible.

- *Anticholinergic drugs* are often ineffective. Unlike in acute akathisia, beta-blockers do not work in tardive akathisia.

- Reports on *opiates* are conflicting.

- *Dopamine-depleting agents* may be considered.

- *Electroconvulsive therapy* may be effective for intractable, functionally impairing akathisia.

■ Restless legs syndrome (RLS) is a common sensorimotor disorder characterized by discomfort or unusual sensation in the legs (or arms) that is characteristically relieved by movement of the affected limb(s).

○ Recent studies suggest a prevalence between 3% and 15% in the general population. The prevalence is higher in women and increases with age.

○ The updated standardized clinical criteria for the diagnosis of RLS by the International Restless Legs Syndrome Study Group[17] are as follows:

- Desire to move the limbs (with or without paresthesia), and the arms may be involved.

- Urge to move or the unpleasant sensation improves with activity, and symptoms are worse with rest or inactivity.

- The urge to move or the unpleasant sensations are partially or totally relieved with movement.

- The symptoms have a circadian variation, occurring most often in the evening or at night when the patient lies down.

○ There are two distinct types of RLS: primary (idiopathic) and secondary.

- The majority of individuals with *primary* RLS have a positive family history; primary RLS has a high concordance in monozygotic twins; an autosomal dominant mode of inheritance has been proposed.

- *Secondary* RLS is often associated with iron deficiency anemia, pregnancy, end-stage renal disease, or medications such as antidepressants and dopamine blockers.

○ Possible mechanisms of pathophysiology in primary RLS include abnormal iron metabolism and functional alterations in central dopaminergic neurotransmitter systems.

○ Nonpharmacologic treatment of RLS includes improved sleep hygiene, avoidance of alcohol and caffeine, and moderate exercise daily.

- The treatment of secondary RLS includes discontinuing the offending medications and correcting the iron deficiency, in addition to initiating medication.[18]

- *Dopaminergic medications* have the greatest efficacy in RLS.

- All medications used to treat RLS can cause augmentation (ie, the occurrence of more severe symptoms that develop earlier in the day), rebound (ie, recurrence of symptoms in the early morning hours), and/or tolerance. Dopamine agonists are less likely to cause augmentation, but tolerance may develop rapidly.

- *Gabapentin* is second-line therapy for those unable to tolerate dopaminergic agents.

- *Opioids* or *clonidine* may be tried as third-line therapy, and *benzodiazepines* may provide relief.

■ Painful legs and moving toes (PLMT)

○ The motor component of this syndrome is usually confined to the toes but may involve proximal parts of the legs as well.

○ Movements are continuous and stereotyped. Flexion–extension or adduction–abduction of the toes is characteristic.

○ PLMT often disappears with sleep and is relieved by rest and hot or cold water.

○ Sensory symptoms range from mild to excruciatingly painful.

○ There is no subjective desire or urge to move, distinguishing this syndrome from akathisia and RLS.

○ PLMT may be associated with peripheral neuropathy or radiculopathy.

REFERENCES

1. Walker RH. Differential diagnosis of chorea. *Curr Neurol Neurosci Rep.* 2011; 11:385–395.
2. Labbadia J, Morimoto RI. Huntington's disease: underlying molecular mechanisms and emerging concepts. *Trends Biochem Sci.* 2013; 38(8):378–385.
3. Rosenblatt A, Ranen NG, Nance MA, Paulsen JS. *A Physician's Guide to the Management of Huntington's Disease.* 2nd ed. New York, NY: Huntington's Disease Society of America; 1999.
4. Xiang F, Almqvist EW, Huq M, et al. Huntington disease-like neurodegenerative disorder maps to chromosome 20p. *Am J Hum Genet.* 1998; 63:1431–1438.
5. Walker RH, Jankovic J, O'Hearn E, Margolis RL. Phenotypic features of Huntington disease-like 2. *Mov Disord.* 2003; 18:1527–1530.

6. Spitz MC, Jankovic J, Kilian JM. Familial tic disorder, parkinsonism, motor neuron disease, and acanthocytosis—a new syndrome. *Neurology.* 1985; 35:366–377.
7. Witt TN, Danek A, Hein MU, et al. McLeod syndrome: a distinct form of neuroacanthocytosis. *J Neurol.* 1992; 239:302–306.
8. Wheeler PG, Weaver DD, Dobyns WB. Benign hereditary chorea. *Pediatr Neurol.* 1993; 9:337–340.
9. Burke JR, Wingfield MS, Lewis KE, et al. The Haw River syndrome: dentatorubropallidoluysian atrophy in an African-American family. *Nat Genet.* 1994; 7 :521–524.
10. Malandrini A, Fabrizi GM, Bartalucci P, et al. Clinicopathological study of familial late infantile Hallervorden-Spatz disease: a particular form of neuroacanthocytosis. *Childs Nerv Syst.* 1996; 12:155–160.
11. Bhatia KP. Paroxysmal dyskinesias. *Mov Disord*, 2011; 26:1157–1165.
12. Baizabal-Carballo JF, Jankovic J. Movement disorders in autoimmune diseases. *Mov Disord.* 2012; 27:935–946.
13. Nance MA. Therapy in Huntington's disease: where are we? *Curr Neurol Neurosci Rep.* 2012; 12:359–366.
14. Mestre TA, Ferreira JJ. An evidence-based approach in the treatment of Huntington's disease. *Parkinsonism Relat Disord.* 2012; 18:316–320.
15. Jankovic J, Clarence-Smith K. Tetrabenazine for the treatment of chorea and other hyperkinetic movement disorders. *Expert Rev Neurother.* 2011; 11:1509–1523.
16. Edwards TC, Ludvic Z, Limousin P, Foltynie T. Deep brain stimulation in the treatment of chorea. *Mov Disord.* 2012; 27:357–363.
17. Allen RP, Picchietti D, Hening WA, et al. Restless legs syndrome: diagnostic criteria, special considerations, epidemiology: a report from the restless legs syndrome diagnosis and epidemiology workshop at the National Institutes of Health. *Sleep Med.* 2003; 4:101–119.
18. Aurora RN, Kristo DA, Bista SR, et al. The treatment of restless legs syndrome and periodic limb movement disorder in adults—an update for 2012: practice parameters with an evidence-based systematic review and meta-analyses: an American Academy of Sleep Medicine Clinical Practice Guideline. *Sleep.* 2012; 35:1039–1062.

7

MYOCLONUS

DESCRIPTION

- Sudden, brief, shocklike, involuntary movements result from brief contractions (or lapse in contractions) of a muscle or group of muscles.[1]

- When the movement results from a contraction of muscles, it is also termed *positive myoclonus*.

- The movement is called *negative myoclonus* when it results from a transient loss of muscle contraction.

- Friedreich first described myoclonus as a separate entity in a case report in 1881, but it was in 1883 that Lowenfeld used the term *myoclonus* for the first time.

- In 1903, Lundborg proposed a classification scheme for myoclonus: *symptomatic*, *essential*, and *familial*.

- Lindenmulder described the first family with essential myoclonus and drew attention to its occurrence in nondegenerative conditions without metabolic derangements or epilepsy.[2]

PHENOMENOLOGY AND DIFFERENTIAL DIAGNOSIS

- Although myoclonus is quite distinctive in its presentation with "sudden shocklike movements," it may sometimes still be confused with other movement disorders, such as tics, chorea, dystonia, and tremor. It then becomes important to make sure that the phenomenology is consistent with myoclonus (Table 7.1).

CLINICAL APPROACH

- There is no single best way to approach a patient with myoclonus.

- Here is a suggested sequence to follow (Figures 7.1–7.3).

Table 7.1
Clinical Presentation of Myoclonus Compared With Other
Hyperkinetic Movement Disorders

Tics	Myoclonus
Do not interfere with motor acts	May interfere with motor acts
Can be voluntarily suppressed	Cannot be suppressed
Preceded by an internal urge and followed by relief	No urge or relief
Often disappear during sleep	May continue in sleep
Stereotyped and repetitive	May be random or localized
Slower than myoclonus	Faster than tics
Chorea	**Myoclonus**
Not stimulus-sensitive	May be stimulus-sensitive
Movements in constant flow, randomly distributed over body and in time	No sequential movement of body parts
With motor impersistence (fly catcher tongue, milkmaid grip)	No motor impersistence
Slow or impaired Luria three-step test	Normal Luria test (unless associated with encephalopathy/dementia)
Dystonia	**Myoclonus**
Prolonged muscle spasms with twisting and posturing	Sudden brief contraction of muscles that may move a joint
May have sensory trick	No sensory trick
Postural/action tremor	**Myoclonus**
Rhythmic	May be rhythmic or arrhythmic
Frequency usually slower	Usually faster
Fasciculations	**Myoclonus**
Usually do not move a joint	May or may not move a joint

CLASSIFICATION

○ Myoclonus may be classified in several ways: according to distribution, clinical presentation, pathophysiology, or etiology (Table 7.2).

○ Identifying myoclonus by its distribution and/or type may assist in localizing the pathology (Table 7.3A, B).

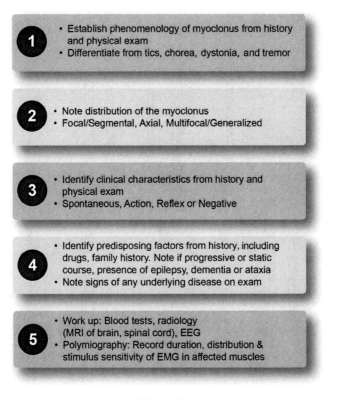

1
- Establish phenomenology of myoclonus from history and physical exam
- Differentiate from tics, chorea, dystonia, and tremor

2
- Note distribution of the myoclonus
- Focal/Segmental, Axial, Multifocal/Generalized

3
- Identify clinical characteristics from history and physical exam
- Spontaneous, Action, Reflex or Negative

4
- Identify predisposing factors from history, including drugs, family history. Note if progressive or static course, presence of epilepsy, dementia or ataxia
- Note signs of any underlying disease on exam

5
- Work up: Blood tests, radiology (MRI of brain, spinal cord), EEG
- Polymiography: Record duration, distribution & stimulus sensitivity of EMG in affected muscles

Figure 7.1
Suggested general approach to myoclonus.

○ After determining the distribution of myoclonus, look for clues to possible underlying pathology (Table 7.4A–C).

SPECIFIC ETIOLOGIES OF MYOCLONUS

▪ Myoclonus with ataxia and epilepsy

▪ Drug-induced myoclonus

○ Myoclonus secondary to underlying conditions accounts for 72% of cases (Figure 7.4).[3]

○ A detailed drug history with identification of all current and recent medications is imperative. Drug-induced myoclonus is especially common in hospitalized patients (Table 7.5).[4]

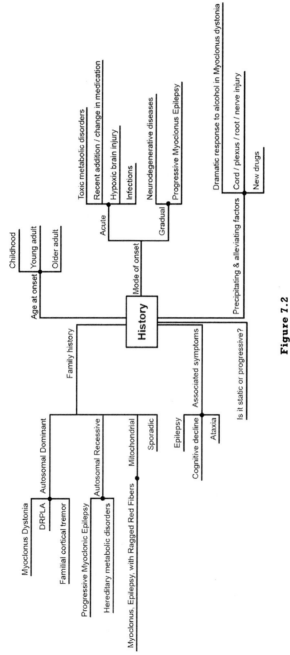

Figure 7.2

Specific questions to ask during the historical assessment of a patient with myoclonus.

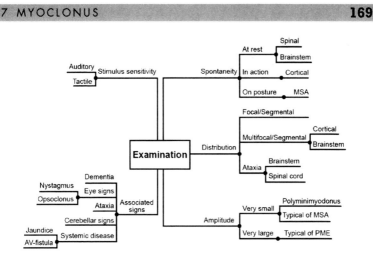

Figure 7.3

Things to look for when examining a patient with myoclonus.

Table 7.2
Methods of Classifying Myoclonus

Distribution	Clinical Presentation	Pathophysiology	Etiology
Focal	Spontaneous	Cortical	Physiologic
Segmental	Action	Focal	Essential
Axial	Reflex	Multifocal	Epileptic
Multifocal	Rhythmic	Generalized	Focal damage
Generalized	Irregular	Epilepsia partialis	Symptomatic
	Negative	continua (EPC)	Storage diseases
		Thalamic	Basal ganglia
		Brainstem	degeneration
		Reticular	Cerebellar
		Startle	degeneration
		Palatal	Dementias
		Spinal	Viral
		Segmental	encephalopathies
		Propriospinal	Metabolic
		Peripheral	encephalopathies
			Toxic
			encephalopathies
			Hypoxia

Table 7.3A
Clinical Description of Myoclonus According to Distribution
Suggesting Location of Pathology

Distribution	Description	Location of Pathology
Focal/Segmental	Confined to a particular region of the body	Peripheral nerve, root, plexus, spinal cord, brainstem, or cortex
Axial	Flexion of neck, trunk, and hips; abduction of arms	Brainstem or spinal cord
Multifocal	Different parts of the body, not necessarily at the same time	Sensory motor cortex or brainstem
Generalized	Whole body affected in a single jerk	Sensory motor cortex or brainstem

Table 7.3B
Clinical Characteristics of Myoclonus and Their Importance

Type of Myoclonus	Clinical Description	Examples
Spontaneous	• May be unpredictable or occur at specific times • May be focal, multifocal, or generalized	• Early morning myoclonus in juvenile myoclonic epilepsy • Hypnic jerks when falling asleep • Palatal myoclonus • Creutzfeldt-Jakob disease
Action	• During active muscle contraction, posture, and movement • Is the most debilitating myoclonus, interferes with gross voluntary movements • May be multifocal or generalized > focal/segmental	• Lance Adams syndrome (posthypoxic myoclonus)
Reflex	• May be focal or generalized, proximal > distal muscles and flexors > active than extensors • May look like a tremor • Stimulus may be somesthetic, visual, or auditory • Somesthetic: tap the face (mentalis zone) for generalized reflex myoclonus, tendon reflex	• Brainstem reflex reticular myoclonus

continued

Table 7.3B (cont.)
Clinical Characteristics of Myoclonus and Their Importance

Type of Myoclonus	Clinical Description	Examples
	• Visual: threatening stimulus or flash stimulation always provokes an underlying generalized myoclonus in sensitive patients • Auditory: common in children, usually provoked by unexpected sounds; differentiate from hyperekplexia • May be very sensitive, self-perpetuate, and simulate spontaneous myoclonus	
Rhythmic	• Focal or segmental • Always spontaneous • Usually slow (1–4 Hz) • Persists in sleep (ask bed partner) • Usually due to focal lesion of spinal cord or brainstem	• Spinal myoclonus • Palatal myoclonus
Negative	• Always during action/posture • Sudden, transient loss of muscle tone in an actively contracting muscle	• Asterixis in hepatic encephalopathy • "Bouncy legs" in Lance Adams syndrome causing falls

Table 7.4A
Possible Etiologies of Focal Myoclonus

Location of Pathology	Type of Myoclonus	Clinical Characteristics	Examples of Disease
Peripheral nerve, plexus, or root		• Usually arrhythmic • Not stimulus-sensitive	Trauma, tumors, radiation
Spinal cord	Spinal segmental myoclonus	• In muscles innervated by adjacent spinal segments • Rhythmic (0.5–3 Hz) • Persists in sleep • Usually not stimulus-sensitive	Multiple sclerosis, inflammatory myelitis, trauma, tumor, vascular lesion

continued

Table 7.4A (cont.)
Possible Etiologies of Focal Myoclonus

Location of Pathology	Type of Myoclonus	Clinical Characteristics	Examples of Disease
Brainstem	Essential palatal myoclonus	• Ear click (tensor veli palatini opens eustachian tube and pulls roof of soft palate) • Stops during sleep • No hypertrophic olivary degeneration (HOD)	Usually younger patients
	Symptomatic palatal myoclonus	• No click (levator veli palatini pulls back of soft palate) • May have pendular vertical nystagmus and even facial, intercostal, and diaphragmatic contractions with palatal myoclonus • Continues in sleep • Ipsilateral cerebellar dysfunction and contralateral HOD	Encephalitis, stroke, trauma, tumor, degenerative disease
Cortex	Epilepsia partialis continua (EPC)	• Usually rhythmic	Stroke, subarachnoid hemorrhage, trauma, tumor, encephalitis, hepatic encephalopathy

Table 7.4B
Possible Etiologies of Axial Myoclonus

Location of Pathology	Type of Myoclonus	Clinical Characteristics	Examples of Disease
Brainstem (brainstem reticular myoclonus)	Reticular reflex	• Generalized axial myoclonic jerks • Stimulus sensitivity greatest over limbs • Spontaneous jerks common	• Hypoxia/anoxia • Metabolic syndromes like uremia, drugs • Brainstem encephalitis: • Multiple sclerosis, viral infection, sarcoidosis, paraneoplastic syndrome

continued

Table 7.4B (cont.)
Possible Etiologies of Axial Myoclonus

Location of Pathology	Type of Myoclonus	Clinical Characteristics	Examples of Disease
	Hyperekplexia (exaggerated startle)	• Blink, facial contortion, neck and trunk flexion, arm abduction and flexion • Fall to the ground with possible injury • Does not habituate • Spontaneous jerks not prominent	• Inherited (autosomal dominant) • Local pathology • Jumping Frenchmen of Maine syndrome • Hysterical jumps
Spinal cord	Propriospinal myoclonus	• Truncal flexion most prominent movement • Spontaneous or stimulus-induced • Worse in supine position and sleep-wake transition • Nonrhythmic • Midthoracic generator with slow spread up and down the cord	• Idiopathic, trauma, psychogenic

Table 7.4C
Possible Etiologies of Multifocal and Generalized Myoclonus

Location of Pathology	Type of Myoclonus	Clinical Characteristics	Examples of Disease
• Sensorimotor cortex o Usually distal, presents more as flexion than as extension movements o Typically stimulus-sensitive	Epileptic myoclonus	• Brief myoclonic, atonic, or tonic seizures • May be positive or negative myoclonus	• Infantile spasms • Lennox-Gastaut syndrome • Cryptogenic and juvenile myoclonic epilepsy
	Progressive myoclonic epilepsy	• Severe myoclonus (spontaneous, action- and stimulus-sensitive)	• Lafora body disease (EPM2) • Neuronal ceroid lipofuscinosis (Batten disease)

continued

Table 7.4C (cont.)
Possible Etiologies of Multifocal and Generalized Myoclonus

Location of Pathology	Type of Myoclonus	Clinical Characteristics	Examples of Disease
		• Severe generalized tonic-clonic seizures • Progressive neurological decline (dementia and ataxia)	• Unverricht-Lundborg disease (EPM1) • Mitochondrial encephalopathies (myoclonic epilepsy with ragged red fibers) • Sialidosis (cherry red spot myoclonus syndrome) • AMRF syndrome • In an adult, consider DRPLA

	Progressive myoclonic ataxia (Ramsay Hunt syndrome)	• Like progressive myoclonic epilepsy but seizures mild/absent
		• Dementia mild/absent
		• Myoclonus and ataxia are the major problems
			• All of the above
			• Spinocerebellar degenerations
			• Rare causes
			  o Celiac disease
			  o Whipple disease
			  o DRPLA
			  o Gaucher disease
			  o Neuroaxonal dystrophy
			  o Biotin-responsive encephalopathy

	Post-anoxic myoclonus (Lance Adams syndrome)	• Spontaneous, action-induced, stimulus-sensitive on recovery from coma • Prominent negative myoclonus of legs causing falls	• Anesthetic accident • Cardiac arrest • Respiratory failure in asthma
		• Myoclonus periodic at long intervals • "Hung up" jerk	• Acute encephalitis • Post-infectious • SSPE • CJD

Brainstem	Opsoclonus-myoclonus (dancing eyes-dancing feet syndrome)	• Opsoclonus: continuous, arrhythmic, large saccades in multiple directions
		• Myoclonus: palate, pharynx, larynx, diaphragm, trunk, and limbs
			• Children (6–18 y)
			  o Neuroblastoma
			  o Autoimmune
			• Adults
			  o Paraneoplastic (breast CA, large-cell lung CA)
			  o Inflammatory (Whipple disease)

	Brainstem encephalitis	• Subacute onset of features • Ataxia, dysarthria, diplopia, nystagmus, ophthalmoplegia, opsoclonus, deafness, and myoclonus	• Infectious • Para-infectious • Paraneoplastic (cancers of the ovary and lung)

continued

Table 7.4C (cont.)
Possible Etiologies of Multifocal and Generalized Myoclonus

Location of Pathology	Type of Myoclonus	Clinical Characteristics	Examples of Disease
Various causes	Myoclonus with dementia	• CBD: stimulus-sensitive with short latency	• CJD • AD • HE • CBD
	Multifocal myoclonus without dementia or epilepsy	• Nonprogressive course • Multifocal myoclonus • No cognitive deficits, seizures, or ataxia • EEG normal	• Essential myoclonus (autosomal dominant)

Abbreviations: AD, Alzheimer disease; AMRF, action myoclonus-renal failure; CA, carcinoma; CBD, corticobasal degeneration; CJD, Creutzfeldt-Jakob disease; DRPLA, dentatorubropallidoluysian atrophy; EEG, electroencephalography; EPM, epilepsy, progressive myoclonic; HE, hepatic encephalopathy; SSPE, subacute sclerosing panencephalitis.

■ Inherited disorders presenting with myoclonus (Table 7.6A–C)[5]

■ Essential myoclonus

○ Essential myoclonus can be hereditary or sporadic (Figure 7.5).

■ Opsoclonus-myoclonus-ataxia syndrome (Table 7.7)[3,6–11]

■ Palatal myoclonus (Figure 7.6)

■ Myoclonus in neurodegenerative extrapyramidal disorders (Figure 7.7)

■ Physiologic myoclonus

○ This occurs as the body's physiologic response to certain external or internal triggers in otherwise healthy individuals and includes hiccups (singultus), hypnic jerks that are abundant in the facial and distal limb muscles, and physiologic startle.

○ These symptoms do not usually need to be treated.

■ Orthostatic myoclonus (OM)

○ A relatively recent observation of myoclonus that occurs on standing[12,13] and in subjects who may or may not have neurodegenerative conditions like Parkinson's disease (PD). It may be even more common than orthostatic tremor.[14]

○ The most frequent symptom was unexplained unsteadiness in a series of patients referred for gait imbalance and tested. OM was diagnosed in 17.2% of the patients.[14]

○ The most frequent comorbid neurological condition was parkinsonism.[14]

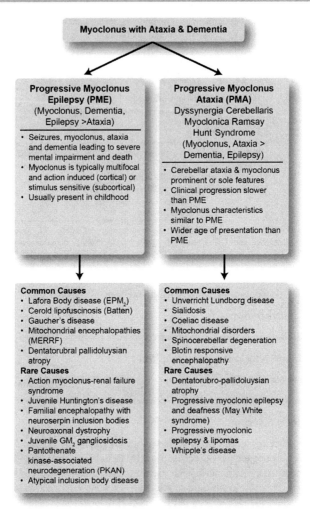

Figure 7.4
Classification of secondary myoclonus associated with epilepsy, dementia, and ataxia.

■ Asterixis (negative myoclonus)

   ○ First described in 1949 by Adams and Foley in hepatic encephalopathy as rhythmic movements of the fingers and occasionally of the arms, legs, and face at 3 to 5 Hz on active maintenance of posture.[15] The term *asterixis* was coined by the same investigators in 1953 when they identified that this movement follows pauses of 200 to 500 msec.[16] The term *negative myoclonus* was coined by Shahani and Young in 1976.[17]

Table 7.5
Drugs and Toxins Associated With Myoclonus

Class	Examples	Comment
Psychiatric medications	Tricyclic antidepressants (TCAs)	Encephalopathy with myoclonus; EEG changes may be confused with those of Creutzfeldt-Jakob disease
	Selective serotonin reuptake inhibitors (SSRIs)	
	Monoamine oxidase Inhibitors (MAOIs)	
	Lithium	Multifocal cortical action myoclonus with normal EEG
	Long-term exposure to neuroleptics	Tardive myoclonus
Anesthetics	Fentanyl	
	Propofol	Transient cortical reflex myoclonus; treatment unnecessary
Anti-infectious agents	Mefloquine	Multifocal myoclonus
	Gatifloxacin	
Antiepileptic drugs	Lamotrigine	
	Gabapentin	
Cardiac medications	Calcium channel blockers	
	Carvedilol	
Narcotics	Morphine	
Contrast media	Intravenous iodinated contrast	Spinal myoclonus may indicate underlying spinal cord lesion
Drug withdrawal	Benzodiazepines Propranolol	
Other neurological medications	Levodopa	
	Amantadine	Cortical myoclonus with EEG changes in one patient[4]
Toxins	Bismuth Dichlorodipheny ltrichloroethane (DDT) Heavy metals Glue sniffing Gasoline sniffing Toxic cooking oil in Spain	

Abbreviation: EEG, electroencephalography.

Table 2.6A

Causes of Myoclonus With Autosomal Dominant Inheritance and Key Features

Disease	Inheritance and Chromosome	Protein	Age at Onset	Major Clinical Features	Helpful Investigations
Essential myoclonus	• Autosomal dominant, variable penetrance • 7q.18	Epsilon-sarcoglycan	Typically < 20 y	• Myoclonus in arms and axial musculature • Worse with action • Marked improvement with alcohol • Benign course • May have dystonia (myoclonus dystonia)	
Hyperekplexia	• Autosomal dominant	Inhibitory glycine receptor, glycine transporter 2	Infancy to adulthood	• Patients jump in response to sound and fall to the ground, injuring themselves • No loss of consciousness	• Classic history with family members • Examination
DRPLA	• Autosomal dominant • 12	Atrophin 1		• Spinocerebellar ataxia • Myoclonus, presumed cortical (uncommon, but causes PMA picture when present) • Epilepsy, chorea, ataxia, parkinsonism, psychosis, and dementia	• History and examination • Genetic testing

Familial nocturnal faciomandibular myoclonus	• Autosomal dominant	• Recurrent tongue biting during sleep • Only in NREM sleep • May be associated with bruxism and PLMS • No seizures	• Typical history • Polysomnography
Familial adult myoclonic epilepsy (FAME)/cortical tremor/benign autosomal dominant familial myoclonic epilepsy (BADFME)	• Autosomal dominant • 8q(5) • 2p • 5p • 3	• Adult-onset tremor before seizures • Action myoclonus (may worsen with age) • Generalized seizures • Good response to antiepileptic drugs • Clinical anticipation in some families	• Clinical (adult-onset myoclonus, then epilepsy) • Family history • Electrophysiology (cortical reflex myoclonus)

Abbreviations: DRPLA, dentatorubropallidoluysian atrophy; PLMS, periodic limb movements of sleep; PMA, progressive myoclonic ataxia.

Table 7.6B
Causes of Myoclonus With Autosomal Recessive Inheritance and Key Features

Disease	Inheritance and Chromosome	Protein	Age at Onset	Major Clinical Features	Helpful Investigations
Sialidoses I, II	Autosomal recessive 6p	Lysosomal sialidase	8–30 y	• Cherry red spot on retina • Dysmorphic	• Alpha-N-acetyl neuraminidase
GM2 gangliosidosis	Autosomal recessive 5q				
Lafora body disease	Autosomal recessive 6q NHLRC1 (EPM2B)	Tyrosine phosphatase (PTP) Laforin (EPM2A)	11–18 y	• Childhood onset: behavioral change, dementia, occipital seizures, and myoclonus • Late onset: benign	• EEG • Lafora bodies (skin, liver, and brain)
Unverricht-Lundborg disease	Autosomal recessive 21q	Cystatin-B	6–15 y	• Myoclonus: severe • Dementia: absent/mild	• Clinical • EEG
AMRF syndrome	Autosomal recessive SCARB2/LIMP2 gene mutation		17–26 y	• Starts with tremor, then action myoclonus; infrequent generalized seizures and cerebellar signs • Possible CMP and PNP • Invariably progresses to renal failure	• History • Proteinuria and renal failure

Ceroid lipofuscinosis (Batten disease)	Autosomal recessive	1p	Palmitoyl protein thioesterase	Late infantile, 2–4 y	• Severe seizures with rapid regression and macular degeneration • Dead by 6–10 y	• EEG, ERG, VER, EM of skin, muscle, rectum, or brain
		11p	Tripeptidyl peptidase 1	Juvenile, 4–10 y	• Visual failure from macular degeneration • Seizures, dementia • Dead by 15–25 y	
		13q	CLN5 gene	Adult	• Behavioral changes and dementia	
		16p	CLN3 gene			

Abbreviations: CMP, cardiomyopathy; EEG, electroencephalography; EM, electron microscopy; EPM, epilepsy, progressive myoclonic; ERG, electroretinography; PNP, peripheral neuropathy; VER, visual evoked responses.

Table 7.6C
Causes of Myoclonus With Autosomal Recessive Inheritance and Key Features

Disease	Inheritance and Chromosome	Protein	Age at Onset	Major Clinical Features	Helpful Investigations
Myoclonic epilepsy with ragged red fibers (MERRF)	Mitochondrial Mitochondrial DNA		5–42 y	Short stature Deafness	Blood and cerebrospinal fluid lactate Muscle biopsy (ragged red fibers) DNA test

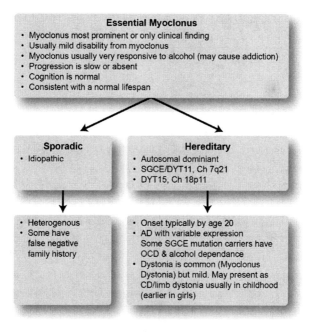

Essential Myoclonus
- Myoclonus most prominent or only clinical finding
- Usually mild disability from myoclonus
- Myoclonus usually very responsive to alcohol (may cause addiction)
- Progression is slow or absent
- Cognition is normal
- Consistent with a normal lifespan

Sporadic
- Idiopathic

Hereditary
- Autosomal dominant
- SGCE/DYT11, Ch 7q21
- DYT15, Ch 18p11

- Heterogenous
- Some have false negative family history

- Onset typically by age 20
- AD with variable expression Some SGCE mutation carriers have OCD & alcohol dependance
- Dystonia is common (Myoclonus Dystonia) but mild. May present as CD/limb dystonia usually in childhood (earlier in girls)

Figure 7.5
Sporadic versus hereditary essential myoclonus.

Negative myoclonus may be classified according to its origin (cortical or subcortical), as epileptic or nonepileptic, or according to the presence or absence of rhythmicity (Figure 7.8).[18–20]

Table 7.7
Opsoclonus-Myoclonus-Ataxia Syndrome

Opsoclonus-Myoclonus-Ataxia Syndrome		
Proposed diagnostic criteria (at least three of four)	Opsoclonus	• Spontaneous, conjugate, involuntary, multidirectional, chaotic eye movements • Persist in fixation, smooth pursuit, and convergence • Persist in sleep and eye closure • Large amplitude and high frequency (10–15 Hz): visual blurring and oscillopsia • Differentiate from nystagmus (a saccade takes eye away from target, not slow movement) and ocular flutter (back-to-back saccades confined to horizontal plane while multidirectional in opsoclonus) • May be absent or delayed in atypical cases
	Myoclonus	• Multifocal • Stimulus-sensitive, provoked by action • Exacerbated by crying, excitement, and stress • May have polyminimyoclonus • May persist in sleep
	Ataxia	• May be severe enough to impair sitting and ambulation • Ataxia may be markedly asymmetric in atypical cases
	Behavioral changes	• Irritability and sleep disturbances • Particularly prominent in children
Age factor	Children	• Usually start with ataxia, followed by irritability • 40%–50% of all cases related to underlying neuroblastoma
	Adults	• 20% of cases paraneoplastic (70% of these from lung and breast cancer)
Associations	Idiopathic	• Majority of patients with OMA syndrome seronegative for all known antineuronal antibodies • Usually presents in 30s and 40s
	Paraneoplastic	• Presents at 6–36 months in children, 60s in adults • Neuroblastoma (40%–50% of children with OMA syndrome have a neuroblastoma, but only 2%–4% of patients with a neuroblastoma develop OMA)

continued

Table 7.7 (cont.)
Opsoclonus-Myoclonus-Ataxia Syndrome

Opsoclonus-Myoclonus-Ataxia Syndrome		
		• Small-cell lung cancer • Breast cancer • Malignant melanoma • Non-Hodgkin lymphoma • Ovarian cancer • Pancreatic cancer • Medullary thyroid cancer
	Parainfectious	• HIV • Post-streptococcal group A • *Mycoplasma pneumoniae* • West Nile virus • Lyme disease • Varicella-zoster virus
	Miscellaneous	• Celiac disease • Allogeneic bone marrow transplant • Hyperosmolar coma
Pathogenesis • No common antineuronal antibody detected • Most patients do not have autoantibodies • May have cellular immune mechanisms • May have a genetic predisposition (15.8% of parents of OMS patients reported autoimmune disorders compared with 2% of controls)[8]	Varieties of autoantibodies detected so far	• Small-cell lung cancer: anti-Hu (ANNA-1), anti-amphiphysin antibody • Breast cancer: anti-Ri (ANNA-2) • Neuroblastoma: anti-Hu, alpha-enolase, IgG class antibody, antibody to neuroblastoma cells and cerebellar granular neurons • Celiac disease: anti-gliadin antibody of IgA subtype, anti-endomysial antibody, and anti-CV2 antibody • Post-streptococcal OMA syndrome: anti-neuroleukin antibody • Cerebellar or brainstem encephalitis: anti-Yo, anti-Ma2
Investigation	Adults: rule out cancer first	• Careful breast and neurological examination • CT of chest, abdomen, and pelvis with contrast • Mammography in female patients • If all above tests negative, consider onconeural antibodies (eg, anti-Hu) • Consider whole-body FDG-PET if high risk for tumor

continued

Table 7.7 (cont.)
Opsoclonus-Myoclonus-Ataxia Syndrome

	Opsoclonus-Myoclonus-Ataxia Syndrome	
	Children: look for neuroblastoma first	• Traditional methods to detect neuroblastoma may be insensitive • 24-hour urine catecholamines quantitative assessment • MIBG scan • Contrast CT/MRI of entire torso if above tests negative • Infectious workup
Therapeutic options and prognosis	Adults	• Paraneoplastic: severe course despite immunotherapy, especially if tumor unresected; complete or partial recovery with resection • Idiopathic: responds better to immunotherapy • Prognosis with paraneoplastic OMA syndrome worse with protracted course; high mortality despite corticosteroids and IV Ig compared with idiopathic disease
	Children 1. Corticosteroids 2. ACTH 3. IV Ig 4. Rituximab	• Paraneoplastic: with neuroblastoma resolves with or without treatment • Combination of corticosteroid or ACTH and monthly IV Ig becoming standard therapy • Relapses at dose tapering very common (75%) and appear to worsen long-term outcome[8] • Early multiple-agent treatment may reduce risk for relapse from 75% to 17%[9] • Substantial developmental and behavioral sequelae, including cognitive, motor, speech, and language deficits • Early treatment may be needed to preserve long-term cognition[11]

Abbreviations: ACTH, adrenocorticotropic hormone; FDG-PET, fluorodeoxyglucose positron emission tomography; IV Ig, intravenous immunoglobulin; MIBG, meta-iodobenzylguanidine; OMA, opsoclonus-myoclonus-ataxia.

Source: Adapted from Refs. 2, 6–11.

Although metabolic derangements and toxins may be the most common causes of asterixis, negative myoclonus may be unilateral in structural diseases affecting the central nervous system (CNS)[21] at levels that include thalamus, parietal lobe, internal capsule, and even the midbrain.[22] A symmetric negative myoclonus does not rule out the presence of a structural lesion on one side (Figure 7.9).[23]

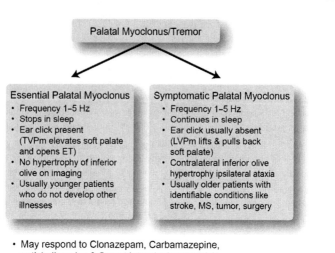

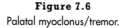

- May respond to Clonazepam, Carbamazepine, anticholinergics & Sumatriptan (only essential)
- Botulinum toxin injection in selected muscles for ear click relief

Figure 7.6
Palatal myoclonus/tremor.

Silent period locked averaging (SPLA) in electromyography (EMG), introduced by Ugawa et al[22] and further described by Shibasaki and Hallet[23], classifies the silent period into three types.

- Type 1: Abrupt cessation and return of background EMG activity without any positive EMG burst at the start. Duration of silent period is between 100 and 200 msec.

- Type 2: Same duration as type 1, but preceded by a brief but variable positive EMG burst. This may be multifocal.

- Type 3: These are shorter in duration and follow typical positive myoclonus.

DIAGNOSTIC WORKUP

- Although an underlying cause is usually discernible from a detailed history and physical examination in most cases, some patients require further investigations ranging from blood work to imaging and electrophysiologic studies. Several investigations need to be considered in the evaluation of a patient with myoclonus (Figure 7.10 and Table 7.8).

- Electrophysiologic analysis of myoclonus

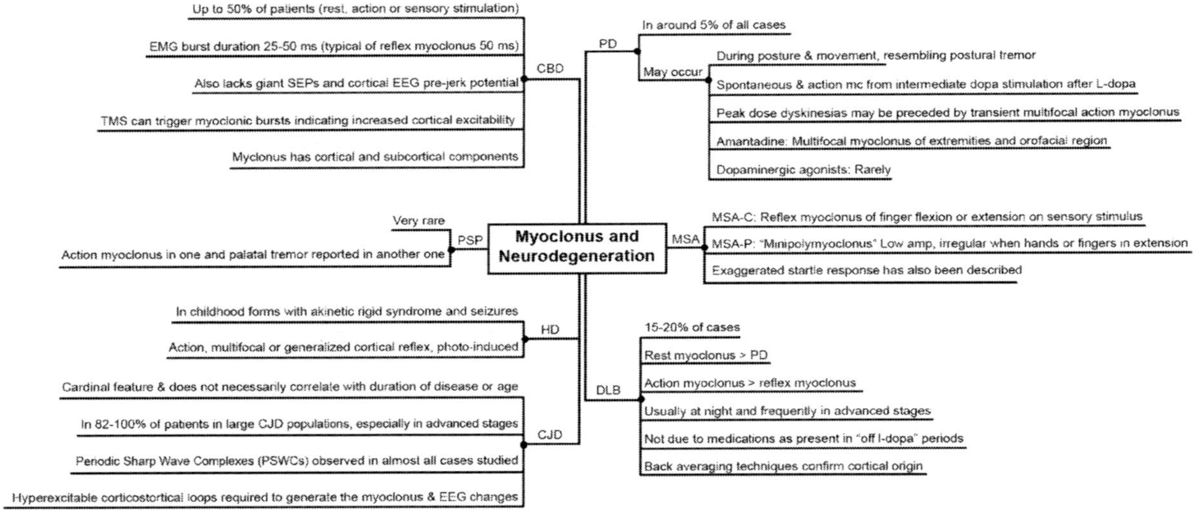
Myoclonus and Neurodegeneration
CBD
Up to 50% of patients (rest, action or sensory stimulation)
EMG burst duration 25-50 ms (typical of reflex myoclonus 50 ms)
Also lacks giant SEPs and cortical EEG pre-jerk potential
TMS can trigger myoclonic bursts indicating increased cortical excitability
Myclonus has cortical and subcortical components
PSP
Very rare
Action myoclonus in one and palatal tremor reported in another one
HD
In childhood forms with akinetic rigid syndrome and seizures
Action, multifocal or generalized cortical reflex, photo-induced
CJD
Cardinal feature & does not necessarily correlate with duration of disease or age
In 82-100% of patients in large CJD populations, especially in advanced stages
Periodic Sharp Wave Complexes (PSWCs) observed in almost all cases studied
Hyperexcitable corticostortical loops required to generate the myoclonus & EEG changes
PD
In around 5% of all cases
May occur
During posture & movement, resembling postural tremor
Spontaneous & action mc from intermediate dopa stimulation after L-dopa
Peak dose dyskinesias may be preceded by transient multifocal action myoclonus
Amantadine: Multifocal myoclonus of extremities and orofacial region
Dopaminergic agonists: Rarely
MSA
MSA-C: Reflex myoclonus of finger flexion or extension on sensory stimulus
MSA-P: "Minipolymyoclonus" Low amp, irregular when hands or fingers in extension
Exaggerated startle response has also been described
DLB
15-20% of cases
Rest myoclonus > PD
Action myoclonus > reflex myoclonus
Usually at night and frequently in advanced stages
Not due to medications as present in "off l-dopa" periods
Back averaging techniques confirm cortical origin

Figure 7.7

Myoclonus in neurodegenerative conditions like Parkinson's disease (PD), multiple systems atrophy (MSA), dementia with Lewy bodies (DLB), corticobasal degeneration (CBD), progressive supranuclear palsy (PSP), Huntington's disease, and Creutzfeldt-Jakob disease (CJD).

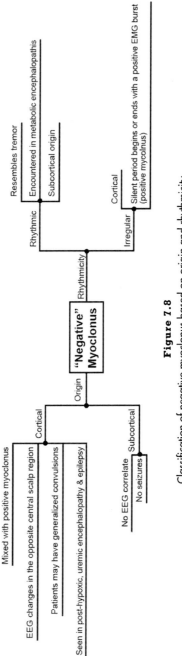

Figure 2.8

Classification of negative myoclonus based on origin and rhythmicity.

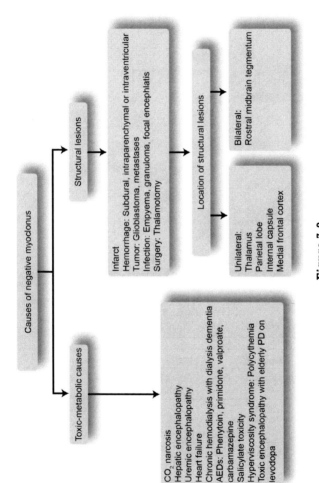

Figure 7.9
Causes of negative myoclonus.

189

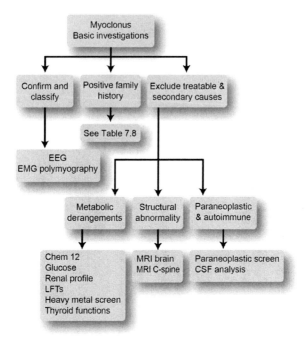

Figure 7.10

Basic investigations to order when evaluating patients with myoclonus.

Table 7.8

Investigations to Consider in a Patient With Myoclonus and a Positive Family History

Pattern of Inheritance	Suspected Condition	Initial Investigations	Confirmatory/ Investigational Tests
Autosomal dominant	Essential myoclonus	EEG, EMG polygraphy	ES
	DRPLA		PCR for CAG triplet repeat expansion for *DRPLA* gene
	Familial nocturnal faciomandibular myoclonus	EEG, EMG showing bursts of activity originating in the masseter muscle and spreading to the orbicularis oris and orbicularis oculi muscles	

continued

Table 7.8 (cont.)
Investigations to Consider in a Patient With Myoclonus and a Positive Family History

Pattern of Inheritance	Suspected Condition	Initial Investigations	Confirmatory/ Investigational Tests
	Familial adult myoclonic epilepsy	EEG, EMG polygraphy showing cortical reflex myoclonus and cortical origin of tremor	
Autosomal recessive	Sialidoses I, II	EMG: myoclonus induced by action or sound High urinary levels of oligosaccharides	Alpha-N-acetyl neuraminidase
	Lafora body disease	EEG: occipital spike-wave discharges, seizures at high-frequency photostimulation Skin biopsy: periodic acid-Schiff–positive Lafora bodies in sweat glands	
	Unverricht-Lundborg disease	EEG MRI of brain: vermian cerebellar atrophy	
	Action myoclonus-renal failure (AMRF) syndrome	Proteinuria and renal failure	SCARB2/LIMP2 gene mutation
	Ceroid lipofuscinosis (Batten disease)	EEG	ERG; VER; EM of skin, muscle, rectum, or brain
Mitochondrial	Myoclonic epilepsy with ragged red fibers (MERRF)	Blood and cerebrospinal fluid lactate Muscle biopsy (ragged red fibers)	

Abbreviations: DRPLA, dentatorubropallidoluysian atrophy; EEG, electroencephalography; EM, electron microscopy; EMG, electromyography; ERG, electroretinography; PCR, polymerase chain reaction; VER, visual evoked responses.

Table 7.9
Different Studies Employed Along With Their Utility in
Diagnosing and Classifying Myoclonus

Technique	Information Obtained
EMG	Diagnosis and classification
EEG, EMG polygraphy	Relationship to cortical activity
Jerk locked back averaging of EEG and EMG	Detection of myoclonus-related cortical activity and its temporal and spatial relationship to myoclonus
Corticomuscular coherence	Relationship of rhythmic oscillations between sensorimotor cortex and muscle discharge
Evoked potentials or magnetic fields	Cortical sensitivity to various stimuli
Paired stimulation evoked potentials and loop reflex	Recovery functions of cortical response and reflex myoclonus
Jerk locked evoked potentials	Cortical excitability change following spontaneous myoclonus
Transcranial magnetic stimulation	Excitability of motor cortex

Abbreviations: EEG, electroencephalography; EMG, electromyography.
Source: Adapted from Ref. 23: Shibasaki H, Hallet M. Electrophysiological studies of myoclonus. *Muscle Nerve.* 2005;31:157–174.

○ Electrophysiologic studies are useful not only in confirming a diagnosis of myoclonus but also in understanding the underlying physiology and thus the possible cause (Table 7.9).[25]

▓ EMG is a direct measure of alpha motor neuron activity. It provides information about the central nervous system activity that generates the movement.

○ It is mainly used for timing information and can be collected from surface electrodes.

○ Myoclonus can be *regular, irregular,* or *periodic.*

● Fast and irregular myoclonus may appear clinically as rhythmic.

○ Antagonist muscle relation can be described as *synchronous* or *asynchronous.*

● Cortical myoclonus produces synchronous activation of the agonist and antagonist muscles of an affected limb.

○ EMG burst duration can also be noted (Table 7.10)

▓ The sequence of activation of different muscles also plays an important role in identifying the source of myoclonus (Table 7.11).[25]

Table 7.10
Electromyographic Burst Duration as a Guide to the Source of Myoclonus

EMG Burst Duration	Implication
Up to 50 msec	Almost exclusively epileptic myoclonus
50–100 msec	Essential myoclonus
100–150 msec	Nonepileptic, possibly psychogenic myoclonus
150–300 msec	Fragments of another movement disorder, such as dystonia

Table 7.11
Sequence of Activation of Muscles as a Clue to the Source of Myoclonus

Type of Myoclonus	Sequence of Activation of Different Muscle Groups
Epileptic myoclonus	• Rostrocaudal activation starting from upper cranial nerves and descending along neuraxis with conduction velocity consistent with pyramidal tract • Synchronous activation of distal antagonist muscles
Reticular reflex myoclonus	• Activation initiating in the sternocleidomastoid then progressing both rostrally and caudally
Nonepileptic myoclonus	• Proximal muscles involved

Source: Adapted from Ref. 23: Shibasaki H, Hallet M. Electrophysiological studies of myoclonus. *Muscle Nerve.* 2005;31:157–174.

- Table 7.12 provides a summary of the electrophysiologic findings in the different types of myoclonus.

TREATMENT

- General guidelines

  ○ Focus first on reversible causes: treatment of metabolic encephalopathy, removal of the offending drug in case of toxicity, excision of an excitable lesion, psychotherapy for psychogenic myoclonus.

  ○ Nonetheless, most causes of myoclonus are not reversible and will need symptomatic therapy. A physiologic classification of the myoclonus may assist in optimal treatment.

  ○ In most instances, multiple trials of drugs in high doses are needed to achieve significant symptomatic benefit.

Table 7.12

Summary of Electrophysiologic Findings in Different Types of Myoclonus

Type of Myoclonus	EEG	EMG Burst	Jerk Locked Back Averaging of EEG	SEPs	C-Reflex	Surface EMG
Cortical	Biphasic discharge in central electrodes	Bursts typically < 75 msec	Biphasic spike at central electrodes Initial positive part of EEG precedes myoclonic EMG discharge	Enlarged	Variable; long C-reflex in cortical reflex myoclonus	Rostrocaudal activation from cranial nerve musculature descending along neuraxis with conduction velocity of pyramidal tract
Subcortical	Generalized spike and wave	Bursts < 100 msec	Time-locked correlate typical	May be enlarged	Some have C-reflex at rest	Cranial nerve muscles activated from nerve XI nucleus up the brainstem, limb, and axial muscles activated in descending order
Segmental	Normal	Bursts typically > 100 msec	No association	Normal	Very short latency incompatible with supraspinal origin	Propriospinal; first muscles usually in thoracic segment, then spread up and down
Peripheral	Normal	Variable duration, irregular discharges	No association	Normal	Normal	Localized to single nerve distribution
Psychogenic	Bereitschafts potentials prior to EMG bursts	Burst typically < 150 msec	Prepotential before EMG burst	Normal	Normal	Variable

Abbreviations: EEG, electroencephalography; EMG, electromyography; SEP, sensory evoked potential.

194

Table 7.13
Treatment of Myoclonus

Type of Myoclonus	First-Line Treatment		Adjuncts		Drugs to Avoid
Cortical	Sodium valproate	• Most effective • Doses up to 1.2 g/d • May cause hepatotoxicity, nausea, hair loss, and tremor	Piracetam	• Large doses required (3.2–4.8 g/d) • Abrupt withdrawal may precipitate worsening, seizures	Phenytoin Carbamazepine Lamotrigine Vigabatrin
	Clonazepam	• Up to 15 mg/d • Tolerance may develop • May cause ataxia and drowsiness (avoided with gradual upward titration) • Abrupt withdrawal may precipitate worsening and seizures	Levetiracetam	• Very potent • 1–3 g/d • Abrupt withdrawal may precipitate worsening • May be combined with valproate and clonazepam	
			Primidone	• Is a metabolite of phenobarbital • Use with caution in elderly as can cause sedation, depression • May be useful as add-on • Target dose of 500–750 mg/g • Contraindicated in porphyria	
			Zonisamide	• Helped in some cases of progressive myoclonic epilepsy	

continued

Table 7.13 (cont.)
Treatment of Myoclonus

Type of Myoclonus	First-Line Treatment	Adjuncts		Drugs to Avoid
Subcortical	Clonazepam	• Useful in hyperekplexia • Partially effective in reticular reflex myoclonus and myoclonus dystonia	Deep brain stimulation (especially in myoclonus dystonia syndrome)	• Bilateral pallidal or thalamic deep brain stimulation may help in severe myoclonus dystonia
Post-hypoxic	Clonazepam Levetiracetam	• Distal upper limb more responsive than proximal lower limb myoclonus		
Spinal	Clonazepam	• Effective in both types of spinal myoclonus • Doses up to 6 mg may be needed in segmental type	Levetiracetam	• Reported to be helpful in spinal segmental myoclonus
Segmental	Botulinum toxin			
Peripheral	Botulinum toxin		Carbamaze-pine Surgery to remove pressure from cranial nerve VII in hemifacial spasms	
Psychogenic jerks	Psychotherapy Physical therapy			

8

ATAXIA

Ataxia is characterized by "unsteadiness" or "clumsiness," which can result from lesions at multiple levels of the neuraxis. Ataxic disorders affect primarily movement, coordination, gait, and balance, and cognition as well.[1] Ataxia is a multifactorial syndrome with a wide etiology involving cortical, cerebellar, thalamic, spinal, and somatosensory pathways.

PATHOPHYSIOLOGY

- **Role of the cortex**

  - Frontal lobe lesions can give rise to what is known as *frontal ataxia.* Frontal ataxia can result in truncal imbalance, gait hesitation, wide-based gait, falls, and disability.[2] Frontal lobe ataxia can also arise from disturbance of frontopontocerebellar tract (Arnold bundle).[3]

- **Role of the cerebellum**

  - The cerebellum modulates functions that are generated in other areas of the brain. As a motor modulator, the cerebellum has two functions:

    - It balances contractile forces of muscles during motor activity.

    - It organizes complex motor actions.

  - Different regions of the cerebellum have different functions. Table 8.1 delineates the functions of the various cerebellar divisions.

  - **Anatomical/functional correlations:** A few brief key anatomical facts are useful in understanding the clinical findings of cerebellar dysfunction (Table 8.2).

  - **Clinical manifestations of cerebellar dysfunction:** Table 8.3 outlines how cerebellar dysfunction parallels cerebellar phylogenetic organization.

Table 8.1
Functional Divisions of the Cerebellum

Phylogenetic Origin	Anatomical Location	Function Modulated
Archicerebellum	**Midline** Flocculonodular lobe	Vestibular function Eye movements
Paleocerebellum	**Midline** Vermis (anterior lobe) Pyramis Uvula Paraflocculus	Muscle tone Axial control Stance Gait
Neocerebellum	**Midline/hemispheres** Middle vermis Cerebellar hemispheres	Movement initiation, planning Fine motor programs Possibly cognition

Table 8.2
Key Functional and Anatomical Facts of Cerebellar Dysfunction

Remember	Because	Implications
Location	The cerebellum is located in close proximity to vital brain structures.	• A swelling of the cerebellum or a cerebellar mass can cause hydrocephalus. • A swelling of the cerebellum or a cerebellar mass can displace other brain structures, causing herniation.
Anatomy	The hemispheres coordinate the arms and legs. The midline coordinates the trunk (balance).	• Lesions in the hemispheres result in limb ataxia. • Lesions in the midline result in gait and balance problems, truncal titubation, and a wide-based gait.
Decussation	The cerebellum features a double decussation.	• Lesions of the left cerebellum affect the left side. • Lesions of the right cerebellum affect the right side.
Function	The cerebellum is a motor modulator.	• Ataxia and gait problems can result not only from lesions of the cerebellum but also from lesions of the input and output pathways. o Spinal sensory afferents (routed mainly through the medulla) o Cortical motor afferents (routed through the pons) o Thalamic output pathways (routed through the midbrain)

Table 8.3
How Cerebellar Dysfunction Parallels Cerebellar Phylogenetic Organization

Region of Lesions	Type of Dysfunction
Midline cerebellar lesions	Impaired axial control, vestibular function, eye movements, balance, and postural stability
Hemispheric cerebellar lesions	Impaired motor planning, control of fine motor movements; impact on cognitive planning, organizing, and sequencing of executive planning functions parallels impact on motor planning and fine motor programs

- **Role of the thalamus**
  - Ventrolateral thalamic lesions can result in contralateral ataxia, dysmetria, rebound, and overshoot phenomena. Most lesions are vascular in nature. These entities can be differentiated from ataxic hemiparesis syndrome, in which hemiparesis persists.[4]

- **Role of the spinal cord**
  - Dorsal column lesions and large-fiber sensorimotor neuropathy can produce somatosensory ataxia. Vitamin B_{12} deficiency and spinal degenerative diseases like Friedreich ataxia can give rise to ataxic gait.[5,6]
  - Strokes affecting the anterior columns of the spinal cord can also give rise to ataxia, in addition to weakness, by affecting the vestibulospinal, reticulospinal, and ventral spinocerebellar tracts.

ETIOLOGY OF ATAXIA

The etiology of ataxia is multifactorial. The cause of primary ataxia can be a genetic disorder. The causes of secondary ataxia include an extensive list of diseases, such as neurodegenerative, infectious, vascular, traumatic, autoimmune, neoplastic, paraneoplastic, toxic, and demyelinating disorders.

Genetic Causes of Ataxia

No aspects of ataxia are more complex than its genetic etiologies.

- **Autosomal dominant cerebellar ataxias**
  - **Episodic ataxia** is a rare genetic entity with autosomal dominant inheritance. Two distinct presentations have been identified, and genetic tests are available.

- In *episodic ataxia 1* (EA1), episodes of ataxia, with gait imbalance and slurring of speech, occur spontaneously or can be precipitated by sudden movement, excitement, or exercise. The attacks generally last from seconds to several minutes and may recur many times per day.

- In *episodic ataxia 2* (EA2), the ataxia lasts hours to days, with interictal abnormalities of eye movement. Exertion and stress commonly precipitate the episodes. EA2 notably is due to a genetic defect in a calcium channel (*CACNA1A*), and different genetic defects of this channel can cause genetically transmitted familial hemiplegic migraine.[7]

  - A CAG repeat in this gene causes a progressive ataxia (spinocerebellar ataxia [SCA]6), and there are overlaps in symptomatology.[8,9]

  - Patients may have migrainous episodes as well as ataxia, and some patients with the SCA6 mutation may present with episodic ataxia.

  - **Acetazolamide may be helpful in the treatment of episodic ataxia.**

- Potential identifiable causes of ataxia in individuals who have a history suggestive of a dominant pedigree have proliferated.

- There are currently 24 identified causes of autosomal dominant ataxia, including seven syndromes caused by CAG repeats encoding a polyglutamine protein domain (SCA1, SCA2, SCA3, SCA6, SCA7, SCA17, and dentatorubropallidoluysian atrophy [DRPLA]). Another five syndromes have other identified genetic causes.[10] The search for the genetic locus and gene product in the remaining 12 are still ongoing. Currently, genetic testing is available for several of these disorders through a variety of sources.

  - Worldwide, approximately 65% of identified families with an autosomal dominant ataxia have SCA1, SCA2, SCA3, SCA6, SCA7, or SCA8. The frequency of individual ataxic syndromes varies from one country to another.[11–17]

  - **SCA3 is the most common form of autosomal dominant cerebellar ataxia, accounting for roughly 21% of identified families** (see also Chapter 5). SCA3 is especially common in Brazil, Germany, and China.

  - SCA1 is more prevalent in Italy and South Africa.

  - DRPLA, a disease with protean manifestations that can present with ataxia, is an uncommon cause of ataxia worldwide.

However, it is more prevalent in Japan and in some areas of the southeastern United States (see also Chapters 5 and 7).

— In approximately 30% of families with ataxia and autosomal dominant inheritance, the genetic cause is unknown.

○ In patients with an onset of ataxia and a family history, autosomal dominant ataxias should be considered. Table 8.4 lists the major known autosomal dominant disorders and their genetic causes. A full discussion of the causes of autosomal dominant ataxia is beyond the scope of this review; however, a few important points are relevant:

  • Some forms of autosomal dominant ataxia cause a "purely ataxic syndrome," whereas in others, spasticity, neuropathy, cognitive changes, dystonia, and parkinsonism may be associated features. The identification of features not part of a purely motor ataxia may be helpful in diagnosing a specific disorder.

  • The genetic testing of unaffected relatives of individuals with a proven autosomal dominant SCA is a complex issue, and in many cases a genetic counselor should be involved before testing is undertaken.

  • Autosomal dominant ataxias that are due to trinucleotide repeats, such as CAG repeats, have the characteristic of *anticipation*, in which later generations may exhibit expansion of the repeat and an earlier onset of the disease. The offspring of male carriers are more likely to have a repeat expansion than are the offspring of female carriers.

  • A special comment is necessary with respect to SCA8. Although most cases of SCA8 appear to be associated with a CTG expansion, CTG expansions in the same region have been shown to occur in some healthy controls. The results of genetic testing in this disorder should therefore be interpreted with particular caution.

■ Autosomal recessive cerebellar ataxias

  ○ Identifiable autosomal recessive causes of ataxia are more common in children, including a host of metabolic abnormalities such as juvenile forms of GM2 gangliosidoses, sulfatide lipidoses, and other syndromes involving the deposition of abnormal metabolic intermediates.[18]

  ○ *Friedreich ataxia* can occur in children and in young adults, and it has occasionally been described in older individuals.

  ○ *Hereditary ataxia with vitamin E deficiency* is recessive and can present with symptoms very similar to those found in Friedreich ataxia.[19,20]

Table 8.4
Autosomal Dominant Cerebellar Ataxias

Name	Gene Product Identified?	Available Test?	Clinical Findings
SCA1	Yes	Yes	Ataxia, spasticity, executive dysfunction
SCA2	Yes	Yes	Ataxia, hyporeflexia, dementia, rare parkinsonism
SCA3	Yes	Yes	Ataxia, spasticity, dystonia, parkinsonism, restless legs syndrome, dementia
SCA4			Ataxia, spasticity, axonal sensory neuropathy
SCA5	Yes	Yes	Typically early-onset ataxia with normal life expectancy
SCA6	Yes	Yes	Ataxia
SCA7	Yes	Yes	Ataxia, pigmentary retinopathy, spasticity
SCA8	Yes	Yes	Ataxia
SCA10	Yes	Yes	Ataxia, epilepsy
SCA11			Ataxia, normal life expectancy, occasional spasticity
SCA12	Yes	No	Ataxia, spasticity
SCA13			Often early-onset (childhood) ataxia (but may occur later) with slow progression and normal life expectancy; mental retardation
SCA14	Yes	Yes	Slowly progressive ataxia with normal life expectancy; myoclonus if childhood onset
SCA15			Ataxia, occasional spasticity
SCA16			Ataxia, normal life expectancy, head tremor
SCA17	Yes	Yes	Ataxia, parkinsonism, dystonia, chorea, psychosis
SCA18			Ataxia, axonal neuropathy
SCA19			Ataxia, dementia, hyporeflexia or hyperreflexia
SCA21			Ataxia, dementia
SCA25			Ataxia, sensory neuropathy
SCA26	No	No	
SCA27 (*FGF14*)	*FGF14*	No	Ataxia, psychiatric abnormalities
DRPLA	Yes	Yes	Ataxia, myoclonus, epilepsy, chorea, psychosis, dementia

Abbreviations: DRPLA, dentatorubropallidoluysian atrophy; FGF, fibroblast growth factor; SCA, spinal cerebellar ataxia.

- ○ *Abetalipoproteinemia* is a recessive cause of vitamin E deficiency, and depending on the severity of the deficit and the related vitamin E deficiency, it may occur in children or adults.

- ○ Table 8.5 lists some of the more frequently seen causes of recessive cerebellar ataxia, as well as the clinical findings.

- **X-linked ataxias**

  - ○ *X-linked ataxia with sideroblastic anemia* can present in childhood with slowly progressive ataxia and sideroblastic anemia. The gene has been identified, but commercial testing is not available.

  - ○ *Fragile X–associated tremor/ataxia syndrome* (FXTAS) is a neurodegenerative disease with predominant ataxia related to the *FMR1* gene. It presents in children.[21]

Table 8.5
Autosomal Recessive Cerebellar Ataxias

Name	Gene Product Identified?	Available Test?	Clinical Findings
Friedreich ataxia	Yes	Yes	Classically, juvenile ataxia with a proprioceptive neuropathy, but a wide variety of presentations described
Hereditary ataxia with vitamin E deficiency	Yes	Yes	Ataxia with proprioceptive neuropathy, low vitamin E level
Abetalipoproteinemia	Yes	Yes	Ataxia with proprioceptive neuropathy, low vitamin E level, abnormal serum lipoproteins
Ataxia with oculomotor apraxia 1 (AOA1)	Yes	No	Slowly progressive childhood-onset ataxia with ocular apraxia, axonal neuropathy, and areflexia
Ataxia–telangiectasia	Yes	Yes	Ataxia, chorea, dystonia, oculomotor apraxia
Autosomal recessive spastic ataxia of Charlevoix-Saguenay	Yes (sacsin)	No	Early-onset ataxia, spasticity, and amyotrophy
Spinocerebellar ataxia with axonal neuropathy (SCAN)	Yes (*TDP1*)	No	Ataxia, axonal neuropathy, hypercholesterolemia, intellectual impairment

- **Mitochondrial ataxias**

  - Ataxia is usually present in disorders associated with mutations in mitochondrial DNA.

  - Genomic mitochondrial defects can result in mitochondrial diseases such as maternally inherited Leigh syndrome (MILS), Kearns-Sayre syndrome, and mitochondrial encephalopathy, lactic acidosis, and strokelike episodes (MELAS), which can cause ataxia.[22]

  - Mitochondrial dysfunction is also increasingly being recognized in recessive forms of cerebellar ataxias.[23,24]

Causes of Secondary Ataxia

Table 8.6 lists common causes of secondary ataxia.

- Some relevant points regarding the causes of secondary ataxia:

  - Vascular lesions, infections (including abscesses), and structural lesions should always be considered in the diagnosis of ataxia, and an imaging study is often warranted.

  - **In an acute setting, strokes and cerebellar masses can be a neurological emergency, and neurosurgical intervention may be required.**

  - Multiple sclerosis, acute demyelinating encephalomyelitis, and the Miller Fisher variant of Guillain-Barré syndrome can all present acutely with ataxia, and all of these should be considered in the diagnosis of acute ataxia. A lumbar puncture is frequently helpful in the diagnosis of autoimmune causes of ataxia.

  - Paraneoplastic ataxia should be evaluated in patients with a subacute to chronic onset of ataxia. Antibodies that are most likely to be elevated in autoimmune cerebellar ataxia include anti-GQ1b (in Guillain-Barré syndrome),[25] anti-Hu, anti-CV2, and anti-CRMP-5.[26] Paraneoplastic ataxia is most closely associated with small-cell cancer of the lung, but other primary tumors that may be associated include thymoma and, rarely, uterine sarcoma. In the case of paraneoplastic syndromes, in addition to an evaluation of paraneoplastic antibodies in the serum, a lumbar puncture may reveal evidence of paraneoplastic antibodies in the cerebrospinal fluid (CSF).

  - Imaging of the chest and neck with contrast-enhanced CT is indicated if a paraneoplastic syndrome is suspected.

  - Case reports in the literature suggest that vitamin B_{12} may occasionally present with chronic ataxia, often related to a loss of proprioception.[27–29]

Table 8.6
Common Causes of Secondary Ataxia

Category	Etiology	Investigation	Treatment
Vascular	Stroke (ischemic and hemorrhagic) Arteriovenous malformation (AVM)	CT, MRI	Medical and surgical
Autoimmune	Multiple sclerosis Acute demyelinating encephalomyelitis Miller Fisher variant of Guillain-Barré syndrome	MRI, LP, serum antibodies	Steroids, immunomodulators
Toxic	Drugs Antiepileptics Neuroleptics Lithium	Serum drug levels	Reduction of drug dosing
Heavy metals	Thallium Lead	Serum and urine levels	Chelation, hemodialysis
Infectious	Bacterial cerebellar abscess Acute cerebellitis Creutzfeldt-Jakob disease (CJD)	MRI, LP	Antibiotics
Metabolic	Vitamin B_{12} deficiency Alcoholic cerebellar degeneration	Vitamin levels	Replacement therapy
Neoplastic	Primary neoplasm Astrocytoma Medulloblastoma Meningioma	CT, MRI	Chemotherapy and surgery
	Metastatic neoplasm Lung Breast Renal	MRI, CT of chest, abdomen, and pelvis	Chemotherapy and surgery
	Paraneoplastic Anti-Hu Anti-CV2 Anti-CRMP-5	Serum antibodies	Intravenous immunoglobulin (IVIG), plasmaphersis, treatment of primary tumor
Neurodegenerative	Multiple system atrophy Progressive supranuclear palsy	CT, MRI	Symptomatic therapy

Abbreviation: LP, lumbar puncture

○ Vitamin E and vitamin B$_{12}$ levels should be checked in all individuals with a new onset of ataxia, as deficiency of these vitamins is a potentially correctable cause of progressive ataxia.

Sporadic Ataxia

Unexplained chronic progressive ataxia in adult patients without a family history is less likely to be genetic (although still possible!).[30]

■ In patients with chronic adult-onset ataxia, a cause of the ataxia may not be found.

■ In a recent German study of 112 patients with chronic progressive ataxia (inclusion criteria were onset after the age of 20 years, progressive course, no identified symptomatic cause, including no evidence of a paraneoplastic process, and no evidence of a family history of ataxia), 58% still had no diagnosis after an extensive workup.

○ In 29% of the cases, patients met the criteria for multiple system atrophy (MSA).

○ Genetic testing revealed an autosomal dominant or recessive ataxia in 13% (SCA1, SCA2, SCA6, or adult-onset Friedreich ataxia was identified during genetic screening in these individuals).

○ In the 58% of patients in whom a diagnosis could not be made, the ataxia tended to have a slower rate of progression than MSA.

CLINICAL EXAMINATION OF THE PATIENT WITH ATAXIA

Table 8.7 outlines simple bedside clinical examination techniques for patients with suspected cerebellar dysfunction. Depending on the severity of the deficit and localization of the lesion, some deficits will be evident on examination, while others may be subtle or not present.

DIAGNOSIS OF ATAXIC SYNDROMES

The diagnosis of ataxic syndromes is becoming increasingly challenging. A complete history and physical examination, neuroimaging, and an extensive laboratory evaluation are required. In many cases, the etiology of ataxia remains uncertain despite a complete workup.

■ Many chronic cerebellar ataxias are genetically determined, and a family history should be obtained. Many genetic ataxic syndromes can feature "anticipation," in which the age at onset is progressively lower in successive generations (a family history may be lacking in some individuals). In some cases, the presentation of a similar syndrome in a sibling despite unaffected

Table 8.7
Examination of the Patient Suspected to Have Cerebellar Dysfunction

Clinical Domain	Examination Technique	Finding With Cerebellar Dysfunction
Eye movements	Observation	Macular square-wave jerks (sudden, spontaneous, unplanned deviations of the eye with corrective saccades back to original position)
	Have patient fix gaze on an object off midline (eg, examiner's finger). Command: "Look at my finger here on the right ... now on the left."	Fixation instability • Involuntary saccades away from object • Corrective saccades back to object Nystagmus (fixation in lateral or vertical gaze) • Fixation interrupted by slow, rolling movements, often toward a neutral position, interrupted by rapid corrective saccades
	Saccade between two objects (eg, examiner's finger and nose) Command: "Look at my finger ... now look at my nose ... finger ... nose."	Dysmetric saccades • Saccade may overshoot or undershoot target, with a correction
	Smooth pursuit of an object through space Command: "Follow my finger through space."	Eyes should move smoothly; saccadic fragmentation of smooth pursuit common in healthy elderly but can also be sign of cerebellar disease
	Caveats	• Vestibular dysfunction may cause nystagmus. • Slight lateral nystagmus is common in healthy adults. • Saccadic pursuit may occur in healthy elderly. • Slowed saccades, inability to generate saccades, and ophthalmoplegia may occur but generally indicate additional brainstem involvement.
Tremor	Finger-to-nose testing and finger chasing, holding hands in horizontal posture	• Usually low-frequency but high-amplitude intention and postural tremor

continued

Table 8.7 (cont.)
Examination of the Patient Suspected to Have Cerebellar Dysfunction

Clinical Domain	Examination Technique	Finding With Cerebellar Dysfunction
Limb coordination	Finger-to-nose testing Finger chasing: examiner moves his/her finger and has the patient try to keep his/her finger behind examiner's finger (mirroring)	• Past pointing (missing examiner's finger) • Excessive corrections • Rebound
	Tapping heel to knee Running heel from knee to shin	• Abnormal speed • Poor precision • Excessive corrections
	Rapid alternating tapping (rapidly tapping palmar and dorsal aspect of hand on thigh)	• Slowed movements with impaired precision • "Painting the leg" rather than tapping the leg
Stance/gait	Observation of casual gait	• Unsteady, wide-based gait • Difficulty with sudden stops or changes in direction • Variable step length • Patients often visually focus on ground
	Tandem gait	More pronounced deficits, "steps to the side" to catch balance
	Stance with eyes closed	"Positive Romberg": abnormal sensory input or reception in the cerebellum • Patients unable to maintain balance with eyes closed
Muscle tone	Evaluation of tone at wrist, elbow, knee, and ankle	Decreased resistance to passive movement
Speech evaluation	Prepared text may be helpful (eg, "The Rainbow Passage")	• Altered articulation of words • Abnormal fluency • Slowed speech • "Scanning dysarthria": words broken into syllables

parents may be an important clue. Patients should be asked about consanguinity (eg, are your parents related in any way?) because this can sometimes point to the possibility of a recessively inherited disorder, such as Friedreich ataxia.

■ Ataxia may occur sporadically in disorders such as MSA, a syndrome that can also present with autonomic instability and parkinsonism. In younger patients, nutritional abnormalities (some genetically related), such as primary vitamin E deficiency, as well as abnormalities in serum lipoproteins leading to fat malabsorption, can cause ataxia, as can mitochondrial disease. In older patients, autoimmune syndromes including paraneoplastic syndromes can result in ataxia. Celiac disease, an autoimmune disease with anti-gliadin antibodies, may result in ataxia.[31] Furthermore, ataxia can be associated with multiple sclerosis as either an acute or a chronic feature of the disease.

■ With the proliferation of potential diagnoses associated with ataxia, clinicians should develop a careful and standardized approach to the diagnosis (Figures 8.1 and 8.2). The time course of the ataxia is an important diagnostic feature, as acute ataxic syndromes frequently are related to acute infectious or to vascular, structural, or metabolic lesions, whereas chronic ataxias are more apt to be related to genetic syndromes or slowly growing mass lesions. Possible flow charts for the evaluation of ataxic syndromes in children and adults are presented next. In some cases, certain genetic syndromes may be more common in a local population or the family history may provide guidance, and appropriate modification of these templates may be necessary.

MANAGEMENT

Acute cerebellar ataxia should be considered a neurological emergency until certain diagnoses have been excluded. Key facts to consider in the management of acute ataxia are the following:

■ In children, metabolic abnormalities can be caused by inborn errors of metabolism, and rapid treatment may be required to prevent permanent brain injury. Acute intoxications in children and adults can be fatal if not treated.

■ Vascular and structural cerebellar lesions, such as strokes, hemorrhages, and neoplasms, can result in swelling that causes herniation or obstruction of CSF flow with hydrocephalus, and neurosurgical intervention may be required.

■ The Miller Fisher variant of Guillain-Barré syndrome can present with ataxia and dysarthria and cause deficits in upper airway function that can impair respiration.

■ In children, physical abuse should always be considered as a potential etiology for trauma.

For patients with chronic ataxia, a complete family history should be obtained. An autosomal dominant pattern of inheritance may be helpful in narrowing the differential diagnosis. There is currently no universal treatment for ataxia.

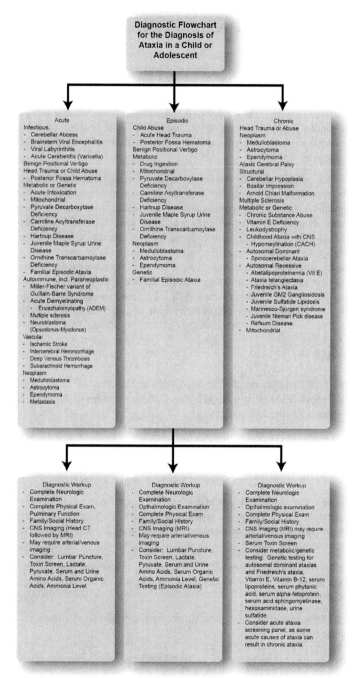

Diagnostic Flowchart for the Diagnosis of Ataxia in a Child or Adolescent

Acute
Infectious:
- Cerebellar Abcess
- Brainstem Viral Encephalitis
- Viral Labyrinthitis
- Acute Cerebellitis (Varicella)
Benign Positional Vertigo
Head Trauma or Child Abuse
- Posterior Fossa Hematoma
Metabolic or Genetic
- Acute Intoxication
- Mitochondrial
- Pyruvate Decarboxylase Deficiency
- Carnitine Acyltransferase Deficiency
- Hartnup Disease
- Juvenile Maple Syrup Urine Disease
- Ornithine Transcarbamoylase Deficiency
- Familial Episodic Ataxia
Autoimmune, incl. Paraneoplastic
- Miller-Fischer variant of Guillain-Barre Syndrome
- Acute Demyelinating Encephalomyopathy (ADEM)
- Multiple sclerosis
- Neuroblastoma (Opsodonus-Myodonus)
Vascular
- Ischemic Stroke
- Intercerebral Hemmorhage
- Deep Venous Thrombosis
- Subarachnoid Hemorrhage
Neoplasm
- Medulloblastoma
- Astrocytoma
- Ependymoma
- Metastasis

Episodic
Child Abuse
- Acute Head Trauma
- Posterior Fossa Hematoma
Benign Positional Vertigo
Metabolic
- Drug Ingestion
- Mitochondrial
- Pyruvate Decarboxylase Deficiency
- Carnitine Acyltransferase Deficiency
- Hartnup Disease
- Juvenile Maple Syrup Urine Disease
- Ornithine Transcarbamoylase Deficiency
Neoplasm
- Medulloblastoma
- Astrocytoma
- Ependymoma
Genetic
- Familial Episodic Ataxia

Chronic
Head Trauma or Abuse
Neoplasm
- Medulloblastoma
- Astrocytoma
- Ependymoma
Alaxic Cerebral Palsy
Structural
- Cerebellar Hypoplasia
- Basilar Impression
- Arnold Chiari Malformation
Multiple Sclerosis
Metabolic or Genetic
- Chronic Substance Abuse
- Vitamin E Deficiency
- Leukodystrophy
- Childhood Ataxia with CNS Hypomeylination (CACH)
- Autosomal Dominant
  - Spinocerebellar Ataxia
- Autosomal Recessive
  - Abetalipoproteinemia (Vit E)
  - Ataxia telangiectasia
  - Friedreich's Ataxia
  - Juvenile GM2 Gangliosidosis
  - Juvenile Sulfatide Lipidosis
  - Marinesco-Sjorgen syndrome
  - Juvenile Nieman Pick disease
  - Refsum Disease
- Mitochondrial

Diagnostic Workup
- Complete Neurologic Examination
- Complete Physical Exam, Pulminary Function
- Family/Social History
- CNS Imaging (Head CT followed by MRI)
- May require arterial/venous imaging
- Consider: Lumbar Puncture, Toxin Screen, Lactate, Pyruvate, Serum and Urine Amino Acids, Serum Organic Acids, Ammonia Level

Diagnostic Workup
- Complete Neurologic Examination
- Opthalmologic Examination
- Complete Physical Exam
- Family/Social History
- CNS Imaging (MRI)
- May require arterial/venous imaging
- Consider: Lumbar Puncture, Toxin Screen, Lactate, Pyruvate, Serum and Urine Amino Acids, Serum Organic Acids, Ammonia Level, Genetic Testing (Episodic Ataxia)

Diagnostic Workup
- Complete Neurologic Examination
- Opthalmologic examination
- Complete Physical Exam
- Family/Social History
- CNS Imaging (MRI) may require arterial/venous imaging
- Serum Toxin Screen
- Consider metabolic/genetic testing: Genetic testing for autosomal dominant ataxias and Friedreich's ataxia, Vitamin E, Vitamin B-12, serum lipoproteins, serum phytanic acid, serum alpha-fetoprotein, serum acid sphingomyelinase, hexosaminidase, urine sulfatide.
- Consider acute ataxia screening panel, as some acute causes of ataxia can result in chronic ataxia.

FIGURE 8.1
Diagnostic flowchart for the child or adolescent with ataxia.

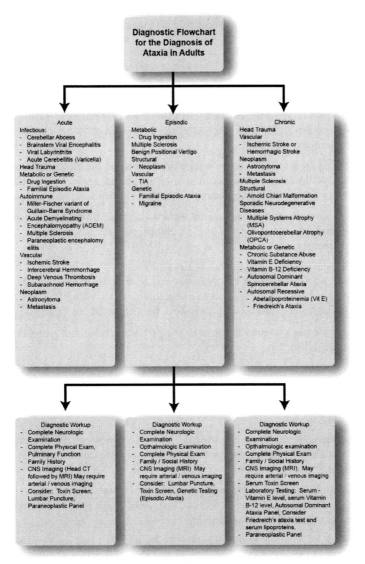

FIGURE 8.2

Diagnostic flowchart for the adult with ataxia.

- In some cases (paraneoplastic ataxia or ataxia due to an autoimmune disease, structural abnormality, nutritional deficiency, or metabolic abnormality), identification of the underlying cause of ataxia may also identify a treatment modality.

- In many cases, treatment is supportive and includes physical therapy, occupational therapy, and speech therapy for patients with dysarthria and dysphagia. A baseline speech and swallowing evaluation by a speech pathologist should be performed in most cases, even if there is no overt swallowing deficit.

■ In the case of the genetically linked ataxias, genetic counseling is an important part of management, and testing of unaffected family members should be performed only with much care after full information has been provided to family members.

■ Several agents have been inconsistently reported to mitigate ataxia amantadine, l-5-hydroxytryptophan, ondansetron, physostigmine, branched-chain amino acid therapy, gabapentin, piracetam, buspirone, and varenicline.

■ Baclofen may reduce associated leg spasticity. GABAergic agents such as clonazepam, beta-blockers, and primidone, may reduce associated cerebellar tremors.

■ Surgical ablation or deep brain stimulation surgery of the ventral intermediate nucleus (VIM) of the thalamus may be effective in reducing cerebellar tremor; however, these procedures often do not significantly lessen ataxia, although a few cases with benefit have been reported (eg, SCAs).

Ataxia is a complex entity that can be the presenting feature of many different neurological disorders.

■ The evaluation and management of ataxia should focus first on excluding symptomatic causes.

■ Genetic testing should be considered after reversible causes have been excluded.

■ Ataxia with an acute onset should be considered a neurological and potentially a neurosurgical emergency until structural, vascular, and toxic causes of acute ataxia have been ruled out.

■ In children, reversible causes include a host of metabolic lesions that should be considered, and referral to a pediatric neurologist may be appropriate if initial evaluations are not fruitful.

■ In adults, vitamin E and occasionally vitamin B_{12} deficiency are rarely a cause of chronic progressive ataxia and should not be overlooked in the diagnostic workup.

■ After a careful symptomatic workup, testing for genetic causes of ataxia should be considered.

■ In patients with an identified genetic cause, unaffected family members should be tested with caution, and the participation of a genetic counselor is often helpful.

■ After symptomatic causes have been corrected, management is typically supportive but may include physical, occupational, and speech therapy.

REFERENCES

1. Globas C, Bosch S, Zuhlke CH, et al. The cerebellum and cognition. Intellectual function in spinocerebellar ataxia type 6 (SCA6). *J Neurol*. 2003; 250(12):1482–1487.
2. Thompson PD. Frontal lobe ataxia. *Handb Clin Neurol*. 2012; 103:619–622.
3. Terry JB, Rosenberg RN. Frontal lobe ataxia. *Surg Neurol*. 1995; 44(6):583–588.
4. Solomon DH, Barohn RJ, Bazan C, et al. The thalamic ataxia syndrome. *Neurology*. 1994; 44(5):810–814.
5. Chevis CF, da Silva CB, D'Abreu A, et al. Spinal cord atrophy correlates with disability in Friedreich's ataxia. *Cerebellum*. 2013; 12(1):43–47.
6. Crawford JR, Say D. Vitamin B_{12} deficiency presenting as acute ataxia. *BMJ Case Rep*. 2013.
7. Ophoff RA, Terwindt GM, Vergouwe MN, et al. Familial hemiplegic migraine and episodic ataxia type-2 are caused by mutations in the Ca2+ channel gene CACNL1A4. *Cell*. 1996; 87:543–552.
8. Frontali M. Spinocerebellar ataxia type 6: channelopathy or glutamine repeat disorder? *Brain Res Bull*. 2001; 56:227–231.
9. Abele M, Burk K, Schols L, et al. The aetiology of sporadic adult-onset ataxia. *Brain*. 2002; 125(pt 5):961–968.
10. Schöls L, Bauer P, Schmidt T, et al. Autosomal dominant cerebellar ataxias: clinical features, genetics, and pathogenesis. *Lancet Neurol*. 2004; 3:291–304.
11. van de Warrenburg BP, Sinke RJ, Verschuuren-Bemelmans CC, et al. Spinocerebellar ataxias in the Netherlands: prevalence and age at onset variance analysis. *Neurology*. 2002; 58:702–708.
12. Silveira I, Miranda C, Guimaraes L, et al. Trinucleotide repeats in 202 families with ataxia: a small expanded (CAG)n allele at the SCA17 locus. *Arch Neurol*. 2002; 59:623–629.
13. Brusco A, Gellera C, Cagnoli C, et al. Molecular genetics of hereditary spinocerebellar ataxia: mutation analysis of spinocerebellar ataxia genes and CAG/CTG repeat expansion detection in 225 Italian families. *Arch Neurol*. 2004; 61(5):727–733.
14. Bryer A, Krause A, Bill P, et al. The hereditary adult onset ataxias in South Africa. *J Neurol Sci*. 2003; 216:47–54.
15. Tang B, Liu C, Shen L, et al. Frequency of SCA1, SCA2, SCA3/MJD, SCA6, SCA7, and DRPLA CAG trinucleotide repeat expansion in patients with hereditary spinocerebellar ataxia from Chinese kindreds. *Arch Neurol*. 2000; 57:540–544.
16. Saleem Q, Choudhry S, Mukerji M, et al. Molecular analysis of autosomal dominant hereditary ataxias in the Indian population: high frequency of SCA2 and evidence for a common founder mutation. *Hum Genet*. 2000; 106:179–187.
17. Moseley ML, Benzow KA, Schut LJ, et al. Incidence of dominant spinocerebellar and Friedreich triplet repeats among 361 ataxia families. *Neurology*. 1998; 51:1666–1671.
18. Berman P. Ataxia in children. *Int Pediatr*. 1999; 14(1):44–47.
19. Stocker A. Molecular mechanisms of vitamin E transport. *Ann N Y Acad Sci*. 2004; 1031:44–59.
20. van de Warrenburg BPC, Sinke RJ, Kremer B. Recent advances in hereditary spinocerebellar ataxias. *J Neuropathol Exp Neurol*. 2005; 64(3):171–180.
21. Hagerman P. Fragile X-associated tremor/ataxia syndrome (FXTAS): pathology and mechanisms. *Acta Neuropathol*. 2013; 126(1):1–19.
22. Zeviani M, Simonati A, Bindoff LA, et al. Ataxia in mitochondrial disorders. *Handb Clin Neurol*. 2012; 103:359–372.

23. Girard M, Lariviere R, Parfitt DA, et al. Mitochondrial dysfunction and Purkinje cell loss in autosomal recessive spastic ataxia of Charlevoix-Saguenay (ARSACS). *Proc Natl Acad Sci U S A.* 2012; 109(5):1661–1666.

24. Murad NA, Cullen JK, McKenzie M, et al. Mitochondrial dysfunction in a novel form of autosomal recessive ataxia. *Mitochondrion.* 2013; 13(3):235–245.

25. Paparounas K. Anti-GQ1b ganglioside antibody in peripheral nervous system disorders: pathophysiologic role and clinical relevance. *Arch Neurol.* 2004; 61:1013–1016.

26. Bataller L, Dalmau J. Paraneoplastic neurologic syndromes. *Neurol Clin N Am.* 2003; 21:221–247.

27. Miller MA, Martinez V, McCarthy R, et al. Nitrous oxide "whippit" abuse presenting as clinical B_{12} deficiency and ataxia. *Am J Emerg Med.* 2004; 22(2):124.

28. Morita S, Miwa H, Kihira T, et al. Cerebellar ataxia and leukoencephalopathy associated with cobalamin deficiency. *J Neurol Sci.* 2003; 216(1):183–184.

29. Facchini SA, Jami MM, Neuberg RW, et al. A treatable cause of ataxia in children. *Pediatr Neurol.* 2001; 24(2):135–138.

30. Abele M, Burk K, Schols L, et al. The aetiology of sporadic adult-onset ataxia. *Brain.* 2002; 125(pt 5):961–968.

31. Abele M, Schöls L, Schwartz S, et al. Prevalence of antigliadin antibodies in ataxia patients. *Neurology.* 2003; 60:1674–1675.

9

TICS

DEFINITION

A tic is an involuntary movement or vocalization that is usually of sudden onset, brief, repetitive, and stereotyped, but nonrhythmic. Tics frequently imitate normal behavior, often occurring during normal activity and without alteration of consciousness. A tic is usually associated with a premonitory "buildup" sensation or feeling of discomfort that is often localized to the affected area. Usually, the individual experiences a sensation of relief once the tic has occurred. Unlike most movement disorders, tics can persist during sleep.

Tics can be classified as motor or vocal. Motor tics are associated with movements, whereas vocal tics are associated with sounds. Sometimes, the distinction between a motor tic and a vocal tic may be difficult because the noise may result from a muscle contraction.

Tics can also be categorized as simple or complex, depending on the manifestation (Table 9.1).

Simple motor tics involve only a few muscles, usually restricted to a specific body part. They can be clonic (abrupt in onset and rapid), tonic (isometric contraction of the involved body part), or dystonic (sustained abnormal posture).[1] Examples of simple motor tics include the following:

- Eye blinking

- Shoulder shrugging

- Facial grimacing

- Neck stretching

- Mouth movements

- Jaw clenching

Simple vocal tics consist of sounds that do not form words, such as these:

- Throat clearing

- Grunting

Table 9.1
Simple Versus Complex Tics

Type	Characteristics	Examples
Simple motor tics	Only one body region involved, only a few muscles used	Eye blinking, shoulder shrugging, facial grimacing, neck stretching, spitting, hair combing
Simple vocal tics	Sounds that do not form words	Throat clearing, grunting, coughing, sniffing
Complex motor tics	Multiple body regions involved	Jumping, kicking, squatting, abnormal body posturing, echopraxia, copropraxia
Complex vocal tics	Pronunciation of words or sentences, repetition of other people's words	Coprolalia, palilalia, formed words, echolalia

- Coughing
- Sniffing
- Blowing
- Squeaking

Complex motor tics consist of movements involving multiple muscle groups and have a deliberate character, frequently resembling normal movements or gestures. They usually last longer than simple tics. Examples of complex motor tics include these:

- Jumping
- Kicking
- Squatting
- Holding the body in an atypical position
- Imitating other people's gestures (echopraxia)
- Vulgar or obscene gesturing (copropraxia)

Complex vocal tics consist of pronounced words or sentences. Examples include the following:

- Repetition of other people's words (echolalia)
- Repetition of a last word or parts of a word (palilalia)
- Verbalizing profanities (coprolalia)

CHARACTERISTICS OF TICS

■ Tics are commonly associated with a premonitory sensation or feeling of discomfort that is usually relieved by performing a specific activity.

■ Tics can be suppressed, but suppression usually requires concentration on the part of the affected individual and results in a buildup of an uncomfortable sensation that is relieved when the tic occurs.

■ Typically, tics do not disrupt volitional movement, unlike other abnormal movements, such as those of chorea and myoclonus, which may share some of the features of tics.

■ There can also be **tic blocking,** during which there is a sudden stoppage of movement.

■ The severity of tics usually waxes and wanes, and the affected individual experiences episodes of repeated tics alternating with tic-free periods that may last from minutes to hours.[2]

■ Involvement in activities that require a great deal of attention or concentration usually diminishes the frequency of tics, whereas tics tend to occur more often during periods of stress or fatigue.

■ The classification of tic disorders is based on the type(s) of tics and duration of symptoms. The Tourette Syndrome Classification Study Group classification of idiopathic tic disorders appears in Table 9.2.[3]

■ However, there are many behavioral/psychiatric manifestations of Tourette syndrome (TS), and these are often more disabling than tics.

  ○ Two behavioral features commonly associated with TS are attention-deficit/hyperactivity disorder (ADHD) and obsessive–compulsive disorder (OCD).

  ○ The incidence of ADHD in TS ranges from 50% to 75%, and ADHD is the most commonly reported comorbidity. OCD may be seen in 30% to 60% of patients with TS.

  ○ The symptoms of ADHD begin aproximately 2.5 years before the onset of TS, whereas OCD generally appears after the onset of tics.[4]

  ○ Other symptoms seen in TS are listed in Table 9.3.

EPIDEMIOLOGY, PATHOGENESIS, AND PATHOPHYSIOLOGY

■ Tics usually begin during childhood. The average age at the onset of symptoms ranges from 5.6 to 6.4 years. On average, tics become most severe at the age of 10 years and then decrease in frequency to the point that by age 18, half of patients who have had tics are free of them.[5] The incidence of TS

Table 9.2
Classification of Idiopathic Tic Disorders

Tourette Syndrome	• Multiple motor AND one or more vocal tics at some time but not required to be concurrent. • Tics occur over more than 1 year, multiple times a day, nearly daily or intermittently. • Location, frequency, complexity, and severity of tics fluctuate over time. • Onset before age 21. • Symptoms cannot be attributed to other conditions.
Chronic Multiple Motor Tic or Phonic Tic Disorder	• Multiple motor OR vocal tics present at some time. • Tics occur over more than 1 year, multiple times a day, nearly daily or intermittently. • Location, frequency, complexity, and severity of tics fluctuate over time. • Onset before age 21. • Symptoms cannot be attributed to other conditions.
Chronic Single Tic Disorder	• Same as chronic multiple motor tic or phonic tic disorder except single vocal OR motor tic.
Transient Tic Disorder	• Single or multiple motor and/or vocal tics. • Tics occur over at least 2 weeks but for less than 12 consecutive months. • Daily or nearly daily tics. • No history of Tourette syndrome or chronic tic disorder. • Onset before age 21. • Diagnosis can be made only in retrospect.

Source: Adapted from Ref. 3: The Tourette Syndrome Classification Study Group. Definitions and classification of tic disorders. *Arch Neurol.* 1993; 50:1013–1016.

Table 9.3
Other Symptoms Associated With Tourette Syndrome

Attention-deficit/hyperactivity disorder	Short temper
Obsessive–compulsive disorder	Oppositional defiant behavior
Confrontation	Mania
Violence	Agoraphobia
Anger	Simple phobia
Depression	Social phobia
Personality disorder	Problems with discipline
Inattention	Disinhibition
Poor impulse control	Self-injurious behavior

is higher in males, with a male-to-female ratio of 4.3:1.[6] Tics rarely begin in adulthood, and when they do, they are most frequently recurrences of tics that occurred during childhood.[7] Underlying causes must be strongly considered in adult-onset tics.

- The prevalence of tic disorders shows a dramatic variation that is probably a result of the studied populations along with the diagnostic criteria and methodology used in different studies.

- For all tic disorders, the prevalence may be as high as 4.2%.[8] The prevalence of transient tic disorder has been reported to range from 4% to 24%, and the prevalence of TS is 3%.[9]

- The exact origin of tics and TS is unknown, but it has been hypothesized that the corticostriatothalamocortical circuitry is involved, particularly the caudate nucleus.

- Abnormalities in several neurotransmitter systems, particularly dopamine,[10] have been linked to the etiology of the syndrome.

- Despite contradictory findings in functional MRI studies, other modalities have detected metabolic derangement in the orbitofrontal cortex, dorsolateral prefrontal cortex, supplementary motor areas, cingulate gyrus, sensorimotor cortex, and basal ganglia, consistent with the idea that TS is both a motor and a behavioral disorder.[11]

- Immunologic mechanisms have been proposed and are controversial. Some reports link TS, ADHD, and OCD to previous infection with group A beta-hemolytic streptococci.

- The occurrence of TS in family clusters suggests that TS has a genetic/familial basis (53% pairwise concordance observed for TS in monozygotic twins, in contrast to 8% observed for dizygotic twins).

- Multiple investigators have suggested a mutation with autosomal dominant inheritance and reduced penetrance, and numerous candidate genes have been proposed. However, to date there have been no significant linkage findings.

EVALUATION

- The diagnosis of tics and TS is a clinical one. Many other movements can resemble tics, and these are listed in Table 9.4.[12]

- No blood work or imaging studies will confirm the diagnosis.

- Once the diagnosis is suspected, the patient should be screened for behavioral symptoms, and treatment should be initiated if necessary.

- Review the patient's current medications because some may induce tics, including antidepressant medications and anticonvulsive agents.

■ If a neurological abnormality is found on examination, further workup should be undertaken to evaluate for causes of secondary tics (Table 9.5).[13]

Table 9.4
Differential Diagnosis of Tics

Movement/Behavior	Definition	Examples	Comments
Akathisia	Sensation of excessive restlessness resulting in constant movement of affected body parts, with relief obtained by moving	Leg movements, leg rubbing, walking, face rubbing, inability to sit still	Associated with exposure to dopamine receptor blockers (tardive akathisia), no diurnal fluctuation
Compulsive behavior	Repetitive and ritualistic movements that usually are a response to psychological need	Hand washing, repetitive cleaning, organizing in a particular manner	Seen in normal individuls or those with developmental delay. Obsessive thoughts may also be present
Mannerism	Particular voluntary movement, usually associated with a gesture or other particular movements	Rubbing hair after removing hat, extending little finger when holding a cup; movements may have a purpose	Nonpathologic action that can often be a distinguishing feature of an individual
Myoclonus	Sudden, brief, involuntary muscle jerk	May involve any body part, nonsuppressible	Myoclonus can resemble simple motor tics but is nonsuppressible and often random
Punding	Stereotypical motor behaviors characterized by an intense fascination with repetitive handling and examination of mechanical objects	Picking at oneself, taking watches and radios apart, sorting and arranging common objects (eg, lining up pebbles, rocks, or other small objects)[12]	Originally described in amphetamine users, now often reported in patients with Parkinson's disease as a dopaminergic-induced complication May be socially disruptive, responds to medication readjustment

continued

Table 9.4 (cont.)
Differential Diagnosis of Tics

Movement/Behavior	Definition	Examples	Comments
Restless legs syndrome	Uncomfortable sensation, usually in lower extremities, occurring or worsening in the afternoon or evening and relieved by movement	Various symptoms described by patients (eg, cramp, spasm, numbness, tingling, crawling sensation)	The circadian nature suggests the diagnosis. Improvement with dopamine agonist or narcotics
Seizure	Involuntary movement that may or may not be associated with alteration of conciousness	Action varies depending on body region affected, electroencephalogram helpful for diagnosis	Nonsuppressible
Stereotypy	Repetitive, purposeless movements	Rocking, shuddering, clapping, flapping, facial movements	Seen in normal children, also autism, developmental delay, and pervasive developmental disorder

Table 9.5
Causes of Secondary Tics

Precipitants
Carbon monoxide intoxication
Drugs: stimulants, anticonvulsants, anticholinergics, antidepressants, cocaine, neuroleptics
Genetic, chromosomal, developmental disorders
Head trauma
Huntington's disease
Infections: encephalitis, neurosyphilis, Creutzfeldt-Jakob disease
Neuroacanthocytosis
Schizophrenia
Stroke

Source: Adapted from Ref. 13: Fahn S, Jankovic J. *Principles and Practice of Movement Disorders.* Philadelphia, PA: Elsevier; 2007.

TREATMENT (FIGURE 9.1)

- Most patients with mild symptoms will benefit from education regarding the diagnosis and what to expect from the condition.

- Parents as well as teachers should be instructed to create a suitable environment for the affected individual, and it should be explained to them this is not a volitional behavior.

- Giving the child the opportunity to "release" the tics by providing him or her with a scheduled break may be all that is needed. The same may be effective for adults in the work environment.

- Pharmacologic treatment for tics may not be needed unless they cause severe interference with school, work, or social development. Often education, couseling, and behavior modification/therapy are sufficient.

If medical therapy is necessary, the following should be considered:

- The focus of medical therapy should be on decreasing the impairment created by the tics rather than on attempting to suppress them completely.

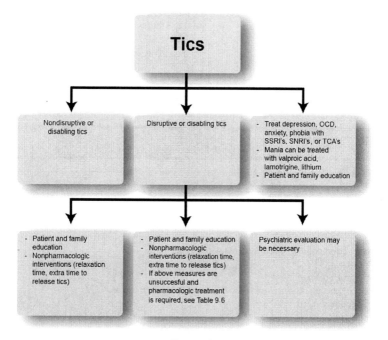

Figure 9.1
Approach to the management of the patient with tics.

- Therapy should be instituted with the potential side effects taken into consideration.

- The most bothersome symptoms should be targeted first.

- Therapy should be started at low doses and titrated to the lowest effective dose.

- Medications require adequate trials.

Table 9.6
Medications Commonly Used for the Treatment of Tics in Tourette Syndrome

Generic Name	Dosing (mg/d)	Adverse Effects	Comments
Risperidone	0.25–6 mg 1 or 2 times daily	TD, dizziness, sedation, akathisia, EPS	Begin with 0.25 mg at bedtime, increase every 3 days by 0.25 mg to benefit or side effects, risk for EPS >6 mg/d.
Haloperidol	0.5–5 mg 2 or 3 times daily (adults) 0.05–0.075 mg/kg 2 or 3 times daily (children)	Sedation, TD, EPS, NMS, galactorrhea, akathisia	Monitor for EPS.
Olanzapine	2.5–20 mg daily	Weight gain, EPS, sedation, diabetes mellitus, NMS, TD	Monitor for EPS and glucose.
Pimozide	1–10 mg/d	EKG changes, weight gain, EPS, sedation, TD	Check EKG at baseline, then periodically (prolongation of QT interval).
Quetiapine	25–800 mg/d	Weight gain, dizziness, drowsiness, hypotension, EPS	
Fluphenazine	1–10 mg/d	Sedation, TD, EPS, NMS, galactorrhea, akathisia	Better tolerated than haloperidol in some reports.

continued

Table 9.6 (cont.)
Medications Commonly Used for the Treatment of Tics in Tourette Syndrome

Generic Name	Dosing (mg/d)	Adverse Effects	Comments
Clonidine	0.05–0.6 mg 1 or 2 times daily	Sedation, hypotension, rebound hypertension with discontinuation, confusion	Start with low dose, monitor for hypotension, avoid abrupt withdrawal.
Tetrabenazine	Start at 25 mg/d	Depression, suicidality, parkinsonism, somnolence, NMS, orthostatic hypotension	Available only through specialty pharmacy.
Clonazepam or other benzodiazepines	Depending on the benzodiazepine	Sedation, tolerance, cognitive impairment	Should not be used as first-line treatment; start with a low dose if possible.

Abbreviations: EKG, electrocardiogram; EPS, extrapyramidal syndrome; NMS, neuroleptic malignant syndrome; TD, tardive dyskinesia.

- Dopamine receptor blockers are the mainstay of treatment for tics and TS (Table 9.6).

  - Side effects include sedation, parkinsonism, and risk for tardive dyskinesia. Some can cause QT prolongation, so electrocardiographic monitoring is necessary.

  - These are the only medications for TS approved by the Food and Drug Administration (FDA).

  - Haloperidol and pimozide are probably the most widely used medications and provide benefit in to up to 80% of patients.

  - Fluphenazine has also been reported to be beneficial for tics, among others, in patients who cannot tolerate haloperidol.

- Atypical antipsychotics have been reported to be beneficial and may be associated with a lower incidence of side effects in comparison with the typical antipsychotics.

  - Aripiprazole, risperidone, and ziprasidone have been reported to decrease the severity and frequency of tics in multiple reports.

- Tetrabenazine, a monoamine-depleting and dopamine receptor–blocking drug, is now available in the United States. It is currently FDA-approved only for Huntington's disease, so treatment of tics would be an off-label use.

○ Its efficacy for reducing tics has been demonstrated in multiple studies, without the same risks for tardive dyskinesia.

■ Benzodiazepines, in particular clonazepam, can be helpful and there is no risk for tardive dyskinesia.

■ Other treatments reported to be beneficial in reducing the frequency of tics in patients with TS include the following:

○ Nicotine

○ Mecamylamine, a nicotinic acetylcholine antagonist

○ Tetrahydrocannabinol

○ Baclofen

○ Botulinum toxin treatment of the muscles involved in the tics

○ Clonidine and guanfacine

○ Ondansetron

■ Reports of improvement after deep brain stimulation (DBS) in patients with medically refractory TS have been published, although there does not seem to be consensus on the best target for electrode placement. Although still in the experimental phase, DBS may be a viable option for patients with medically refractory TS. It now has received a Humanitarian Device Exemption from the FDA.

■ Particular attention should be paid to the associated behavioral features because they may become the most disabling aspect of the disease. Treatment for depression, anxiety, and OCD with a selective serotonin reuptake inhibitor (SSRI) or clomipramine may be required and may be all that is needed. ADHD should be treated accordingly.

REFERENCES

1. Jankovic J. Tourette syndrome. Phenomenology and classification of tics. *Neurol Clin.* 1997; 15(2):267–275.
2. Peterson BS, Leckman JF. The temporal dynamics of tics in Gilles de la Tourette syndrome. *Biol Psychiatry.* 1998; 44(12):1337–1348.
3. The Tourette Syndrome Classification Study Group. Definitions and classification of tic disorders. *Arch Neurol.* 1993; 50:1013–1016.
4. Shapiro AK, Shapiro SE, Young JG, Feinberg TE. *Gilles de la Tourette Syndrome.* 2nd ed. New York, NY: Raven Press; 1988.
5. Leckman JF, Zhang H, Vitale A, et al. Course of tic severity in Tourette syndrome: the first two decades. *Pediatrics.* 1998; 102(1 pt 1):14–19.
6. Freeman RD, Fast DK, Burd L, et al. An international perspective on Tourette syndrome: selected findings from 3,500 individuals in 22 countries. *Dev Med Child Neurol.* 2000; 42(7):436–447.

7. Chouinard S, Ford B. Adult onset tic disorders. *J Neurol Neurosurg Psychiatry.* 2000; 68(6):738–743.

8. Costello EJ, Angold A, Burns BJ, et al. The Great Smoky Mountains Study of Youth. Goals, design, methods, and the prevalence of DSM-III-R disorders. *Arch Gen Psychiatry.* 1996; 53(12):1129–1136.

9. Mason A, Banerjee S, Eapen V, et al. The prevalence of Tourette syndrome in a mainstream school population. *Dev Med Child Neurol.* 1998; 40(5):292–296.

10. Kurlan R. Tourette's syndrome: current concepts. *Neurology.* 1989; 39(12):1625–1630.

11. Adams JR, Troiano AR, Calne DB. Functional imaging in Tourette's syndrome. *J Neural Transm.* 2004; 111(10–11):1495–1506.

12. Fernandez HH, Friedman JH. Punding on L-dopa. *Mov Disord.* 1999; 14(5):836–838.

13. Fahn S, Jankovic J. *Principles and Practice of Movement Disorders.* Philadelphia, PA: Elsevier; 2007.

10

SLEEP-RELATED MOVEMENT DISORDERS

Although most movement disorders typically disappear during sleep, some persist, and some even occur almost exclusively while the patient is asleep or falling asleep. Movement disorders that occur during sleep should be distinguished from mimickers (Figure 10.1).[1,2]

MOVEMENT DISORDERS THAT OCCUR ONLY DURING SLEEP/FALLING ASLEEP AND DISAPPEAR DURING WAKEFULNESS

REM Sleep Behavioral Disorder (RSBD)

- Sleep with rapid eye movements (REM sleep) is the stage of sleep in which dreaming occurs. It is associated with ocular movements and atonia of the other somatic muscles.

- In RSBD, muscle atonia is absent, thereby enabling the patient to unwarily "act out his or her dreams."

- The patient can wake up and injure himself or herself or, more commonly, a bed partner.

- **Polysomnography (PSG) showing excessive chin muscle tone and limb jerking during REM sleep is needed for a definitive diagnosis.**[3]

- RSBD may precede by several years a synucleinopathy (eg, Parkinson's disease, dementia with Lewy bodies, or multiple systems atrophy), and its presence in a middle-aged man implies a 52.4% risk for the development of Parkinson's disease or dementia at 12 years.[4]

- Medications commonly associated with RSBD are selective serotonin reuptake inhibitors, monoamine oxidase inhibitors, and tricyclic antidepressants.[5]

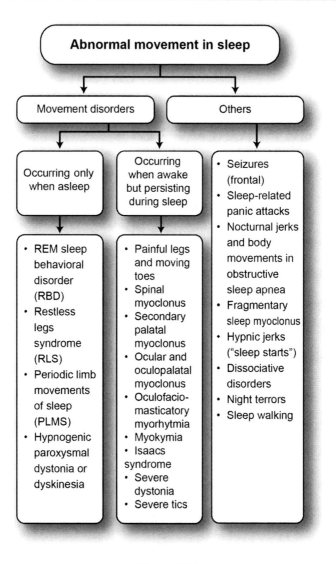

Figure 10.1
Differential diagnosis of abnormal movement in sleep.
Source: From Refs. 1, 2.

■ Treatment may not be necessary if symptoms are mild or intermittent, but it will be needed if the behavior is violent and dangerous for either the patient or the bed partner.

■ Clonazepam is the first-line medication, with doses from 0.5 to 3 mg taken every evening most often used. One evening dose of 3 to 12 mg of melatonin or 0.5 to 1.25 mg of pramipexole can also be tried.[6]

Restless Legs Syndrome (RLS)

■ RLS is now considered the most frequent movement disorder.[2]

■ It is characterized by a deep, ill-defined sensation of discomfort or dysesthesia in the legs that arises during prolonged rest or when the patient is drowsy and trying to fall asleep (Table 10.1).[7] Wayne Hening coined the acronym URGE as a convenient reminder of the key features of RLS (Table 10.2).[8]

Table 10.1
Essential Diagnostic Criteria for Restless Legs Syndrome

1	An urge to move the legs, usually accompanied or caused by uncomfortable and unpleasant sensations in the legs. (Sometimes the arms or other body parts are involved in addition to the legs.)
2	The urge to move or unpleasant sensations begin or worsen during periods of rest or inactivity such as lying or sitting.
3	The urge to move or unpleasant sensations are partially or totally relieved by movement, such as walking or stretching, at least as long as the activity continues.
4	The urge to move or unpleasant sensations are worse in the evening or night than during the day or only occur in the evening or night. (When symptoms are very severe, the worsening at night may not be noticeable but must have been previously present.)

Source: From Ref. 7: Allen RP, Picchietti D, Hening WA, Trenkwalder C, et al; Restless Legs Syndrome Diagnosis and Epidemiology workshop at the National Institutes of Health; International Restless Legs Syndrome Study Group. Restless legs syndrome: diagnostic criteria, special considerations, and epidemiology. A report from the restless legs syndrome diagnosis and epidemiology workshop at the National Institutes of Health. *Sleep Med.* 2003; 4(2):101–119.

Table 10.2
The URGE Acronym for Restless Legs Syndrome

U: Urge to move the legs, usually associated with unpleasant leg sensations.
R: Rest induces symptoms.
G: Getting active (physically and mentally) brings relief.
E: Evening and night make symptoms worse.

- The discomfort is often described as crawling, creeping, pulling, itching drawing, or stretching, among others. True pain is rare.

- Supportive clinical features of RLS include a family history and a good initial response to low doses of levodopa or a dopamine receptor agonist.

- The physical examination is generally normal and does not contribute to the diagnosis, except for comorbid conditions or causes of secondary RLS.

- RLS is generally a condition of middle to old age, but at least one-third of patients experience their first symptoms before the age of 20. If the patient is older than 50 years at symptom onset, the symptoms often develop abruptly and severely, whereas if the patient is younger than 50 years, the onset is often more insidious. Symptoms usually worsen with age.[8]

- The prevalence of RLS among the first-degree relatives of people with RLS is 3 to 5 times greater than the prevalence in people without RLS. An autosomal dominant genetic transmission is suspected, but no single causal gene has been identified.

- Periodic limb movements in sleep (PLMS) occur in 85% of patients with RLS. The clinical spectrum may also include myoclonic jerks, more sustained dystonic movements, or stereotypic movements that occur while the patient is awake.[2]

- RLS can be divided into primary and secondary forms.

  ○ Primary RLS is idiopathic and frequently familial, and it starts at a younger age.

  ○ Secondary, or symptomatic, RLS is associated with iron deficiency anemia, pregnancy, or end-stage renal disease, and also with chronic myelopathies, peripheral neuropathies, gastric surgery, chronic lung disease, and some drugs (Figure 10.2).

- The diagnosis of RLS is clinical. PSG is not necessary. The differences between RLS and akathisia are listed in Table 10.3. RLS must also be distinguished from the syndrome of painful legs and moving toes (see below).

- The treatment of secondary RLS requires addressing its cause (stopping the offending medication, correcting iron deficiency, treating uremia, etc).

- **Dopamine agonists are the first-line pharmacotherapy. They are associated with less risk for augmentation** (defined as an increase in the severity of symptoms, a shift in the time when symptoms start to earlier in the day, a shorter latency to the start of symptoms during rest, and sometimes the spread of symptoms to other body parts) than levodopa, which is also effective.[2,8]

- Gabapentin and gabapentin enacarbil are second-line therapy and can be especially beneficial in cases of painful RLS.[9,10]

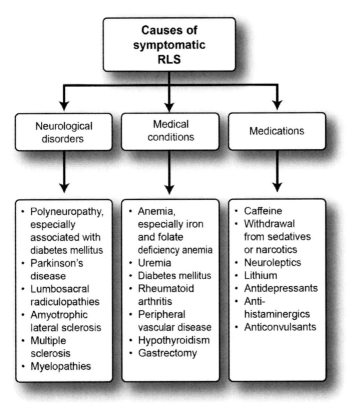

Figure 10.2

Causes of symptomatic restless legs syndrome.

Source: From Ref. 1: Bhidayasiri R. Movement disorders. In: Bhidayasiri R, Waters MF, Giza C, eds. Neurological Differential Diagnosis: A Prioritized Approach. Hoboken, NJ: Wiley-Blackwell; 2005: 203–239.

- A recent study found pregabalin to be beneficial with less risk of augmentation than pramipexole.[11]

- Opiates and benzodiazepines can be used as third-line therapy.

- The off-label use of an antiepileptic drug, such as topiramate, can be considered in cases of refractory RLS, especially if it is painful.[12]

- Iron infusion must be reserved for severe cases unresponsive to other therapies and associated with low plasma levels of ferritin. A high-dose intravenous infusion of iron dextran (1,000 mg) or iron sucrose (5 infusions of 200 mg each over 3 weeks) can be used, the former being more effective but carrying a higher risk for anaphylactic shock. Patients receiving ferritin should

Table 10.3
Restless Legs Syndrome Versus Akathisia

Features	Restless Legs Syndrome	Akathisia
Definition	See Tables 10.1 and 10.2.	Inner restlessness, fidgetiness with jittery feeling, or generalized restlessness
Occurs as a side effect of neuroleptics	Less common	More common
Disease course	Chronic and progressive	Can be acute, chronic, or tardive
Character of restlessness	Tossing, turning in bed, floor pacing, leg stretching, leg flexion, foot rubbing, need to get up and walk	Swaying and rocking movements, crossing and uncrossing the legs, shifting body positions, inability to sit still; resembles mild chorea
Schedule	Mostly in the evening or at night	Mostly during the day
Worsening factor	Inactivity or rest.	Anxiety or stress
Alleviating factor	Moving the legs, walking	Moving around, walking

Source: Adapted from Ref. 1: Bhidayasiri R. Movement disorders. In: Bhidayasiri R, Waters MF, Giza C, eds. *Neurological Differential Diagnosis: A Prioritized Approach.* Hoboken, NJ: Wiley-Blackwell; 2005:203–239.

be monitored closely during therapy to avoid hemochromatosis. Oral iron does not seem to be effective except to correct an iron deficiency anemia.[7]

Periodic Limb Movements of Sleep (PLMS) (Table 10.4)

■ PLMS can affect one or both legs.

■ Movements are brief (1–2 seconds).

  ○ Dorsiflexion of big toe and foot.

  ○ Flexion of hip and knee also possible. The movement then resembles a flexion reflex.

  ○ Occurs every 20 seconds, for minutes or hours.

■ Can wake up bed partner and may cause a sleep disturbance in the patient, who then experiences excessive daytime drowsiness.

■ The diagnosis is confirmed by PSG. PLMS usually occurs during stages I and II of sleep and decreases in stages III and IV. Unusual in REM sleep.

■ Occasionally seen in an awake, drowsy patient.[2]

■ Although PLMS can be seen alone, RLS occurs in 30% of cases of PLMS.

Table 10.4
Periodic Movements of Sleep

- Brief (lasting 1–2 seconds) jerks in one or both legs
- Occur in runs (every 20 seconds) for minutes to hours
- Initial jerk followed by tonic spasm
- Dorsiflexion of big toe and foot (or flexion of whole leg)
- Occurs during light sleep (stages I and II)
- Occasionally seen in an awake, drowsy patient
- Usually asymptomatic, may wake sleeping partner or, less often, the patient
- Prevalence increases with age: younger than 30 years, rare; 30 to 50 years, 5%; older than 50 years, 29%

Source: Adapted from Ref. 2: Fahn S, Jankovic J, Hallet M, eds. *Principles and Practice of Movement Disorders.* 2nd ed. Philadelphia, PA: Elsevier; 2011.

- When the condition is isolated, patients are usually asymptomatic and do not require treatment. If needed, the treatment is the same as for RLS (see above).

Hypnogenic Paroxysmal Dystonia or Dyskinesia

- Occurs as a paroxysm during sleep and last only a few minutes.

- Hypnogenic dystonia can be complex and is characterized by sustained contractions, similar to those occurring in torsion dystonia.

- Patients who have hypnogenic paroxysmal dyskinesia can present with bilateral tonic posturing and gross proximal limb movements.

- The movements may or may not awaken the patient.

- Longer (2–50 minutes) attacks occur in a minority of individuals with paroxysmal hypnogenic dyskinesia and do not respond to medication.

- Antiepileptic drugs seem to be effective treatment.

- Multiple studies, including video electroencephalography (EEG), have demonstrated that most of these short- and long-acting events, historically described as "movement disorders," were in fact frontal lobe seizures.[2]

MOVEMENT DISORDERS OCCURRING DURING WAKEFULNESS BUT FREQUENTLY PERSISTING DURING SLEEP

Painful Legs and Moving Toes

- The toes of one foot or both feet are in continual flexion–extension with abduction–adduction, associated with a continuous deep pain in the ipsilateral leg.

- Movements are stereotyped, sinusoidal, and athetoid, with a frequency of 1 to 2 Hz. They may occasionally involve more proximal parts of the legs.[13]

- There is a sensory component described as deeply aching, burning, throbbing, crushing, or tearing. It may occasionally be mild or even absent.

- The leg pain is much more troublesome to the patient than are the constant movements and usually precedes them.

- Usually, adults are affected.

- Unlike in RLS, there is no urge to move, and movement does not relieve the symptoms.

- On examination, there is frequent hyperpathia or allodynia of the painful region.

- In the vast majority of the cases, the condition is secondary to a lesion in the lumbar roots or peripheral nerves, including neuropathy, root compression, herpes zoster, and cauda equina lesions, as well as minor trauma to the legs.

- An analogous disorder, "painful arms and moving fingers," has also been described and appears to be secondary to brachial plexus and cervical root lesions.[14]

- **Pain is the major source of disability and is very hard to treat. Antiepileptic drugs, such as carbamazepine and gabapentin,[15] can be tried as well as amitriptyline, nerve or epidural blocks, epidural cord stimulation, transcutaneous electrical nerve stimulation (TENS) units, and guanethidine infusions. Botulinum toxin injections can mitigate both movement and pain in some patients.[2]**

Myoclonus

- Myoclonic jerks are sudden, brief, shocklike involuntary movements caused by muscular contractions (*positive myoclonus*) or inhibitions (*negative myoclonus*).

- Myoclonic jerks are usually irregular (arrhythmic) but can be rhythmic, such as in palatal myoclonus or ocular myoclonus, with a rate of approximately 2 Hz.

- Rhythmic myoclonus is typically due to a structural lesion of the brainstem or spinal cord (and is therefore also called segmental myoclonus), but not all cases of segmental myoclonus are rhythmic.

- Myoclonus is detailed in Chapter 7. Here, we discuss only the types of myoclonus that usually persist during sleep.

SPINAL MYOCLONUS

- Spinal myoclonus is secondary to lesions of the spinal cord and/or peripheral nerves.

- Causes include peripheral nerve tumors, trauma, or radiation and spinal cord trauma, tumors, vascular lesions, multiple sclerosis, and myelitis.

- Spinal myoclonus is rhythmic (0.5–3 Hz) and confined to muscles innervated by a few spinal segments. It persists during sleep.

- It is usually not stimulus-sensitive.

- Clonazepam is the most effective treatment.[2]

SECONDARY PALATAL MYOCLONUS

- Palatal myoclonus (also known as palatal tremor) consists of rhythmic palatal movements at about 1.5 to 3 Hz.[16]

- There are two forms: *essential palatal myoclonus* and *symptomatic (secondary) palatal myoclonus* (Figure 10.3).

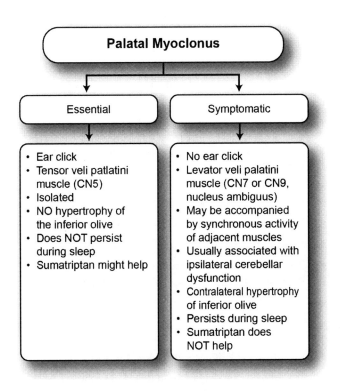

Figure 10.3
Essential versus symptomatic palatal myoclonus.

○ Essential palatal myoclonus

- There is no evident cause.

- It affects only the palate.

- **The only symptom is ear clicking secondary to contraction of the tensor veli palatini muscle, which elevates the roof of the soft palate and opens the eustachian tube.**

- The ear clicking does *not* persist during sleep.

- Patients are younger.

- Treatment is with clonazepam, anticholinergics, carbamazepine, or botulinum injection in the tensor veli palatini muscle. Sumatriptan may help.[2]

○ Secondary palatal myoclonus

- Secondary to a brainstem lesion such as stroke, encephalitis, multiple sclerosis, tumor, trauma, or degenerative disease.

- The brainstem lesion results in denervation and hypertrophy of the inferior olive, which can be seen on brain MRI.

- **There usually is no ear clicking. The palatal movements are secondary to contractions of the levator veli palatini, which lifts and pulls back the soft palate.**

- Secondary palatal myoclonus is frequently not limited to the palate; the eyes, face, tongue, and larynx, and even the head, trunk, intercostal muscles, and diaphragm, can also be involved, depending on the underlying lesion.

- The movements usually are synchronous, bilateral, and symmetric, occurring between 100 and 150 times per minute.

- These movements persist during sleep.

- Patients are older.

- Treatment is with clonazepam, anticholinergics, carbamazepine, or botulinum injection in the levator veli palatini muscle. Sumatriptan does not help.[2]

OCULAR MYOCLONUS

- Rhythmic vertical oscillations occur at a rate of 2 Hz.

- Ocular myoclonus is due to a lesion in the dentato-olivary pathway.

- It can be associated with secondary palatal myoclonus and is treated similarly.

Oculofaciomasticatory Myorhythmia

- Myorhythmia

  - Myorhythmia is a movement that is slow in frequency (<3 Hz), prolonged, rhythmic, or repetitive, without the sharp square-wave appearance of a myoclonic jerk.[2]

  - It is slower than most tremors (parkinsonian, essential, cerebellar).

- Most frequent are *oculofaciomasticatory* myorhythmias.

  - They are typically seen in Whipple disease.

  - Slow-moving, repetitive, synchronous, and rhythmic contractions occur in ocular, facial, masticatory, and other muscles.[17]

  - *Ocular myorhythmia:* continuous, 1-Hz, horizontal, pendular, vergence oscillations of the eyes, usually of small amplitude, without divergence beyond the primary position. Divergence and convergence occur at the same speed. There is no pupillary miosis during these movements.

  - Movements in the face, jaw, and skeletal muscles occur at about at the same frequency but may be somewhat quicker and more like rhythmic myoclonus.[2]

  - Vertical supranuclear ophthalmoplegia is frequently present.

  - Central nervous system Whipple disease is treated with antibiotics, typically 2 g of ceftriaxone given intravenously daily for 2 weeks followed by oral trimethoprim/sulfamethoxazole for 1 to 2 years. There is no clear symptomatic treatment for myorhythmia.

Myokymia

- Myokymia is characterized by fine, persistent quivering or wavelike rippling of muscles ("live flesh").

- On electromyography (EMG), groups of motor unit discharges, especially doublets and triplets, occur at a regular rhythm.

- Myokymia is most commonly seen in facial muscles. Most facial myokymias are due to pontine lesions, particularly multiple sclerosis and less often pontine glioma.[2]

  - When due to multiple sclerosis, the myokymia tends to abate after weeks or months.

  - When due to a pontine glioma, it may persist indefinitely and can be associated with facial contracture.

- There is no well-defined symptomatic treatment for myokymia.

- Myokymia is also a feature of neuromyotonia (see below).

Neuromyotonia and Isaacs Syndrome

- Neuromyotonia

  - Syndrome of failure of muscle relaxation with myokymia and fasciculations.

  - Originates in the peripheral nerve (not the muscle).

  - High-frequency discharges (150–300 Hz) on EMG.

  - Clinically manifests as continuous muscle activity causing stiffness and cramps.

  - The best known neuromyotonic disorder is Isaacs syndrome.

- Isaacs syndrome

  - Isaacs syndrome has multiple other names: "continuous muscle fiber activity," "myokymia with impaired muscle relaxation," "pseudomyotonia and myokymia."

  - Gradual onset of the following:

    - Muscle stiffness at rest

    - Continuous twitching (fasciculation) or rippling (myokymia) of muscles

    - Cramps following voluntary contractions due to delay in muscle relaxation (pseudomyotonia); no percussion myotonia[2]

  - Pain is rare, but muscle aching is common.

  - Muscle contraction is predominantly distal, but proximal and cranial muscles can be affected. Involvement can be focal and mimic focal dystonia.[18]

  - **On EMG, the hallmark is the presence of continuous motor unit activity that persists during sleep.** Fasciculations, myokymia, and neuromyotonia are present. Prolonged high-frequency after-discharges following nerve stimulation, voluntary contraction, or muscle percussion are characteristic. Nerve conduction study (NCS) can shows signs of associated peripheral neuropathy.

  - The serum creatine phosphokinase (CPK) is increased.

  - The condition may be inherited or sporadic. It can be isolated or associated with many types of inherited, inflammatory, or metabolic peripheral neuropathies.

- Isaacs syndrome can also be paraneoplastic. A search for a remote neoplasm is required.

  ○ Sporadic cases appear to be autoimmune in nature, most frequently associated with voltage-gated potassium ion channels (VGKCs).[19,20]

  ○ Symptomatic treatment is with carbamazepine and phenytoin.[2] Focal neuromyotonia can be treated with injection of botulinum toxin.[21] Plasmapheresis or intravenous immunoglobulin may be effective when the disorder is autoimmune.[22,23]

  ○ Neuromyotonia without malignancy or peripheral neuropathy may be relatively benign.

Dystonia

- Involuntary phasic or tonic muscle contractions lead to an irregular tremor or abnormal posture.

- Dystonia is discussed in Chapter 5.

- Although dystonia usually resolves with sleep, it may persist during sleep in severe cases.

Tics

- Involuntary, repetitive, nonrhythmic movement or vocalization preceded by an urge to perform the action and followed by a feeling of relief.

- Tics are discussed in Chapter 9.

- Although tics usually resolve with sleep, they may persist during sleep in severe cases.

REFERENCES

1. Bhidayasiri R. Movement disorders. In: Bhidayasiri R, Waters MF, Giza C, eds. *Neurological Differential Diagnosis: A Prioritized Approach.* Hoboken, NJ: Wiley-Blackwell; 2005:203–239.
2. Fahn S, Jankovic J, Hallet M, eds. *Principles and Practice of Movement Disorders.* 2nd ed. Philadelphia, PA: Elsevier; 2011.
3. Eisensehr I, von Lindeiner H, Jäger M, Noachtar S. REM sleep behavior disorder in sleep-disordered patients with versus without Parkinson's disease: is there a need for polysomnography? *J Neurol Sci.* 2001; 186:7–11.
4. Postuma RB, Gagnon JF, Vendette M, Fantini ML, et al. Quantifying the risk of neurodegenerative disease in idiopathic REM sleep behavior disorder. *Neurology.* 2009; 72:1296–1300.
5. Mayers AG, Baldwin DS. Antidepressants and their effect on sleep. *Hum Psychopharmacol.* 2005; 20(8):533–559.

6. Mehanna R, Ondo W. Sleep problems in Parkinson's disease patients. *Neurodegener Dis Manag.* 2011; 1(4):307–321.

7. Allen RP, Picchietti D, Hening WA, Trenkwalder C, et al; Restless Legs Syndrome Diagnosis and Epidemiology workshop at the National Institutes of Health; International Restless Legs Syndrome Study Group. Restless legs syndrome: diagnostic criteria, special considerations, and epidemiology. A report from the restless legs syndrome diagnosis and epidemiology workshop at the National Institutes of Health. *Sleep Med.* 2003; 4(2):101–119.

8. Trenkwalder C, Paulus W. Restless legs syndrome: pathophysiology, clinical presentation and management. *Nat Rev Neurol.* 2010; 6(6):337–346.

9. Garcia-Borreguero D, Larrosa O, de la Llave Y, Verger K, et al. Treatment of restless legs syndrome with gabapentin: a double-blind, cross-over study. *Neurology.* 2002; 59(10):1573–1579.

10. Walters AS, Ondo WG, Kushida CA, Becker PM, et al; XP045 Study Group. Gabapentin enacarbil in restless legs syndrome: a phase 2b, 2-week, randomized, double-blind, placebo-controlled trial. *Clin Neuropharmacol.* 2009; 32(6):311–320.

11. Allen RP, Chen C, Garcia-Borreguero D, Polo O, et al. Comparison of pregabalin with pramipexole for restless legs syndrome. *N Engl J Med.* 2014 Feb 13;370(7):621–631.

12. Sommer M, Bachmann CG, Liebetanz KM, Schindehütte J, et al. Pregabalin in restless legs syndrome with and without neuropathic pain. *Acta Neurol Scand.* 2007; 115(5):347–350.

13. Alvarez MV, Driver-Dunckley EE, Caviness JN, Adler CH, et al. Case series of painful legs and moving toes: clinical and electrophysiologic observations. *Mov Disord.* 2008; 23(14):2062–2066.

14. Supiot F, Gazagnes MD, Blecic SA, Zegers de Beyl D. Painful arm and moving fingers: clinical features of four new cases. *Mov Disord.* 2002; 17(3):616–618.

15. Villarejo A, Porta-Etessam J, Camacho A, González de la Aleja J, et al. Gabapentin for painful legs and moving toes syndrome. *Eur Neurol.* 2004; 51(3):180–181.

16. Deuschl G, Toro C, Hallett M. Symptomatic and essential palatal tremor. 2. Differences of palatal movements. *Mov Disord.* 1994; 9:676–678.

17. Tison F, Louvet-Giendaj C, Henry P, Lagueny A, et al. Permanent bruxism as a manifestation of the oculo-facial syndrome related to systemic Whipple's disease. *Mov Disord.* 1992; 7(1):82–85.

18. Jamora RD, Umapathi T, Tan LC. Finger flexion resembling focal dystonia in Isaacs' syndrome. *Parkinsonism Relat Disord.* 2006; 12(1):61–63.

19. Newsom-Davis J, Buckley C, Clover L, Hart I, et al. Autoimmune disorders of neuronal potassium channels. *Ann N Y Acad Sci.* 2003; 998:202–210.

20. Rueff L, Graber JJ, Bernbaum M, Kuzniecky RI. Voltage-gated potassium channel antibody-mediated syndromes: a spectrum of clinical manifestations. *Rev Neurol Dis.* 2008; 5(2):65–72.

21. Hobson DE, Kerr P, Hobson S. Successful use of botulinum toxin for post-irradiation unilateral jaw neuromyotonia. *Parkinsonism Relat Disord.* 2009; 15(8):617–618.

22. Hayat GR, Kulkantrakorn K, Campbell WW, Giuliani MJ. Neuromyotonia: autoimmune pathogenesis and response to immune modulating therapy. *J Neurol Sci.* 2000; 181(1-2):38–43.

23. Alessi G, De Reuck J, De Bleecker J, Vancayzeele S. Successful immunoglobulin treatment in a patient with neuromyotonia. *Clin Neurol Neurosurg.* 2000; 102(3):173–175.

III

Psychiatric Approach to Movement Disorders

11

THE PSYCHIATRIC ASSESSMENT

INTRODUCTION

- Psychiatric disorders are frequently encountered in patients with movement disorders and often mask or exacerbate neurological complaints.

- Conducting a psychiatric interview can be a daunting task for many physicians, who are accustomed to a more "hands-on" approach to the patient examination.

- It is critical for every physician working with these patients to have the basic skills required to assess psychiatric symptoms in order to screen for and measure the severity of emotional distress.

- The longitudinal monitoring of psychiatric problems will assist in the treatment of the underlying neurological condition.

THE PSYCHIATRIC INTERVIEW

- The first step in any interview is to establish rapport and develop therapeutic alliance with the patient. This is achieved by a number of fundamental interventions:

  - Establish a comfortable environment with minimal distractions.
  - Display a receptive posture and face the patient.
  - Maintain eye contact.
  - Remain calm and avoid reaction.
  - Acknowledge and normalize (if appropriate) the patient's concerns.

- In most cases, it is helpful to begin the visit by first discussing the "medical" or neurological concerns. These are typically easier for patients to discuss before more sensitive emotional or behavioral topics are approached.

■ The transition from gathering a "medical" history to obtaining a psychiatric history should be undertaken carefully and with empathy in order to allow the patient to experience the interviewer's genuine interest. An abrupt or hasty "review of symptoms" of psychiatric disorders will yield only superficial data. Several ways to make this transition include the following:

   ○ "It seems as if you have been struggling for some time with (medical condition); how does that make you feel?"

   ○ "How did you cope when you discovered you had (medical condition)?"

   ○ "Your quality of life seems to have been affected by the diagnosis of (medical condition). Can you tell me more about that?"

   ○ "It is normal for people with (medical condition) to experience (psychological symptom). Have you experienced anything like this?"

■ External factors, such as a family history of psychosocial burden, play an influential role in the development of psychiatric conditions.

■ Table 11.1 lists sample questions that may be asked during a psychiatric assessment.

Table 11.1
Sample Questions to Ask in the Psychiatric Assessment
of a Patient With Parkinson's Disease

- When was the onset of Parkinson's disease (PD) symptoms? How was PD diagnosed?
- What type of motor symptoms developed, and how quickly did they progress?
- Which PD medications have been tried to date?
- Have there been any adverse medication side effects, such as hallucinations, psychosis, and/or impulse control difficulties?
- Are there frequent on–off fluctuations that trigger distress?
- How did the patient initially cope with the diagnosis?
- What is the level of acceptance of the diagnosis?
- What functional limitations have occurred as result of the motor symptoms?
- What is the current level of socialization?
- Are there any cognitive changes or concerns?
- How have family/occupational demands been affected by the symptoms?
- Are there feelings of being a burden to the family?
- Has the patient had any thoughts of not wanting to live? Suicidal thoughts?
- Is there a history of psychiatric difficulties before the diagnosis of PD?
- Has the patient ever received formal psychiatric care or treatment?
- What are the patient's goals regarding treatment?
- Is the patient optimistic about his or her future?

MENTAL STATUS EXAMINATION

- The Mental Status Examination (MSE) is a comprehensive evaluation of the patient's current state of psychiatric functioning, based on the examiner's observations and responses directly elicited from the patient.

- Documenting a thorough and descriptive MSE is important in accurately capturing a patient's current mental state, which will assist not only in the diagnosis and management of the underlying psychiatric condition but also in the longitudinal monitoring of a patient's stability.

- The components of the MSE are listed in Table 11.2.

Table 11.2
Components of a Mental Status Examination

Domain	Description/Examples
Orientation	Intact, disoriented, confused
Attention	Alert, engaged, awake, drowsy, lethargic, sedated, sleepy
Appearance	Well nourished, well groomed, well dressed, unkempt, malodorous, obese, tired, cachectic, pale
Behavior	Gentle, confrontational, hostile, combative, passive, apathetic, restless, relaxed, casual
Attitude	Agreeable, pleasant, cooperative, difficult, threatening, suspicious, shy, resigned, assertive, stubborn
Speech	Appropriate rate and tone, underproductive, spontaneous, rapid, slow, overly inclusive, slurred, rambling, soft, incoherent
Mood	Usually taken directly from the patient's report ("depressed," "anxious," "irritated," "angry," "good")
Affect	Usually derived from the examiner's observations (mood-congruent, mood-incongruent, restricted, blunted, flat, labile, intense, bright, serious, animated, aloof, worried)
Thought process/form	Linear, goal-directed, ruminative, circumstantial, loose, tangential, disorganized
Thought content	Paranoid, delusional, grandiose, nihilistic, somatically preoccupied, religiously preoccupied, magical thinking
Suicidality and homicidality	Presence of any suicidal/ homicidal thinking, intent, and/or plan
Insight and judgment	Intact, limited, good, fair, appropriate, impaired
Memory	Status of remote memory, recent memory, and immediate memory
Fund of knowledge	Appropriate, above average, below average, developmentally appropriate
Impulse control	Intact, poor, unpredictable

Special Situations: Asking About Suicide

- As a result of the progressive impact of most movement disorders on functioning and quality of life, it is critical to ask about suicide at every visit.

- Be direct! Ask patients if they have thoughts about suicide. Practitioners should not fear that asking someone about suicide will trigger suicide.

- Although the word *suicide* can be dramatic and intense, using it nonjudgmentally and openly will make patients feel more comfortable discussing it.

- If suicidal ideation is endorsed, ask about the patient's level of intent to act on these thoughts or whether there is a plan. Inquire about any access to weapons or a past history of suicide attempts or violence that may elevate the risk.

- Inquire about any protective factors that may prevent someone from acting on suicidal thoughts, such as children or spirituality/religion.

- Evidence of imminent intent and/or plan should trigger acute intervention and stabilization, such as psychiatric hospitalization.

Special Situations: Asking About Trauma

- Asking about *exposure* to trauma (including emotional, verbal, physical, and sexual abuse and domestic violence) should be part of an initial neurological evaluation; however, the clinician should avoid pushing the patient to recount details of the trauma (ie, giving a trauma narrative).

- Many patients may deny trauma altogether in an effort to avoid talking about the experience or to avoid triggering symptoms of posttraumatic stress disorder (PTSD).

- Rarely, patients may volunteer too much detail about a history of trauma, not realizing the possibility for psychiatric decompensation, which may include the following:

  - Emotional dysregulation

  - Self-harm behaviors

  - Intrusive thoughts, memories, nightmares, or flashbacks

- If a patient begins to divulge an excessive trauma history too early in treatment, it is best to respectfully (while validating the patient's honesty) change the course of the interview. It may be helpful to offer a referral to an experienced mental health provider to further address/manage the psychological trauma.

DIAGNOSIS

- Psychiatric diagnoses are defined by the *Diagnostic and Statistical Manual of Mental Disorders, Fifth Edition (DSM-5)*.[1] Tables 11.3 through 11.8 briefly highlight some of the psychiatric conditions that may be encountered in patients with movement disorders.

- It is important to keep in mind that many of the diagnostic descriptions/criteria may somewhat differ when seen in patients with neurological conditions. For example, patients with neurodegenerative disorders may display changes in somatic symptoms (eg, sleep, appetite, concentration, energy) that may be a product of the neurological condition and not necessarily a primary psychiatric condition.

Table 11.3
Mood Disorders

Major Depressive Disorder	• Two-week period of change in functioning with depressed mood and/or loss of interest in pleasurable activities • Other symptoms: sleep disturbance, appetite change, concentration difficulties, fatigue, agitation/retardation, excessive guilt, and/or suicidal thinking
Persistent Depressive Disorder (Dysthymia)	• Two-year period of depressed mood for more days than not (1 year for children) • Other symptoms: sleep disturbance, appetite change, concentration difficulties, fatigue, low self-esteem, feelings of hopelessness
Bipolar Disorder (Mania/Hypomania)	• Distinct period of elevated, expansive, or irritable mood (1 week for mania, 4 days for hypomania) • Common symptoms: inflated self-esteem, insomnia, pressured speech, racing thoughts, distractibility, and/or risk-taking behaviors
Mood Disorder with Anxious Distress	• Criteria met for specific mood disorder (Major Depressive Disorder, Persistent Depressive Disorder, Bipolar Disorder) • Accompanied by feeling keyed up, tense, and unusually restless; difficulty concentrating; having catastrophic fears and/or a feeling of losing control
Disruptive Mood Dysregulation Disorder	• Severe recurrent temper outbursts • Grossly out of proportion to situation • Diagnosis made after age 6 or before age 18

Table 11.4
Anxiety Disorders

Generalized Anxiety Disorder	• Six-month period of excessive anxiety or worry over multiple situations • Accompanying symptoms: restlessness, fatigue, mind going blank, muscle tension, irritability, and/or sleep disturbance
Social Anxiety	• Marked fear about social situation(s) • Worry about scrutiny from others, being humiliated or embarrassed • Anxiety is out of proportion to threat of situation
Phobias	• Marked fear about specific object or situation • Anxiety is out of proportion to actual danger
Panic Disorder	• Abrupt surge of intense fear or discomfort • Common symptoms: palpitations, sweating, shaking, sensations of shortness of breath, nausea, dizziness, fear of losing control or dying • Persistent concern about future attacks
Agoraphobia	• Marked fear or anxiety about using public transportation, being in open/enclosed spaces, standing in line, being in a crowd, and/or being away from home alone

Table 11.5
Obsessive–Compulsive, Impulse Control, and Addictive Disorders

Obsessive–Compulsive Disorder	• Intrusive thoughts, urges, or images ("obsession") • Repetitive behaviors or mental acts performed to neutralize anxiety ("compulsion") • Behaviors are time-consuming or functionally impairing
Obsessional Jealousy	• Nondelusional preoccupation with partner's perceived infidelity
Intermittent Explosive Disorder	• Recurrent behavioral outbursts (verbal or physical) • Grossly out of proportion to precipitator
Impulse Control Disorder, unspecified	• Failure to resist an impulse, drive, or temptation to perform an act that is harmful to the self or to others

Table 11.6
Psychotic, Trauma-Related, and Stressor-Related Disorders

Schizophrenia	• Six-month presence of two or more of the following: delusions, hallucinations, disorganized speech, disorganized behavior, or diminished emotional expression • Functionally impairing symptoms
Delusional Disorder	• One-month duration of delusional thinking • Outside the context of the delusion, behavior is not obviously bizarre, odd, and/or functionally impairing
Posttraumatic Stress Disorder (PTSD)	• Exposure to serious threat, injury, or violence • Combination of reexperiencing phenomena, avoidance behavior, negative alterations in mood or thought, and hyperarousal symptoms
Adjustment Disorder	• Development of emotional or behavioral symptoms in response to stressor within 3 months of the onset of stressor

Table 11.7
Somatic Symptom Disorder and Related Disorders

Somatic Symptom Disorder	• Distressing somatic symptoms • Excessive thoughts, feelings, or behaviors related to somatic symptom • Disproportionate and persistent thoughts about the seriousness of somatic symptom • Persistently high levels of anxiety related to health or symptoms
Illness Anxiety Disorder	• Preoccupation with having a serious illness • Minimal, if any, evidence of somatic symptoms • High level of anxiety about health
Functional Neurological Symptom Disorder (Conversion Disorder)	• Symptom of altered motor or sensory function • Incompatibility between the symptom and recognized neurological condition • Symptom types: weakness/paralysis, abnormal movement, swallowing, speech, attacks/seizures, sensory loss, mixed symptoms

Table 11.8
Neurodevelopmental and Neurocognitive Disorders

Attention-Deficit/ Hyperactivity Disorder (ADHD)	• Persistent pattern of inattention and/or hyperactivity–impulsivity • Inattention: careless mistakes, poor concentration, distractible, disorganized, forgetful • Hyperactivity/impulsivity: fidgety, restless, talkative, intrusive, impatient • Symptoms occur in more than one setting
Mild Neurocognitive Disorder	• Modest cognitive decline in one or more cognitive domains • Deficits do not interfere with independence
Major Neurocognitive Disorder	• Significant cognitive decline in one or more cognitive domains • Deficits interfere with independence

TREATMENT

See Tables 11.9 through 11.11.[2,3]

Table 11.9
Medications Commonly Used to Treat Depression and Anxiety

Generic Name	Brand Name	Usual Total Daily Dosing Range[a]	Approved Indication(s)[2]	Off-Label Psychiatric Uses[a]
Selective serotonin reuptake inhibitors (SSRIs)				
Citalopram	Celexa	10–40 mg (doses >20 mg contraindicated >60 y/o)	Major Depression	Anxiety Disorders
Escitalopram	Lexapro	5–20 mg	Major Depression, GAD	Anxiety Disorders
Fluoxetine	Prozac	10–80 mg	Major Depression, OCD, Panic Disorder	
Fluvoxamine	Luvox	25–300 mg	OCD	Major Depression, Anxiety Disorders
Paroxetine	Paxil, Paxil CR	10–60 mg (CR: 12.5–50 mg)	Major Depression, OCD, PTSD, Anxiety Disorders	
Sertraline	Zoloft	25–200 mg	Major Depression, OCD, PTSD, Anxiety Disorders	

continued

Table 11.9 (cont.)
Commonly Used to Treat Depression and Anxiety

Generic Name	Brand Name	Usual Total Daily Dosing Range[a]	Approved Indication(s)[2]	Off-Label Psychiatric Uses[a]
Serotonin–norepinephrine reuptake inhibitors (SNRIs)				
Desvenlafaxine	Pristiq	50–100 mg	Major Depression	Anxiety Disorders
Duloxetine	Cymbalta	20–120 mg	Major Depression, GAD, neuropathic pain, fibromyalgia	
Venlafaxine	Effexor XR	37.5–300 mg	Major Depression, Anxiety Disorders	
Benzodiazepines				
Alprazolam	Xanax	0.25–8 mg	Anxiety Disorders	
Clonazepam	Klonopin	0.25–4 mg	Anxiety Disorders, seizures	Insomnia, sleep disorders
Diazepam	Valium	2–40 mg	Anxiety Disorders, convulsive disorders, muscle spasms	Insomnia, sleep disorders
Lorazepam	Ativan	0.5–8 mg	Anxiety Disorders	
Others				
Amitriptyline	Elavil	10–150 mg	Major Depression	Insomnia
Bupropion	Wellbutrin SR, Wellbutrin XL	SR: 50–400 mg XL: 150–450 mg	Major Depression	Apathy, inattention
Buspirone	Buspar	15–60 mg	Anxiety Disorders	
Clomipramine	Anafranil	12.5–250 mg	OCD	
Gabapentin	Neurontin	100–2,400 mg	Partial seizures, post-herpetic neuralgia	Anxiety
Mirtazapine	Remeron	7.5–45 mg	Major Depression	Anxiety Disorders
Trazodone	Desyrel	25–300 mg	Major Depression	Insomnia
Vilazodone	Viibryd	10–40 mg	Major Depression	

Abbreviations: GAD, Generalized Anxiety Disorder; OCD, Obsessive–Compulsive Disorder; PTSD, Posttraumatic Stress Disorder.

[a]Based on author experience in the population of patients with movement disorders.

Source: Adapted from Ref. 2: *Physicians' Desk Reference.* 67th ed. Montvale, NJ: PDR Network; 2013.

Table 11.10
Medications Commonly Used to Treat Irritability, Impulsivity, and Psychosis

Generic Name	Brand Name	Usual Total Daily Dosing Range[a]	Approved Indication(s)[2]	Off-Label Psychiatric Uses[a]
Mood stabilizers				
Carbamazepine	Tegretol	250–1,000 mg	Epilepsy	Mania
Lamotrigine	Lamictal	12.5–300 mg	Bipolar disorder, epilepsy	Irritable depression
Lithium	Lithobid	300–1,800 mg	Mania	Impulse control
Topiramate	Topamax	25–300 mg	Epilepsy	Anxiety, irritability
Valproate	Depakote	250–2,000 mg	Mania, epilepsy	Impulse control
Conventional ("typical") antipsychotics (avoid in parkinsonian states!)				
Fluphenazine	Prolixin	2.5–10 mg	Psychotic disorders	Aggressive behavior, impulse control, hallucinations, delusions
Haloperidol	Haldol	0.5–10 mg	Schizophrenia, tic disorders	Aggressive behavior, impulse control, hallucinations, delusions
Perphenazine	Trilafon	4–16 mg	Schizophrenia	Hallucinations, delusions
Pimozide	Orap	1–8 mg	Tics in Tourette syndrome	Hallucinations, delusions
Trifluoperazine	Stelazine	2–12 mg	Schizophrenia, acute anxiety	Hallucinations, delusions
Atypical antipsychotics (may worsen parkinsonism in parkinsonian disorders)				
Aripiprazole	Abilify	2–20 mg	Schizophrenia, acute mania, augmentation of depression	Impulse control, hallucinations, delusions
Asenapine	Saphris	5–20 mg	Schizophrenia, acute mania	Hallucinations, delusions
Clozapine	Clozaril	12.5–200 mg	Schizophrenia	Tardive dyskinesia, hallucinations, delusions
Iloperidone	Fanapt	2–16 mg	Schizophrenia	Hallucinations, delusions

continued

Table 11.10 (cont.)
Medications Commonly Used to Treat Irritability, Impulsivity, and Psychosis

Generic Name	Brand Name	Usual Total Daily Dosing Range[a]	Approved Indication(s)[2]	Off-Label Psychiatric Uses[a]
Lurasidone	Latuda	20–80 mg	Schizophrenia, bipolar depression	Hallucinations, delusions
Olanzapine	Zyprexa	2.5–20 mg	Schizophrenia, acute mania	Aggressive behavior, impulse control, hallucinations, delusions
Quetiapine	Seroquel	12.5–400 mg	Schizophrenia, acute mania	Insomnia, anxiety, hallucinations, delusions
Risperidone	Risperdal	0.5–8 mg	Schizophrenia, acute mania	Aggressive behavior, impulse control, hallucinations, delusions
Ziprasidone	Geodon	20–160 mg	Schizophrenia, acute mania	Hallucinations, delusions

[a]Based on author experience in the population of patients with movement disorders.

Source: Adapted from Ref. 2: *Physicians' Desk Reference*. 67th ed. Montvale, NJ: PDR Network; 2013.

Table 11.11
Medications Used to Treat Attention-Deficit/Hyperactivity Disorder (ADHD)

Generic Name	Brand Name	Dose Range	
		Adults	Children and Adolescents
Stimulants			
Amphetamine/ dextroamphetamine	Adderall	5–60 mg	3–5 mg until optimal response obtained; 2.5–40 mg (> 6–11 y/o) 5–60 mg (≥ 12 y/o)
	Adderall XR	5–60 mg	5–30 mg (6–12 y/o) 5–40 mg (≥ 12 y/o)
Dextroamphetamine	Dexedrine Dextrostat	5–60 mg	5–40 mg (> 6 y/o)
	Dexedrine Spansule	5–60 mg	5–40 mg (> 6–11 y/o) 5–60 mg (≥ 12 y/o)

continued

Table 11.11 (cont.)
Medications Used to Treat Attention-Deficit/Hyperactivity Disorder (ADHD)

Generic Name	Brand Name	Dose Range	
		Adults	Children and Adolescents
Lisdexamfetamine	Vyvanse	20–70 mg	20–70 mg (≥ 6 y/o)
Methylphenidate	Ritalin	5–60 mg	2.5–60 mg (> 6 y/o)
	Methylin	5–60 mg	2.5–60 mg (> 6 y/o)
	Metadate ER	20–60 mg	20–60 mg (> 6 y/o)
	Methylin ER	20–60 mg	20–60 mg (> 6 y/o)
	Ritalin SR	20–60 mg	20–60 mg (> 6 y/o)
	Metadate CD	20–60 mg	10–60 mg (> 6 y/o)
	Ritalin LA	20–60 mg	20–40 mg (> 6 y/o)
	Concerta	18–72 mg	18–54 mg (6–12 y/o) 18–72 mg (13–17 y/o)
	Daytrana transdermal patch	10–30 mg	10–30 mg (> 6 y/o)
	Quillivant oral solution	20–60 mg	10–60 mg (> 6 y/o)
Dexmethylphenidate	Focalin	5–20 mg	2.5–20 mg (> 6 y/o)
	Focalin XR	5–40 mg	5–30 mg (> 6 y/o)
Nonstimulant medications			
Guanfacine[a]	Tenex	Not FDA-approved	0.5 mg per dose up to 2 mg/d (27–40 kg) 0.5–1 mg per dose up to 3 mg/d (40.5–45 kg) 1 mg per dose up to 4 mg/d (> 45 kg)
	Intuniv	Not FDA-approved	1–4mg (> 6 y/o)
Clonidine	Catapres	Not FDA-approved	0.003–0.005 mg/kg/d–0.1 mg per dose up to 0.3 mg/d (27–45 kg) 0.003–0.005 mg/kg/d–0.1 mg per dose up to 0.3 mg/d (> 45 kg)
	Kapvay	Not FDA-approved	0.1–0.4 mg (> 6 y/o)

continued

Table 11.11 (cont.)
Medications Used to Treat Attention-Deficit/Hyperactivity Disorder (ADHD)

Generic Name	Brand Name	Dose Range	
		Adults	Children and Adolescents
Atomoxetine	Strattera	10–100 mg	0.5–1.4 mg/kg (> 6 y/o)
Modafinil[a]	Provigil	100–400 mg	Not FDA-approved

[a]Based on author experience in the population of patients with movement disorders.

Source: Adapted from Ref. 3: Pliszka S; AACAP Work Group on Quality Issues. Practice parameter for the assessment and treatment of children and adolescents with attention-deficit/hyperactivity disorder. *J Am Acad Child Adolesc Psychiatry.* 2007; 46(7):894–921.

REFERENCES

1. American Psychiatric Association. *Diagnostic and Statistical Manual of Mental Disorders, Fifth Edition.* Arlington, VA: American Psychiatric Association Publishing; 2013.
2. *Physicians' Desk Reference.* 67th ed. Montvale, NJ: PDR Network; 2013.
3. Pliszka S; AACAP Work Group on Quality Issues. Practice parameter for the assessment and treatment of children and adolescents with attention-deficit/hyperactivity disorder. *J Am Acad Child Adolesc Psychiatry.* 2007; 46(7):894–921.

12

PSYCHIATRIC ISSUES IN PARKINSON'S DISEASE

INTRODUCTION

- Psychiatric complications associated with Parkinson's disease (PD) are common. They represent a special challenge to the practitioner because many of the psychiatric syndromes do not merely *co-occur* with PD but often are predictable consequences of responsible treatment of the underlying neurological condition.[1]

- Cavalier treatment of the psychiatric complications may result in poor control of motor symptoms, increased dysfunction, and decreased quality of life, particularly in late or burdensome disease.

- Some psychiatric syndromes in PD are associated with the disease itself:

  - Depression and anxiety

  - Cognitive impairment

  - Apathy

- Other psychiatric symptoms may be associated with the treatment of PD:

  - Impulse control disorders

  - Psychosis

  - Irritability/agitation/dysphoria (eg, "off" periods, treatment withdrawal)

- Dopaminergic circuits in the mesolimbic and mesocortical areas play important roles in reward, affective control, and impulsivity. Disruption of these circuits by cell loss or therapy may therefore have tremendous effects on behavior, affect, personality, and thought content.[2]

- Nonmotor-related symptoms of PD are prominent and an important target of therapy. Sixty-seven percent of such symptoms are related to the psychiatric domain (anxiety in 56%, insomnia in 37%, poor concentration in 31%, and major depression in 22.5%).[3]

EXAMINATION OF THE PATIENT

- An evaluation of the patient with PD starts with a careful examination of the patient's reported psychiatric symptoms and a complete mental status examination (see Chapter 11).

  - Careful elucidation of the patient's psychiatric symptoms and performance on the mental status examination will guide the diagnosis (Table 12.1).

- A dramatic or unexpected worsening of motor control after the addition of a neuroleptic medication should prompt adjustment of the dose, consideration of an alternative, or optimization of antiparkinsonian medications.

DEPRESSION AND ANXIETY

- The incidence of depression and anxiety is greater in patients with PD than in age-matched controls. Depression and anxiety are the result of complex psychological and neurobiological factors.[4]

- The psychiatric burden is not thought to stem solely from the functional decline associated with progressive motor dysfunction or the diagnosis of PD itself.

- Depression in PD follows a bimodal distribution, with the psychiatric burden peaking around the time of symptom onset/diagnosis and with the loss of independence in late disease.

- Fortunately, the depression in PD is often mild.

  - However, several core and associated symptoms of depression (eg, fatigue, apathy, sleep disruption, psychomotor retardation, weight loss) are intrinsic to PD, so that the diagnosis can be tricky at times.

  - There have been isolated reports of increased suicidality among patients who underwent deep brain stimulation surgery of the subthalamic nucleus, although a direct correlation remains unclear.

- The noradrenergic, dopaminergic, and serotoninergic pathways are thought to be implicated in depression in PD.[2]

Table 12.1
Important Aspects of Psychiatric Phenomena

Symptom	Associated Phenomena
Low mood, anhedonia, hopelessness	Depression
Lack of motivation and initiative	Apathy, abulia
Impairment in planning/attention, poor orientation, memory, behavioral disturbances	Executive dysfunction/dementia of Parkinson's disease
Early or prominent visual hallucinosis	Lewy body dementia
Frank psychosis	Dementia, medication-induced effect
Hypersexuality, poor impulse control, disinhibition	Dopamine dysregulation syndrome, frontal lobe dysfunction

- Generalized anxiety disorder, panic disorder, social phobia, phobic disorder, agoraphobia, and obsessive–compulsive disorder (OCD) have all been described in PD.

- Just like depression, anxiety can be part of the "premotor" manifestations of PD, and it can be another nonmotor manifestation of wearing off.

Treatment of Depression and Anxiety

- Depression in patients with PD should be a target of focused therapy because studies have shown that depression in this population is a major determinant of quality of life. The modality of treatment should be tailored to the severity of the depressive symptoms.

- For mild depression associated with PD, nonpharmacologic approaches may be most indicated. These include the following:

  ○ Supportive psychotherapy

  ○ Cognitive behavioral therapy

- In moderate to more advanced depression, pharmacotherapy is often indicated.

- Certain phenomena of the "off period," such as paroxysmal anxiety and panic, may not respond well to antidepressant and anxiolytic therapy but can respond to dopaminergic adjustments that minimize wearing-off periods.

- The strongest evidence for the treatment of depression in PD has been reported with the tricyclic antidepressants (TCAs).[5] However, these agents may be poorly tolerated because of their anticholinergic effects and arrhythmogenic properties, particularly at higher doses.

- Selective serotonin reuptake inhibitors (SSRIs) may mitigate symptoms of depression and anxiety in patients with PD, with minimal worsening of movement symptoms.

- In a recent study examining venlafaxine XR and paroxetine in depression in PD, equal efficacy was found between the two classes.[6] This was the largest randomized, placebo-controlled clinical trial of commonly used antidepressant medications for the treatment of depression in PD, had the longest observation period, and was the first to evaluate a serotonin–norepinephrine reuptake inhibitor (SNRI).

- When pharmacotherapy has been ineffective or poorly tolerated, or when depression in PD is severe, *electroconvulsive therapy* (ECT) and *transcranial magnetic stimulation* (TMS) may be helpful, although the evidence of efficacy for TMS in PD is still being investigated.

- It is important to mention that certain PD medications, such as dopamine agonists and monoamine oxidase (MAO) inhibitors, have demonstrated partial antidepressant effects in patients with PD, even when they are not being used for their prokinetic properties. However, they are not typically used as the sole treatment for depression in PD.

- There is a remarkable paucity of randomized clinical trials examining the pharmacologic management of anxiety in PD.

  - However, based on clinical experience, the agents that are effective in the treatment of primary anxiety disorders (eg, SSRIs and benzodiazepines) also appear to be effective in PD-related anxiety.

APATHY

- Just as the symptoms of depression are sometimes hard to distinguish from those of PD itself (ie, masked facies, psychomotor slowing, poor appetite), differentiating among depression, the symptoms of PD, and apathy may be challenging.

- Apathy is associated with symptoms of poor motivation and initiative, without depressed mood, anhedonia, or hopelessness.

  - Apathy can be part of a depressive syndrome or occur on its own.

- Apathy appears to correlate well with more severe depression and greater functional impairment in patients with PD, and it may be a predictor of dementia in the absence of depression.[7]

Treatment of Apathy

- There is also a paucity of randomized clinical trials examining the treatment of apathy in PD.

- The antidepressants commonly used to treat depression in PD, such as SSRIs, are generally ineffective treatment options for apathy.

- Occasionally, optimization of the treatment of motor symptoms with dopamine agonists and levodopa to maximize "on" states may alleviate apathy.

- Psychostimulants such as amphetamine salts and methylphenidate may be effective in the treatment of apathy, although the response is often incomplete and variable.

- Bupropion may also show some benefit, with a minimal risk for worsening movement symptoms.

COGNITIVE IMPAIRMENT

- Subtle cognitive impairment, particularly with frontal lobe features in the domains of executive function and planning, is frequently associated with PD and may appear early in the course. It may include less severe (although clear) memory difficulties and visuospatial difficulties.

- Frank dementia, on the other hand, is less commonly associated with PD and accounts for approximately 10% to 20% of cases. One large, longitudinal epidemiologic study reported that approximately 30% of nondemented patients with PD developed dementia within 4 years, and 80% after 8 years.[8]

- Reported risk factors for the development of dementia in PD include the following:

  ○ Preexisting cognitive impairment

  ○ Peripheral vascular disease (PVD)

  ○ Hypertension

  ○ Older age

  ○ Greater disease burden

  ○ Hallucinations

- The development of cognitive impairment and, in particular, frank dementia is often associated with a decline in mental status and psychosis. These are poor prognostic indicators and predict a greater likelihood of nursing home admission and early mortality.

- The presence of dementia and psychosis is perhaps the greatest limiting factor in the optimal use of antiparkinsonian agents.

Treatment of Cognitive Disorders

- The development of cognitive impairment in a patient being treated for PD should prompt a careful evaluation of the patient's medical status and any underlying factors (systemic or focal infections, respiratory insufficiency, metabolic factors, changes to the environment, and offending medications, such as sedatives and anticholinergic agents).

- Antiparkinsonian medications often require adjustment in this context because patients with cognitive decline and dementia are more sensitive to their side effects (ie, anticholinergic agents, dopamine agonists).

  - Every attempt should be made to simplify anti-PD medications by tapering "adjunctive medications" (eg, anticholinergics, MAO-B inhibitors, and amantadine, followed by dopamine agonists and catechol O-methyltransferase [COMT] inhibitors if necessary) (Table 12.2).

  - Patients who have PD with dementia may ultimately be most effectively managed on levodopa alone.

- The cholinesterase inhibitors are indicated for mild to moderate dementia in PD, and the efficacy data are generally considered robust, although gastrointestinal side effects may limit their use.[9]

- Memantine has shown a small beneficial effect over placebo and appears to be well tolerated in this context.

Table 12.2
Order of Taper or Elimination of Antiparkinsonian Medications

1. Anticholinergic agents
2. Amantadine
3. Monoamine oxidase (MAO) inhibitors
4. Dopamine agonists
5. Catechol O-methyltransferase (COMT) inhibitors
6. Levodopa

PSYCHOSIS

- Hallucinations are thought to be the most common treatment-related psychiatric complication of PD.

  - About 50% of patients with PD will develop at least one psychotic episode.

  - In several cross-sectional epidemiologic studies, 20% to 40% of patients with PD have been found to have hallucinations.

- Risk factors for the development of hallucinations include a combination of extrinsic and intrinsic factors, such as cognitive impairment, older age, longer duration of disease, medication effects, delirium, environmental changes, and/or poor visual acuity.[10]

- Most hallucinations associated with PD are visual, in stark contrast to those associated with primary psychotic disorders like schizophrenia, wherein auditory hallucinations are much more prominent. Furthermore, insight is often preserved early on, when cognitive functioning is usually intact.

- Visual hallucinations tend to be formed images of a person or animal, although other objects and vivid scenes are possible. "Minor" hallucinations, such as brief perceptual disturbances in the peripheral visual field, are also sometimes reported.

- Delusions are fixed, false beliefs. They occur in patients who have PD with cognitive decline (and to a lesser degree in those without dementia). The delusions are often persecutory in nature, although they may sometimes involve themes of jealousy and infidelity.

- The development of PD psychosis is one of the greatest risk factors for long-term care placement.

  - Moreover, patients living in long-term care settings who have PD with psychosis have been found to have a higher mortality rate than do those without psychosis.

Treatment of Psychosis

- When psychotic symptoms are mild, nonthreatening, and/or when insight is relatively preserved, education and reassurance may often be used in favor of pharmacologic treatment. When insight is lost or delusions become threatening, treatment is indicated, and an assessment of safety is paramount.

- Psychosis in association with fluctuations in the sensorium should prompt a careful evaluation of underlying factors associated with delirium, and efforts should be made to eliminate them.

- Tapering or elimination of antiparkinsonian medications, starting with the most recently added medications, is a first step. Usually, those most likely to contribute to confusion are tapered first (see Table 12.2).[10]

  - If at all possible, patients with PD who are psychotic should be on levodopa alone for their motor symptoms.

- When psychotic symptoms persist despite the careful elimination of antiparkinsonian medications (or when such elimination is limited by worsening motor symptoms), neuroleptic medications are often indicated.

- Low-potency second-generation (ie, "atypical") antipsychotic medications like quetiapine and clozapine may be of substantial benefit.[9]

  - Because of the possibility that clozapine will cause life-threatening agranulocytosis (in fewer than 1% of patients using it), patients require monitoring of the complete blood cell count weekly for the first 6 months, every other week for the next 6 months, and monthly thereafter.

  - **Clozapine should be stopped immediately when the absolute neutrophil count is below 1,500/mm^3 and the white blood cell count is below 3,000/mm^3.**

- Higher-potency second-generation agents (ie, risperidone and olanzapine) and first-generation ("typical") antipsychotics should be avoided when possible because they are often associated with unacceptable motor-related side effects in patients who have PD and dementia with Lewy bodies (DLB), including worsening parkinsonism and acute dystonia.

- There are insufficient data on the safety of the newer atypical antipsychotic medications in patients with PD.

- **More importantly, all antipsychotic medications carry a black box warning regarding increased mortality, especially when they are used in elderly persons with cognitive impairment.**

- Pimavanserin, a nonantipsychotic agent that works on serotonin (5-HT) 2A receptors, has been reported in a well-designed randomized clinical trial to mitigate psychosis in PD without worsening its motor symptoms.

IMPULSE CONTROL DISORDERS

- The impulse control disorders (ICDs) are a family of neuropsychiatric conditions whose central feature is the uncontrollable need to engage in repetitive behaviors, often to a maladaptive degree.

- It is critical to discover and treat ICDs and compulsive behaviors because their consequences for patients and families may be devastating.

- Because of their intimate relationship with dopamine replacement therapy, ICDs may represent a tremendous burden in and of themselves and may also limit the optimal control of motor symptoms, leading to poorer functional outcomes and a greater overall disease burden.

- The four most prominent treatment-associated ICDs include compulsive gambling, hypersexuality, binge eating, and uncontrollable spending. Table 12.3 sets forth some impulse control and compulsive behaviors.

- ICDs are found in almost 14% of patients being treated for PD, with pathologic gambling and compulsive spending accounting for the largest percentage of cases.[11]

Table 12.3
Impulse Control Disorders and Compulsive Behaviors

Impulse Control Disorders	Examples
Problem gambling	Excessive or new lottery ticket buying
	Excessive or new casino gambling
	Risky or new investment
Hypersexuality	Excessive or new use of pornography
	Compulsive masturbation
	Novel or inappropriate sexual demands
	Exhibitionism, solicitation of prostitution
Binge eating	Excessive food intake in one sitting
	Craving for sweets
Excessive spending	Drive to obtain unneeded items
	Reckless generosity
Compulsive Behaviors	**Examples**
Hobbyism	Intensive attention to a hobby
Punding	Compulsive need to engage in meaningless rituals, such as assembling and disassembling objects, arranging and rearranging items
Walk-a-bout	Aimless or nonpurposeful walking for extended periods of time
Dopamine dysregulation syndrome	A dependence-like overuse of dopaminergic medications beyond the need to control motor symptoms despite side effects

- ICDs are most prominent in patients taking dopamine agonists such as pramipexole and ropinirole, and they may be enhanced when any of these is taken in conjunction with levodopa.

- Levodopa therapy alone is generally not associated with an increase in ICDs except at very high doses. However, levodopa is commonly associated with the related dopamine dysregulation syndrome (see below).

- Patients are often unwilling to discuss the occurrence of or increased urge to engage in impulsive behaviors such as hypersexuality and unrestrained gambling (although an attentive spouse or family member may bring it to the physician's attention).

- Certain ICDs may be idiosyncratic and specific to a particular patient's tendencies (eg, kleptomania, reckless generosity, hoarding) and therefore difficult to uncover with general screening. This may be particularly true of "hobbyism" and other dopamine dysregulation disorders.

- Dopamine dysregulation syndrome is characterized by intense cravings for dopaminergic agents (particularly levodopa) and often present with addictive behaviors and tendencies.

Treatment of Impulse Control Disorders and Compulsive Behaviors

- Patients with preexisting or comorbid ICDs, as well as those with substance use disorders (eg, alcohol or opiate dependence or abuse), OCD, or tic disorders, are probably at a greater risk for the development of treatment-related ICDs and compulsive behaviors.

- Either dopamine agonists should be avoided in these patients, if possible, or the patients should be closely monitored to detect and avoid the occurrence of ICDs.

- In most patients, tapering and/or discontinuing dopamine agonist agents will mitigate or eliminate ICDs and compulsive behaviors.

- Generally, dopamine agonist therapy should be tapered slowly to reduce the risk for dopamine agonist withdrawal symptoms, or DAWS (eg, irritability, agitation, and dysphoria). Transition to levodopa is generally indicated in these situations.

- A patient with dopamine dysregulation syndrome may require transition from levodopa to a dopamine agonist.[12]

- When dysregulated behaviors (impulsive, compulsive, and/or addictive tendencies) persist despite the elimination of dopaminergic agents, there is little evidence available for management. Anecdotal reports have demonstrated variable benefit from atypical antipsychotics, naltrexone, and/or mood stabilizers.

REFERENCES

1. Gallagher DA, Schrag A. Psychosis, apathy, depression and anxiety in Parkinson's disease. *Neurobiol Dis.* 2012; 46:581–589.
2. Blonder LX, Slevin JT. Emotional dysfunction in Parkinson's disease. *Behav Neurol.* 2011; 24(3):201–217.
3. Barone P, Antonini A, Colosimo C, et al. The PRIAMO study: a multicenter assessment of nonmotor symptoms and their impact on quality of life in Parkinson's disease. *Mov Disord.* 2009; 24(11):1641–1649.
4. Weintraub D, Burn D. Parkinson's disease: the quintessential neuropsychiatric disorder. *Mov Disord.* 2011; 26(6):1022–1031.
5. Seppi K, Weintraub D, Coelho M, et al. The Movement Disorder Society Evidence-Based Medicine Review Update: Treatments for the non-motor symptoms of Parkinson's disease. *Mov Disord.* 2011; 26(suppl 3):S42–S80.
6. Richard IH, McDermott MP, Kurlan R, et al. A randomized, double-blind, placebo-controlled trial of antidepressants in Parkinson disease. *Neurology.* 2012; 78(16):1229–1236.
7. Dujardin K, Sockeel P, Delliaux M, et al. Apathy may herald cognitive decline and dementia in Parkinson's disease. *Mov Disord.* 2009; 24:2391–2397.
8. Aarsland D, Andersen K, Larsen JP, et al. Prevalence and characteristics of dementia in Parkinson's disease: an 8-year prospective study. *Arch Neurol.* 2003; 60:387–392.
9. Connolly BS, Fox SH. Drug treatments for the neuropsychiatric complications of Parkinson's disease. *Expert Rev Neurother.* 2012; 12(12):1439–1449.
10. Hindle, JV. The practical management of cognitive impairment and psychosis in the older Parkinson's disease patient. *J Neural Transm.* 2013; 120:649–653.
11. Weintraub D, Koester J, Potenza MN, et al. Impulse control disorders in Parkinson's disease: a cross-section study of 3090 patients. *Arch Neurol.* 2010; 67:589–595.
12. Goetz CG. New developments in depression, anxiety, compulsiveness, and hallucinations in Parkinson's disease. *Mov Disord.* 2010; 25(suppl 1):S104–S109.

13

PSYCHIATRIC ISSUES IN HUNTINGTON'S DISEASE

INTRODUCTION

- Huntington's disease (HD) is a neuropsychiatric disorder characterized by impairments in movement, emotional regulation, and cognitive functioning.

- Psychiatric disorders are a frequently encountered and longitudinal problem in HD.[1,2]

- The psychiatric and cognitive symptoms may often be more challenging to manage than the movement disorder itself and lead to a greater decline in quality of life for both patients and caregivers.[3]

- The average age at the onset of HD is typically identified as 40 years; however, this refers to the emergence of physical deficits (ie, chorea). In many patients with HD, the psychiatric and cognitive deficits present much earlier.

- There are complicated family dynamics that are important to consider in evaluating the psychiatric vulnerability of any patient with HD.

- Dysexecutive syndrome in HD is a complex group of behaviors resulting from the manifestation of psychiatric and cognitive deficits (Figure 13.1).

GENETIC TESTING

- Genetic counseling is a critical component of the genetic testing process.

- All patients should ideally be seen by a mental health provider before testing, to be evaluated for their emotional and cognitive capacity to receive and understand the results of genetic testing.

- **Predictive testing for minors is not routinely recommended.**

- Common acute emotional reactions associated with a positive test result include sadness, anger, anxiety, agitation, shock, tearfulness, and hopelessness.

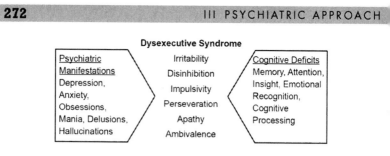

Figure 13.1
Psychiatric and cognitive deficits in Huntington's disease leading to dysexecutive syndrome.

■ Family dynamics may become altered by a positive or negative test result. For example, parents may feel guilt about passing the gene on to their offspring, children with a positive gene may display anger toward the parent or an unaffected sibling, and unaffected individuals may experience relief and gratitude about not passing the gene on to subsequent generations.

COGNITIVE DYSFUNCTION

■ Cognitive deficits usually begin in a gradual fashion, initially affecting the speed of cognitive processing and compromising executive functions, such as organization, planning, attention, and multitasking. Visuospatial dysfunction, decline in working memory, and learning impairments are other frequently seen cognitive deficits.[4]

■ Inattention and distractibility can be accentuated by motor abnormalities, such as restlessness and chorea.

■ Cortical impairments, such as aphasia, amnesia, and agnosia, are rarely seen in HD. Language comprehension also remains fairly unaffected.

■ Cognitive inflexibility, inability to appreciate negative consequences, lack of self-awareness, and failure to read social cues and facial expressions are other features that may be encountered in HD and contribute to abnormal behavioral reactions.[5]

■ Cognitive dysfunction may be the consequence of or exacerbated by overlapping psychiatric symptoms, such as depression and anxiety, or it may be the result of treatment-related adverse effects (ie, sedation).

■ The Montreal Cognitive Assessment (MOCA) is a useful screening instrument in detecting HD-related cognitive changes. Deficits in the serial 7s exercise of the Mini-Mental Status Examination (MMSE) are another change seen in early HD.

Treatment of Cognitive Dysfunction

- There are no significant pharmacologic interventions to change the course of cognitive decline.

- Efforts should be directed at reducing any medications that may be contributory while incorporating interventions that center around environmental adjustments, such as these:

  - Minimizing distractions

  - Implementing routines and structure

  - Creating reminder lists

  - Allowing extended time to complete tasks

DEPRESSION AND APATHY

- The estimated lifetime prevalence of depression in HD is 30% to 70%.[3]

- Patients are susceptible to depression at any point in the course of HD, even if the symptoms are relatively mild and cause minimal functional impairment. As in other degenerative conditions, hopelessness may also surface after a significant change in quality of life (ie, loss of job, loss of driving privileges, increased falls).

- Tetrabenazine, an approved treatment for chorea in HD, carries a boxed warning regarding its propensity to cause depression and suicidal thinking.

- **Suicide rates are significantly higher in patients with HD than in the general population;[6] therefore, acute changes in mood and/or an increase in hopelessness should be taken seriously, trigger an immediate assessment, and never be considered a normal reaction.**

- Physicians should be aware of how many at-risk children a patient may have and be watchful for changes in mood if these children elect to undergo genetic testing. A positive test result may trigger guilt, self-directed anger, and/or thoughts of self-harm in the affected parent.

- Apathy, defined as a loss of motivation or initiation, appears to worsen with disease progression. Apathy is typically associated with a neutral mood, although it can occur in a patient with depression, which will accentuate the loss of motivation and lack of spontaneity.

- Depression may be difficult to detect or evaluate later in the disease process because of the presence of apathy and impairments in speech and/or cognition. Severe depression may be complicated by hallucinations and delusions.

Treatment of Depression and Apathy

* The primary treatment for depression includes the commonly prescribed first-line antidepressants used in the general population, such as selective serotonin reuptake inhibitors (SSRIs), in combination with supportive psychotherapy early in the disease (or pre-manifestation stages), when the ability to communicate is still preserved.

* Most of the antidepressants commonly prescribed in the general population are effective and well tolerated in HD.

* Sedating antidepressants, such as mirtazapine and trazodone, may be useful in the management of depression-related insomnia.

* Adjustments in the doses of fluoxetine and paroxetine should be made cautiously in patients taking tetrabenazine because the former agents are potent inhibitors of cytochrome P450 (CYP) 2D6 and may inadvertently cause fluctuations in tetrabenazine levels.

* Bupropion may be worthwhile in those with significant anhedonia, psychomotor retardation, and/or apathy for its clinically activating effects. Regarding the same point, its stimulating effects may exacerbate irritability or insomnia.

* Tricyclic antidepressants (TCAs) should be used with caution in HD because of its propensity to cause anticholinergic effects and therefore exacerbate cognitive deficits. Clomipramine may be necessary for resistant cases of obsessive worry or perseveration. In those exhibiting significant impulsivity and/or a high risk for suicide, TCAs should be avoided.

* Patients taking monoamine oxidase (MAO) inhibitors must adhere strictly to a tyramine-free diet, so that the use of these agents in patients with cognitive deficits may be precluded.

* Psychostimulants may be a helpful augmentation strategy to improve motivation in patients with apathy and/or depression.

* Electroconvulsive therapy may be used in severe cases, particularly patients who have a psychotic depression or display significant psychomotor retardation that may compromise nutritional status.[7]

ANXIETY AND PERSEVERATION

* Anxiety may be an early manifestation in HD as individuals cope with the uncertainty of their gene status and anticipate future illness. As physical symptoms surface, anxiety may be a reaction to changes in changes in efficiency, functionality, and quality of life.

- Obsessive and/or compulsive behavior (OCB) is frequently observed in HD, although it may not present as the classic "obsessive–compulsive disorder" seen in the general population.[4] For example, patients typically have obsessive worry and compulsive tendencies that may not be linked (ie, behaviors are not necessarily conducted to mitigate an obsession).

- Perseveration, or fixation on the same thought or behavior, may be exacerbated by anxiety. Perseverative tendencies may be difficult to distinguish from OCB, but the affected individual commonly appears to have trouble disengaging from a recently completed activity or conversation (ie, is "stuck").

Treatment of Anxiety and Perseveration

- Anxiety is primarily treated with commonly prescribed first-line anxiolytics for maintenance, such as SSRIs or serotonin–norepinephrine reuptake inhibitors (SNRIs).

- Most of the antidepressants commonly prescribed in the general population have anxiolytic properties. They are well tolerated in patients with HD and useful in the management of pervasive anxiety complaints.

- Clomipramine may be a useful intervention for OCB if patients are unresponsive to initial treatment.[8]

- Discrete episodes or symptoms of anxiety, such as panic attacks, intermittent restlessness, obsessive worry, and/or perseveration, may be effectively managed with low-dose benzodiazepines on an as-needed basis. Those benzodiazepines with a relatively short half-life will have fewer cumulative cognitive effects than agents with a longer half-life.

- Benzodiazepines may also be ideal for those who exhibit anxiety-induced worsening of their movement disorder (ie, chorea, dystonia, rigidity).

- For more severe or resistant cases, augmentation with low-dose atypical antipsychotics may be helpful.

- The ability to incorporate behavioral strategies will depend on the patient's cognitive status.

MANIA, IRRITABILITY, AND IMPULSIVITY

- Mania has been reported to occur in patients with HD, but at a relatively lower rate than depression. Commonly observed manic symptoms (more likely as a result of frontal lobe dysfunction) include insomnia, distractibility, impulsivity, irritable mood, and risk-taking behaviors, such as substance abuse and hypersexuality.

- Substance abuse may exacerbate mood disorders, impulsivity, and cognitive deficits, and therefore every patient with HD should be screened for substance abuse.

- Manic symptoms of grandiosity, an expansive or elated mood, and tangentiality are less frequently observed in HD.

- Impulsivity is a major contributor to falls, accidents, and poor decision making, which may result in significant morbidity and mortality.

- Irritability is a frequently encountered problem in HD, usually resulting from cognitive compromise, that affects frustration tolerance and the ability to appreciate another person's point of view.

- Impulsivity and irritability may lead to verbal or physical aggression, prompting the need for additional caregiver assistance and/or nursing home placement.

Treatment of Mania, Irritability, and Impulsivity

- SSRIs and antipsychotics are effective initial interventions for reducing psychomotor agitation and aggression; they also improve impulse control and frustration tolerance.[9]

- Identifying and anticipating environmental triggers, minimizing unexpected schedule changes, and reducing confrontation may be helpful caregiver strategies to diffuse irritability and avoid aggression.

- Anticonvulsants, such as valproic acid, may be effective in the management of mood lability, mania, irritability, and impulsivity, as well as in the management of certain comorbid conditions, such as myoclonus and seizures, which are seen in juvenile HD.[10]

- Lithium has been shown to be effective in the management of impulsivity in persons without HD. The evidence of its effectiveness in HD, however, is limited.

PSYCHOSIS

- Psychosis, defined as a loss of touch with reality, may sometimes be observed in patients with HD. Symptoms may consist of perceptual disturbances (ie, hallucinations) and/or delusional thinking, such as paranoia.

- Disorganized thoughts, such as thought blocking, or erratic behavior may be an indication of underlying psychosis and may contribute to accidents and injury.

- An acute change in behavior or thought process should prompt investigations for a medical etiology, such as infection or metabolic derangements.

Visual hallucinations are typically more indicative of an acute physiologic disturbance than of HD psychosis.

Treatment of Psychosis

- See Figure 13.2 for an overview of the treatment approach to the psychiatric manifestations of HD.

- Typical and atypical antipsychotics are the mainstay of treatment. The choice depends on the presence and extent of other, accompanying motor and nonmotor symptoms.

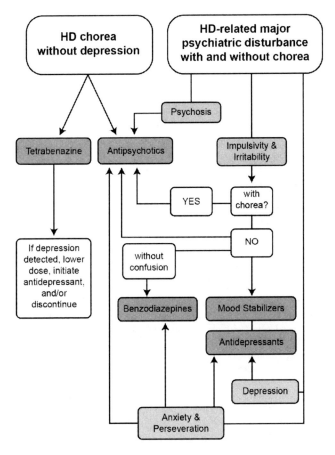

Figure 13.2
Summary of the treatment approach in Huntington's disease.

- Antipsychotic agents are widely used for both the motor and nonmotor symptoms of HD.[11]

- Although conventional antipsychotics (ie, haloperidol) have long been used in the management of chorea in HD, atypical antipsychotics have gained popularity because of their better tolerability and their capacity to control, or augment the treatment of, a spectrum of psychiatric disturbances.

- Antipsychotics are useful not only for the management of positive psychotic symptoms, such as delusions and hallucinations, but also for the control of irritability and aggression.[9]

- For patients requiring a comprehensive treatment strategy targeting chorea, in addition to psychiatric and/or behavioral management, risperidone or olanzapine may be an ideal initial agent of choice.[10]

- High-potency antipsychotics should be avoided in those exhibiting evidence of parkinsonism or other hypokinetic movements, usually appreciated in later stages. Quetiapine and clozapine may be better choices in these circumstances.

REFERENCES

1. Thompson JC, Harris J, Sollom AC, et al. Longitudinal evaluation of neuropsychiatric symptoms in Huntington's disease. *J Neuropsychiatry Clin Neurosci.* 2012; 24:1.
2. Reedeker W, van der Mast RC, Giltay EJ, et al. Psychiatric disorders in Huntington's disease: a 2-year follow-up study. *Psychosomatics.* 2012; 53:220–229.
3. Anderson K. Huntington's disease. *Handb Clin Neurol.* 2011;100:15–21.
4. Nance M, Paulsen JS, Rosenblatt A, et al. *A Physician's Guide to the Management of Huntington's Disease.* 3rd ed. New York, NY: Huntington's Disease Society of America; 2011.
5. Eddy CM, Sira Mahalingappa S, Rickards HE. Is Huntington's disease associated with deficits in theory of mind? *Acta Neurol Scand.* 2012; 126(6):376–383.
6. Hubers AA, Reedeker N, Giltay EJ, et al. Suicidality in Huntington's disease. *J Affect Disord.* 2012; 136:550–557.
7. Cusin C, Franco FB, Fernandez-Robles C, et al. Rapid improvement of depression and psychotic symptoms in Huntington's disease: a retrospective chart review of seven patients treated with electroconvulsive therapy. *Gen Hosp Psychiatry.* 2013; 35(6):678.e3–e5.
8. Anderson K, Craufurd D, Edmondson MC, et al. An international survey-based algorithm for the pharmacologic treatment of obsessive–compulsive behaviors in Huntington's disease. *PLoS Curr.* 2011; 3:RRN1261.
9. Groves M, van Duijn E, Anderson K, et al. An international survey-based algorithm for the pharmacologic treatment of irritability in Huntington's disease. *PLoS Curr.* 2011; 3:RRN1259.
10. Killoran A, Biglan KM. Therapeutics in Huntington's disease. *Curr Treat Options Neurol.* 2012; 14:137–149.
11. Reilmann R. Pharmacological treatment of chorea in Huntington's disease—good clinical practice versus evidence-based guideline. *Mov Disord.* 2013; 28(8):1030–1033.

14

PSYCHIATRIC ISSUES IN TOURETTE SYNDROME

INTRODUCTION

- Tourette syndrome (TS) is considered to be a neuropsychiatric illness. Studies have shown that up to 88% of individuals display psychiatric comorbidity or psychopathology.[1] Up to 36% have more than one psychiatric comorbidity.[2]

- The presence of a psychiatric comorbidity correlates with a worse prognosis, exposure to more medications, and a greater degree of functional impairment.

- The age of onset of motor or phonic tics coincides with the onset of the most common psychiatric comorbidities, such as obsessive–compulsive disorder (OCD) and attention-deficit/hyperactivity disorder (ADHD).

- It is commonly thought that these psychiatric illnesses share neural circuitry with tic disorders

- The severity of the symptoms associated with tics can be influenced by environmental changes or stresses.

- Effectively managing a tic disorder includes understanding the psychiatric/psychological aspects that are commonly seen with this illness.

TICS AND BEHAVIOR

- Tics themselves are categorized as either motor or vocal manifestations. Their characteristics include fluctuating symptomatology over time, suppressibility followed by rebound, suggestibility, and they are preceded by premonitory sensations. Multiple psychiatric symptoms can present in a similar manner (Table 14.1).

Table 14.1
Psychiatric Differential Diagnosis for Tics

Movement Type	Description	Examples	Corresponding Illnesses in Psychiatry
Stereotypy	Repetitive, simple movements that can be voluntarily suppressed. Often rhythmic and usually confined to upper extremity. There is no premonitory urge, but movements occur with stress or excitement.	Waving Rocking back and forth Hand flapping Punding	• Autism spectrum disorders • Intellectual disabilities • Stereotypic movement disorder • Schizophrenia • Frontotemporal dementia • Amphetamine or methamphetamine use in healthy children throughout preschool years
Dystonia (secondary)	Involuntary sustained or intermittent muscle contractions resulting in twisting or repetitive movements.	Torticollis Buccolingual crisis Oculogyric crisis Facial grimacing	Acute dystonia encountered after exposure to high-potency neuroleptics in • Schizophrenia • Autism spectrum disorders
Compulsions	Persistent and repetitive acts that do not lead to reward or pleasure. Aimed at reducing internal psychic stress or urges. They can be simple or complex rituals including both movements and vocalizations.	Rituals that are bizarre in nature, occur at inappropriate times, or are of inappropriate duration, such as repetitive hand washing or checking locks; excessive hoarding, eating, picking, counting, or sexualized behaviors	• Obsessive–compulsive disorder • Paraphilias • Impulse control disorders
Mannerisms	Idiosyncratic or peculiar movements or vocalizations. They are not consciously produced and are suppressible without psychic anxiety.	Snapping knuckles Tapping a foot Greeting everyone with a handshake	Autism
Akathisia	Unpleasant sensation of internal restlessness manifesting as an inability to remain still.	Pacing Repetitive limb shaking	• Medication-induced • Serotonin syndrome
Psychogenic movements	Presentation can be similar to that of biological tics. Do not occur during sleep or relaxation but worsen with stress.	Repetitive movements or vocalizations similar to tics	• Somatoform disorders • Reactions to emotional stress • Can occur along with biological tic disorders

- Distinguishing between tics and other motor or vocal symptoms may be difficult, but a careful history of the movements or vocalizations may aid the clinician in distinguishing one from another.[3]

- Persons with tic disorders may display behavioral symptoms even without psychiatric comorbidities, such as hyperarousal states manifesting as anxiety, hyperactivity, and even self-injurious behaviors.

PSYCHIATRIC COMORBIDITIES

Attention-Deficit/Hyperactivity Disorder

- ADHD is a neurobehavioral disorder that affects 3% to 9% of children. It is characterized by symptoms of hyperactivity, impulsivity, and inattention.

- Children can exhibit symptoms of either inattention or hyperactivity, or they can meet the criteria for both. Symptoms must be present before the age of 11 years[4] and must affect the individual in multiple settings (home, school, work, day care).

- The frequency of ADHD in clinic samples of children with tic disorders is estimated at 50% to 70%.[1] Conversely, up to 20% of children with ADHD present with a comorbid tic disorder.

- Studies suggest that the combination of a tic disorder plus ADHD results in greater overall impairment than either a tic disorder or ADHD alone.

- A comprehensive treatment program for a patient with a tic disorder and comorbid ADHD should include cognitive behavioral therapy plus psychoeducational and psychosocial interventions, along with a consideration of medications.

- There is strong evidence to support the use of habit reversal training in individuals with TS and comorbid ADHD, and such training should be considered before and along with medication management.

TREATMENT OF ATTENTION-DEFICIT/HYPERACTIVITY DISORDER

- Stimulants (methylphenidate, dexmethylphenidate, dextroamphetamine, lisdexamfetamine, and mixed amphetamine salts) are widely recognized as first-line pharmacologic treatments of ADHD.

- Multiple studies comparing the efficacy of stimulants have shown few differences between methylphenidate and mixed amphetamine salt preparations.

- Available evidence indicates that 70% of children with ADHD will show a positive response to a stimulant trial and that approximately half of the nonresponders will show a positive response to a trial of an alternative stimulant.

- Other medications used for the treatment of ADHD include alpha-2-adrenoceptor agonists, atomoxetine, bupropion, and tricyclic antidepressants.

- Stimulants, alpha-2-adrenoceptor agonists, atomoxetine, and partial dopamine agonists have been studied in individuals with comorbid tic disorders and ADHD. Stimulants may produce a transient worsening of tics upon initiation of the medication.

- However, recent well-designed, controlled clinical trials have not indicated chronic exacerbation of tics in persons treated with stimulants.[5,6]

- Alpha-2-adrenoceptor agonists activate presynaptic autoreceptors in the locus ceruleus and reduce norepinephrine release and turnover. These medications have been shown to be beneficial in reducing tics as well as hyperactivity and impulsivity in individuals with ADHD.

- In a randomized, controlled study comparing clonidine, methylphenidate, and placebo, clonidine appeared to be most helpful for impulsivity and hyperactivity and methylphenidate for inattention.

- Atomoxetine is a novel nonstimulant medication used to treat ADHD. It acts by blocking presynaptic norepinephrine reuptake.

- In one setting, atomoxetine was effective in treating both tics and ADHD in patients affected with both. In that study, significant increases were observed in pulse rate and nausea, and decreases in appetite and body weight.[7]

Obsessive–Compulsive Disorder

- OCD is the second most common comorbidity in patients with TS. It is characterized by intrusive thoughts that produce uneasiness, apprehension, fear, or worry, and by repetitive behaviors aimed at reducing the associated anxiety.[4]

- Approximately 20% to 30% of individuals with TS have an additional diagnosis of OCD. OCD is commonly accompanied by another psychopathology, such as depression, anxiety, ADHD, or aggression.

- TS and OCD share several characteristics. Both are characterized by a juvenile or young adult onset, a waxing and waning course, and the presence of repetitive behaviors associated with premonitory urges.

- It can be difficult to distinguish compulsive behaviors from tics, and some individuals will display both. It is possible at times to distinguish compulsive behavior when the patient is able to explain that the ritualistic physical or mental affect serves to reduce intrusive thoughts or images rather than an uncomfortable feeling. However, this distinction is not easily made.[8]

- Obsessions commonly reported by individuals with TS include sexual, religious, aggressive, and symmetric themes.

TREATMENT OF OBSESSIVE–COMPULSIVE DISORDER

- For individuals with OCD, the cognitive behavioral therapy model of exposure and response prevention is the recommended nonpharmacologic treatment of choice.

- Medications used to treat OCD include selective serotonin reuptake inhibitors (SSRIs) and clomipramine. There is also evidence to support using antipsychotic agents as an augmentation strategy for treatment-resistant OCD. However, there is currently little evidence to support the use of medications to treat comorbid TS and OCD.

Autism Spectrum Disorders

- Autism spectrum disorders (ASDs) are typically characterized by social deficits, communication difficulties, stereotyped or repetitive behaviors and interests.[4] TS and ASD share several clinical and behavioral features, including speech abnormalities, such as echolalia and palilalia, and repetitive movements.

- In one study, approximately 5% of the participants with TS had comorbid ASD, and if these illnesses were found together, there was a significant increase in additional comorbidities; conversely, approximately 20% of individuals with ASD displayed tics.[9]

- Stereotypical behavior is common in individuals with ASD and may be difficult to distinguish from tics.

TREATMENT OF AUTISM SPECTRUM DISORDERS

- Applied behavioral analysis and facilitated communication therapy are the first-line treatments for individuals with ASDs.[10]

- Currently, only two medications (aripiprazole and risperidone) are approved by the Food and Drug Administration to treat aggressive behaviors in individuals with ASDs. No evidence is available at this time regarding the effect of these medications when ASD is comorbid with a tic disorder.[10]

Depression

- Depression is characterized by sadness, loss of pleasure and interest in activities, changes in sleeping and/or eating habits, concentration difficulties, thoughts of death or dying, inappropriate and intense feelings of guilt or diminished self-worth, and perceptual disturbances if severe.[4]

■ Individuals with TS have reported more depressive symptoms than age-matched controls. In one study, 60% of children met the diagnostic criteria for major depressive disorder.[11] An important differential and consideration in patients with depressive disorders is the concept of demoralization.

■ Children with TS tend to have a heightened awareness of how they are different from their peers, and they frequently experience frustration or feelings of incompetence regarding controlling their symptoms, which may lead to demoralization.

TREATMENT OF DEPRESSION

■ Demoralization may be mitigated when the patients are placed in environments in which they are protected from harassment or adverse consequences of their symptoms, which may include changes in peer interactions, support systems, and educational interventions.[12]

■ In contrast to demoralization, biological mood disorders tend to persist despite environmental changes and are usually associated with more neurovegetative symptoms (eg, changes in sleep, appetite, and/or energy). The biological mood symptoms should be addressed in parallel with tic control.

■ Psychotherapy, including cognitive behavioral therapy and interpersonal therapy, has been shown to be effective in mild to moderate depression. Medications such as SSRIs have shown utility in moderate to severe depression and can be used in combination with psychotherapy.

■ Depression may occur in the setting of bipolar disorder, which includes manic mood states. Mania can be described as an abnormally and persistently elevated, expansive, or irritable mood. It is associated with such symptoms as grandiosity, euphoria, and irritability; decreased need for sleep; increased talkativeness; distractibility; and excessive involvement in pleasurable activities.[4]

■ Children and adolescents tend to exhibit irritability and aggression rather than euphoria. Few studies have looked at the prevalence or management of mania in individuals with comorbid tic disorders.

■ Of note, both traditional mood stabilizers (lithium, antiepileptic medications) and antipsychotic medications, especially second-generation antipsychotic medications, have been shown to be effective in reducing symptoms of mania or depression associated with a bipolar affective disorder. Specifically, second-generation antipsychotics may be useful in managing both tics and mood symptoms.

Anxiety

- The relationship between tic disorders and anxiety disorders is not well understood. Separation anxiety disorder, generalized anxiety disorder, and social phobia are all thought to be comorbid with tic disorders.

- Anxiety symptoms have been noted in 16% to 80% of individuals with tics and are not correlated with the severity of tics.

TREATMENT OF ANXIETY

- Anxiety can be managed with either cognitive behavioral therapy or SSRI medication with good success. There are limited data on the management of anxiety disorder when it is associated with tics.

- One older study demonstrated benefit and a reduction of non-OCD anxiety along with a reduction of tics with the use of benzodiazepines, but the results have not been duplicated.[13]

Aggression

- Aggressive symptoms and TS are strongly associated and are often seen with family stress, impaired personal and/or occupational functioning, psychiatric hospitalizations, and alternative school or residential placements.

- Aggression may be either reactive (impulsive) or proactive (predatory). It may range from mild temper tantrums to extreme irritability and can include oppositional behaviors, such as bullying and cruelty to animals.

- Aggressive symptoms are fairly common in individuals with TS, occurring approximately 37% of the time.[1]

- Aggression is more likely to occur when an individual with TS has a psychiatric comorbidity (eg, ADHD, OCD).

TREATMENT OF AGGRESSION

- In most cases, the effective management of aggression and TS necessitates a combination of both pharmacologic and psychosocial interventions.[14]

- The impulsive type of aggression appears more likely to respond to pharmacologic and psychosocial interventions that target irritability, impulsivity, and arousal, whereas controlled, proactive, predatory aggression is addressed with behavioral therapy, such as anger management, dialectical behavioral therapy, and relapse prevention programs.[15]

- Multiple classes of medication have been used to target aggression, including the following: serotonin agonists, SSRIs, mixed serotonin–norepinephrine reuptake inhibitors (SNRIs), lithium, anticonvulsants, anxiolytics, first- and second-generation antipsychotics, alpha-2 agonists, beta-blockers, opiate antagonists, and dopamine agonists.

- Mood stabilizers have been shown to be effective in individuals displaying explosive outbursts.

- Risperidone and aripiprazole have been studied for the treatment of aggression in children with cognitive impairments in ASD with demonstrated efficacy. Both of these medications have also been shown to be effective in the treatment of aggression in children with TS.

- Psychostimulants are beneficial for reducing aggression symptoms associated with ADHD. Alpha-2 agonists alone or in combination with a stimulant have been shown to reduce aggressive behaviors in children with conduct disorder or oppositional defiant disorder.

- Beta-blockers such as propranolol have been reported to be effective in reducing aggression in patients with dementia, personality disorders, and traumatic brain injuries.[14]

Pediatric Autoimmune Neuropsychiatric Disorders Associated With Streptococcal Infections

- Pediatric autoimmune neuropsychiatric disorders associated with streptococcal infections (PANDAS) is a diagnosis that Swedo et al proposed in 1998 to describe a new illness characterized by childhood-onset OCD and/or a tic disorder occurring as a postinfectious, autoimmune-mediated phenomenon.[16]

- The diagnostic criteria were developed in 1998 based on findings in 50 patients who had an onset or exacerbation of tics or OCD symptoms after a group A beta-hemolytic streptococcal infection.

- Five diagnostic criteria were proposed:
  - OCD and/or chronic tic disorder
  - Age at onset between 3 years and puberty
  - Abrupt onset of symptoms and course characterized by recurrent exacerbations and remissions
  - Relationship between streptococcal infection and onset and/or exacerbations of clinical symptoms
  - Neurological abnormalities during an exacerbation

- After more than a decade of studies, the diagnosis of PANDAS remains controversial.

■ At this time, it is recommended that the management of symptoms in suspected cases of PANDAS be targeted to the specific symptomatology of tics or OCD with conventional treatment methods.

REFERENCES

1. Freeman RD, Fast DK, Burd L, et al. An international perspective on Tourette syndrome: selected findings from 3,500 individuals in 22 countries. *Dev Med Child Neurol.* 2000; 42(7):436–447.
2. Khalifa N, von Knorring AL. Prevalence of tic disorders and Tourette syndrome in a Swedish school population. *Dev Med Child Neurol.* 2003; 45(5):315–319.
3. Sanger TD, Chen D, Fehlings, et al. Definition and classification of hyperkinetic movements in childhood. *Mov Disord.* 2010; 25(11):1538–1549.
4. American Psychiatric Association. *Diagnostic and Statistical Manual of Mental Disorders, Fifth Edition.* Arlington, VA: American Psychiatric Association Publishing; 2013.
5. Bloch MH, Panza KE, Landeros-Weisenberger A, et al. Meta-analysis: treatment of attention-deficit/hyperactivity disorder in children with comorbid tic disorders. *J Am Acad Child Adolesc Psychiatry.* 2009; 48(9):884–893.
6. Roessner V, Robatzek M, Knapp G, et al, A. First-onset tics in patients with attention-deficit-hyperactivity disorder: impact of stimulants. *Dev Med Child Neurol.* 2006; 48(7):616–621.
7. Allen AJ, Kurlan RM, Gilbert DL, et al. Atomoxetine treatment in children and adolescents with ADHD and comorbid tic disorders. *Neurology.* 2005; 65(12):1941–1949.
8. Worbe Y, Mallet L, Golmard JL, et al. Repetitive behaviours in patients with Gilles de la Tourette syndrome: tics, compulsions, or both? *PloS One.* 2010; 5(9):e12959.
9. Burd L, Li Q, Kerbeshian J, et al. Tourette syndrome and comorbid pervasive developmental disorders. *J Child Neurol.* 2009; 24(2):170–175.
10. Rajapakse T, Pringsheim T. Pharmacotherapeutics of Tourette syndrome and stereotypies in autism. *Semin Pediatr Neurol.* 2009; 17(4):254–260.
11. Wodrich DL, Benjamin E, Lachar, D. Tourette's syndrome and psychopathology in a child psychiatry setting. *J Am Acad Child Adolesc Psychiatry.* 1997; 36(11):1618–1624.
12. Gaze C, Kepley HO, Walkup JT. Co-occurring psychiatric disorders in children and adolescents with Tourette syndrome. *J Child Neurol.* 2006; 21(8):657–664.
13. Coffey B, Frazier J, Chen S. Comorbidity, Tourette syndrome, and anxiety disorders. *Adv Neurol.* 1992; 58:95–104.
14. Budman CL. Treatment of aggression in Tourette syndrome. *Adv Neurol.* 2006; 99:222–226.
15. Malone RP, Bennett DS, Luebbert JF, et al. Aggression classification and treatment response. *Psychopharmacol Bull.* 1998; 34(1):41–45.
16. Swedo SE, Leonard HL, Garvey M, et al. Pediatric autoimmune neuropsychiatric disorders associated with streptococcal infections: clinical description of the first 50 cases. *Am J Psychiatry.* 1998; 155(2):264–271.

15

APPROACH TO CONVERSION DISORDER

APPROACH TO THE PATIENT WITH CONVERSION DISORDER

- Patients with medically unexplained symptoms account for a significant proportion of neurological consultations.[1]

- Such symptoms may include abnormal movements, seizure-like episodes, paralysis, sensory loss, and blindness. Unfortunately, there is no common language to describe such phenomena, with many different terms used by neurologists and psychiatrists alike.[2] The term *conversion disorder* (CD), or *functional neurological symptom disorder*, is a unifying diagnosis that can be used to describe neurologically unexplained symptoms.

- **Terms used to describe neurologically unexplained symptoms**

  - Psychogenic

  - Functional

  - Stress-induced

  - Hysterical

EPIDEMIOLOGY OF CONVERSION DISORDER

- Incidence: CD occurs in 4 to 12 per 100,000 population per year[3] and may be seen in both children and adults.

- In children, the prevalence is equal among boys and girls; however, in adults, CD is seen 2 to 5 times more often in women than in men.[4]

- Frequent psychiatric comorbidities include depression, anxiety disorders, post-traumatic stress disorder (PTSD), dissociative disorders, and borderline personality disorder.[5]

HISTORICAL PERSPECTIVE

- Jean-Martin Charcot, a French neurologist, was the first to use the term *functional* to describe symptoms that did not have an organic basis.

- Sigmund Freud was the first to use the term *conversion* to describe a mechanism whereby unwanted experiences, such as trauma, are repressed in the subconscious but then become "converted" to physical symptoms.

- In 1980, the *Diagnostic and Statistical Manual of Mental Disorders, Third Edition (DSM-III)*, required that for the diagnosis of CD psychological factors must be associated with the etiology of symptoms, evidenced by the following: there exists a temporal relationship with an environmental stimulus related to a psychological conflict, the symptom enables the patient to avoid a noxious stimulus, or the symptom allows the patient to get support from the environment that might otherwise not be forthcoming.[6]

- In 2000, the *Diagnostic and Statistical Manual of Mental Disorders, Fourth Edition, Text Revision (DSM-IV-TR)*, retained the criterion of "associated psychological factors" but removed specifiers.[7]

- Presently, the *Diagnostic and Statistical Manual of Mental Disorders, Fifth Edition (DSM-5)*, does not note a requirement for any association with psychological factors.[8]

NEUROBIOPSYCHOSOCIAL MODEL

- Neuroimaging studies in patients with CD suggest the following:

  ○ Increased limbic activity in response to stressful/traumatic stimuli

  ○ Disruption of prefrontal circuits, including premotor areas

  ○ Greater connectivity between the amygdala and motor preparatory areas during states of arousal, suggesting a possible mechanism of abnormal emotional processing interfering with normal motor planning[9]

- Limited studies with voxel-based morphometry (VBM) demonstrated increased thickness of the premotor cortex in patients with hemiparetic CD compared with normal controls,[10] whereas cortical thinning in the motor and premotor regions was observed in patients with nonepileptic seizures compared with normal controls.[11]

DIAGNOSIS

- It remains well accepted that psychological factors play a role in CD; however, such factors may not always be identified or apparent at the time of the initial evaluation or even well into the course of treatment.

- To reflect this, in 2013 *DSM-5* removed the criterion for the presence of known psychological factors and provided the alternative name of functional neurological symptom disorder.[8]

- The diagnosis of CD may be challenging, depending on the type of presenting symptom. Whereas nonepileptic seizures may be easily diagnosed by the absence of video electroencephalographic (EEG) findings, the diagnosis of conversion in a patient presenting with a movement disorder (eg, tremor, myoclonus, dystonia) is more difficult.

- When a patient presents with symptoms that do not fit with a known neurological disorder, it is imperative that all possible medical conditions be ruled out before CD is diagnosed. This may involve collaboration with the patient's primary care physician, internist, or specialist.

- Historical publications have suggested that the incidence of the eventual diagnosis of an actual medical or neurological condition in a patient being treated for CD is quite high, between 30% and 60%.[12] The medical conditions often misdiagnosed as CD are listed in Table 15.1.

- More recent studies, however, have demonstrated a rate of CD misdiagnosis of only 3% to 7%. It is therefore important that physicians be thorough yet do not become preoccupied with the fear of misdiagnosing CD, which risks delay of treatment.[13]

- To complicate the matter, 5% to 15% of patients with CD will have a comorbid organic neurological disorder.[1]

The Use of "Positive Clinical Signs" in the Diagnosis of Conversion Disorder

- Historically, neurologists have used a set of "positive signs" specific to functional disorders to identify patients with CD; however, very few of these commonly used signs have been validated.[12] Results of a recent systematic review of the validity of "positive signs" are shown in Table 15.2.

Historical Approach to the Diagnosis of Psychogenic Movement Disorders

- In 1988, Fahn and Williams developed a set of diagnostic criteria for psychogenic movement disorders (PMDs) to be used in patients with equivocal

Table 15.1
Medical Conditions Often Misdiagnosed as Conversion Disorder

Disorder	Common Symptoms	Diagnostic Test
Transient ischemic attack	Temporary loss of motor or sensory function, intermittent limb shaking, clonic jerking, tonic posturing	Neuroimaging Cerebral angiography Carotid ultrasound Coagulopathy screening
Frontal lobe epilepsy	Bilateral motor activity with preservation of consciousness, lack of postictal confusion; may have "soft signs" of pelvic thrusting, crying	Video EEG Addition of sphenoidal electrodes SPECT
Hypokalemic periodic paralysis (thyrotoxic periodic paralysis is subtype)	Muscle paralysis, acute hypokalemia, hyperthyroidism, commonly precipitated by heavy carbohydrate loads or after exercise	Potassium levels Thyroid function tests
Syncope (cardiac arrhythmia, long QT syndrome, vasovagal response, orthostatic hypotension)	Convulsions, myoclonus, loss of consciousness, auditory and visual hallucinations	Electrocardiography Arrhythmia monitoring Tilt-table testing
Autoimmune encephalitis (ie, limbic encephalitis, paraneoplastic encephalitis)	Dyskinesias, dystonic posturing, seizures, choreoathetoid movements	CSF/serum antibody testing Rule out neoplasm
Creutzfeldt-Jakob disease	Ataxia, neglect, apraxia, aphasia, hemiparesis, myoclonus, mutism, cognitive decline	EEG MRI Brain biopsy CSF 14-3-3 protein

Abbreviations: CSF, cerebrospinal fluid; EEG, electroencephalography; SPECT, single photon emission computed tomography.

Source: Adapted from Refs. 13–16.

or uncertain diagnoses. These criteria have been widely applied by neurologists and movement disorder specialists, although they have not been validated.[18,19]

■   In 2006, Shill and Gerber[20] reorganized the criteria of Fahn and Williams and proposed additional criteria based on disease modeling; however, these too have

Table 15.2
Validated and Nonvalidated "Positive" Clinical Signs in Conversion Disorder

Validated	Not Validated
Hoover sign	Nonpyramidal weakness
Abductor sign	Absent pronator drift
Abductor finger sign	Arm drop test
Spinal injury test	Barré test
Collapsing/give-away weakness	Wrong-way tongue deviation
Co-contraction	Platysma sign
Motor inconsistency	Babinski trunk–thigh test
Midline splitting	Supine catch sign
Splitting of vibration	Sternocleidomastoid test
Nonanatomical sensory loss	Bowlus-Currier test
Inconsistency/changing pattern of sensory loss	Yes–no test
Systematic failure	Gait fluctuation
Dragging, monoplegic gait	Excessive slowness
Chair test	Psychogenic Romberg test
	Walking on ice
	Noneconomic posture
	Sudden knee buckling
	Staggering to obtain support from opposite walls
	Exaggerated swaying without falling
	Astasia–abasia
	Opposite of astasia–abasia
	Sudden side steps
	Cross legs
	Expressive behavior

Source: Adapted from Ref. 17: Daum C, Hubschmid M, Aybek S. The value of 'positive' clinical signs for weakness, sensory and gait disorders in conversion disorder: a systematic and narrative review. *Neurol Neurosurg Psychiatry.* 2014; 85(2):180–190.

significant limitations, including the suggestion that a PMD can be diagnosed without a consideration of neurological phenomenology (Table 15.3).[19,20]

■ Both sets of criteria have demonstrated poor interrater reliability, even among movement disorder specialists.[21]

Table 15.3
Shill-Gerber Diagnostic Criteria for Psychogenic Movement Disorders

Description	Diagnostic Criteria
Clinically proven psychogenic movement disorder[a]	Remits with psychotherapy, or witnessed to remit when the patient feels unobserved, or there is premovement Bereitschaft potential on electroencephalogram (myoclonus only)
[a]*If not clinically proven, then apply levels of certainty.*	
Clinically definite	At least three (3) primary criteria and one (1) secondary
Clinically probable	Two (2) primary criteria and two (2) secondary
Clinically possible	One (1) primary criterion and two (2) secondary, or Two (2) primary and one (1) secondary
Primary criteria: inconsistent with organic disease, excessive pain or fatigue, previous exposure to a disease model, and/or potential for secondary gain	
Secondary criteria: multiple somatizations (other than pain and fatigue) and/or obvious psychiatric disturbance	

■ A survey of 519 movement disorder specialists reported that most clinicians diagnose PMD after excluding a wide range of organic illnesses rather than using inclusionary criteria such as those proposed by Fahn and Williams and by Shill and Gerber.[22]

Ruling Out Factitious Disorder and Malingering

■ It is of paramount importance not to mistake CD for factitious disorder or malingering, both of which are intentionally feigned by the patient (Table 15.4).

■ CD is not voluntary or feigned.

■ Patients with CD are very sensitive to the physician's perception that they may be faking their symptoms.

■ Often, it takes many years before a diagnosis of CD is made. Within that time, a patient will have usually consulted at least one physician who has stated that the patient's symptoms "are not real," implying that the patient is faking the symptoms.

Table 15.4
Distinguishing Conversion From Factitious Disorder and Malingering

Disease State	Involuntary Versus Feigned Symptoms	Conscious Gain
Conversion disorder	Involuntary	Not applicable (any gain unconsciously driven)
Factitious disorder	Feigned (voluntary)	Primary gain (patient drive to play the sick role)
Malingering	Feigned (voluntary)	Secondary gain (external factors, including but not limited to homelessness, seeking medication, evasion of the law, disability)

Neuropsychological testing with the Minnesota Multiphasic Personality Inventory-2 (MMPI-2) Response Bias Scale and Symptom Validity Scale may help distinguish a patient who is probably malingering from one with CD.

ETIOLOGY OF CONVERSION DISORDER

- Although the exact pathobiology remains elusive, many patients with CD have experienced trauma,[23] including but not limited to the following:

  - Verbal, physical, or sexual abuse as a child, an adult, or both

  - Physical or emotional neglect

  - Recent or chronic medical illness

  - Life-changing event

  - Life-threatening situation, such as a motor vehicle accident, natural disaster, or being held at gunpoint

  - Witnessing the life of a loved one being threatened

  - Witnessing a physically violent event, such as murder, rape, or abuse of an animal

- Risk factors for PMDs include the following:

  - Childhood trauma (specifically, emotional abuse and physical neglect)

  - Fear associated with traumatic life events

  - Multiple traumatic episodes[24]

- Risk factors for PMDs differ slightly from those for nonepileptic seizures, which are associated with childhood sexual trauma, poor perception of parental care, and an increased number of life events in the 12 months before symptom onset.[25]

- Therefore, it is critical for movement disorder clinicians to be able to ask about trauma appropriately (see Chapter 11).

- Often, the nature of the conversion symptom is related to the stressor or trauma, as in the following examples:

  - A patient experiences lower extremity paralysis after she is unable to "stand up" to an abusive partner.

  - A patient is no longer able to drive because of severe upper extremity tremor that developed after a motor vehicle accident in which he was unable to swerve quickly enough to avoid an oncoming car. The accident resulted in the death of the other driver.

  - A young, high-achieving athlete develops convulsions on the basketball court soon after entering a high-profile college on an athletic scholarship.

  - A patient becomes blind after watching her three younger siblings burn to death in a fire.

- CD may occur together with PTSD. Physicians working with patients who may have CD should be aware of the criteria for PTSD. Identifying PTSD in this population may

  - Assist in the identification of CD.

  - Facilitate referral to a psychiatrist when a patient is unaccepting of a CD diagnosis yet recognizes that his or her PTSD symptoms require treatment.

TREATMENT

Explaining the Diagnosis to the Patient

- The way in which a CD diagnosis is explained to the patient is of critical therapeutic importance and may affect the patient's adherence to future treatment recommendations.

- Patients want to be given a diagnosis to explain their experience. It is appropriate to use the term *conversion disorder* or *functional neurological symptom disorder* rather than hide the diagnosis or "talk around" the diagnosis, which may convey the idea that CD is something to be ashamed of.

- Use tactful language and a nonaccusatory tone when explaining the diagnosis (Table 15.5).

Table 15.5
Useful Language for Explaining the Diagnosis of Functional Disorder

- Your symptoms do not fit the pattern of a known neurological or medical condition, which is good news.
- It is not uncommon for people to experience symptoms like these.
- These are real symptoms you are experiencing.
- We know you are not faking these symptoms.
- There is a strong connection between the brain, mind, and body.
- Symptoms like these can be your body's way of letting you know to pay attention to something, like _____ (stress, depression, anxiety, something you might be avoiding or ignoring, etc).

There is a paucity of systematic, controlled trials regarding the treatment of CD. Most data are limited to case reports, observational studies, and years of anecdotal evidence.

Psychiatric Evaluation

- Once the diagnosis of CD has been made and communicated to the patient, the next step in treatment is referral for psychiatric evaluation.

- Preferably, this should be to a psychiatrist experienced in conversion or trauma-based disorders. Organizations with resources for finding such clinicians include the following:

  ○ Academy of Psychosomatic Medicine

  ○ International Society for the Study of Trauma and Dissociation

- The patient should be evaluated for psychiatric comorbidities and the best type of psychotherapy determined.

Psychopharmacology

- There is no significant evidence to support the pharmacologic treatment of CD; however, the treatment of psychiatric comorbidities may improve outcomes.

Psychotherapy

- *Cognitive behavioral therapy* (CBT) is a robust, evidence-based form of psychotherapy that aims to identify and challenge distorted cognitions or beliefs that lead to maladaptive behaviors (or in the case of CD, somatic symptoms). CBT is usually performed by a graduate-level psychologist; however, it may also be practiced by psychiatrists and social workers. It is a structured, time-limited treatment that often involves weekly homework assignments for the patient.

- *Psychodynamic psychotherapy* aims to identify and bring into consciousness any subconscious psychological conflicts, traumas, emotions, or cognitions that may be linked to the onset of conversion symptoms. It is believed that the increased insight generated by the integration of subconscious problems with conscious thought leads to a resolution of symptoms.[26]

- *Dialectical behavioral therapy* (DBT) is an evidence-based treatment for borderline personality disorder (often a comorbidity of CD) that encourages more adaptive coping strategies in the form of mindfulness, emotion regulation, distress tolerance, and interpersonal effectiveness. There are no published trials of the use of DBT in CD; however, it has been postulated that improving one's coping mechanisms may decrease the need for the "conversion" of stress into somatic symptoms. As patients with BPD also have high rates of prior trauma,[27] the same set of strategies may be helpful for patients with CD.

- *Hypnosis* may be used on a case-by-case basis; however, this should be performed by a mental health provider who is both licensed in clinical hypnosis and experienced in the treatment of trauma and CD.

Physical Therapy

- A main goal is to remove the patient from the "sick role," which may be unconsciously reinforced by the social support of family and friends.

- Normal patterns of movement can be reestablished.

- Physical therapy may be a more culturally acceptable treatment than psychotherapy and can serve as a bridge to psychotherapy.[28]

REFERENCES

1. Hallet M. Psychogenic movement disorders: a crisis for neurology. *Curr Neurol Neurosci Rep.* 2006; 6:269–271.
2. Mula M. Are psychogenic non-epileptic seizures and psychogenic movement disorders two different entities? When even neurologists stop talking to each other. *Epilepsy Behav.* 2013; 26:100–101.
3. Akagi H, House A. The epidemiology of hysterical conversion. In: Halligan PW, Bass C, Marshall JC, eds. *Contemporary Approaches to the Study of Hysteria: Clinical and Theoretical Perspectives.* Oxford, UK: Oxford University Press; 2001:73–87.
4. Barsky AJ, Stern TA, Greenberg DB, Cassem NH. Functional somatic symptoms and somatoform disorders. In: Stern TA, Fricchione GL, Cassem NH, Jellinek MS,

Rosenbaum JF, eds. *Massachusetts General Hospital Handbook of General Hospital Psychiatry.* 5th ed. Philadelphia, PA: Elsevier; 2004:269–291.

5. Bowman ES, Markand ON. Psychodynamics and psychiatric diagnoses of pseudo-seizure subjects. *Am J Psychiatry.* 1996; 153(1):57–63.

6. American Psychiatric Association. *Diagnostic and Statistical Manual of Mental Disorders, Third Edition.* Washington, DC: American Psychiatric Association Publishing; 1980.

7. American Psychiatric Association. *Diagnostic and Statistical Manual of Mental Disorders, Fourth Edition, Text Revision.* Washington, DC: American Psychiatric Association Publishing; 2000.

8. American Psychiatric Association. *Diagnostic and Statistical Manual of Mental Disorders, Fifth Edition.* Arlington, VA: American Psychiatric Association Publishing; 2013.

9. Voon V, Brezing C, Gallea C, et al. Emotional stimuli and motor conversion disorder. *Brain.* 2010; 133(5):1526–1536.

10. Aybek S, Nicholson TRJ, Draganski B, et al. Grey matter changes in motor conversion disorder. *J Neurol Neurosurg Psychiatry.* 2014; 85(2):236–238.

11. Labate A, Cerasa A, Mula M, et al. Neuroanatomic correlates of psychogenic nonepileptic seizures: a cortical thickness and VBM study. *Epilepsia.* 2012; 53(2):377–385.

12. Gould R, Miller BL, Goldberg MA, Benson DF. The validity of hysterical signs and symptoms. *J Nerv Ment Dis.* 1986;174(10):593–597.

13. Rosebush PI, Mazurek MF. Treatment of conversion disorder in the 21st century: have we moved beyond the couch? *Curr Treat Options Neurol.* 2011; 13:255–266.

14. Caplan JP, Binius T, Lennon VA, et al. Pseudoseizures: conditions that may mimic psychogenic non-epileptic seizures. *Psychosomatics.* 2011; 52(6):501–506.

15. Kung AWC. Thyrotoxic periodic paralysis: a diagnostic challenge. *J Clin Endocrinol Metab.* 2006; 91(7):2490–2495.

16. Mader EC, El-Abassi R, Villemarette-Pittman NR, et al. Sporadic Creutzfeldt-Jakob disease with focal findings: caveats to current diagnostic criteria. *Neurol Int.* 2013; 5(1):e1.

17. Daum C, Hubschmid M, Aybek S. The value of 'positive' clinical signs for weakness, sensory and gait disorders in conversion disorder: a systematic and narrative review. *Neurol Neurosurg Psychiatry.* 2014; 85(2):180–190.

18. Fahn S, Williams DT. Psychogenic dystonia. *Adv Neurol.* 1988; 50:431-455.

19. Voon V, Lang AE, Hallet M. Diagnosing psychogenic movement disorders—which criteria should be used in clinical practice? *Nat Clin Pract Neurol.* 2007; 3(3):134–135.

20. Shill H, Gerber P. Evaluation of clinical diagnostic criteria for psychogenic movement disorders. *Mov Disord.* 2006; 21(8):1163–1168.

21. Morgante F, Edwards MJ, Espay AJ, et al. Diagnostic agreement in patients with psychogenic movement disorders. *Mov Disord.* 2012; 27(4):548–552.

22. Espay AJ, Goldenhar LM, Voon V, et al. Opinions and clinical practices related to diagnosing and managing patients with psychogenic movement disorders: an international survey of movement disorder society members. *Mov Disord.* 2009; 24(9):1366–1374.

23. Roelofs K, Keijsers, GPJ, Hoogduin KAL, et al. Childhood abuse in patients with conversion disorder. *Am J Psychiatry.* 2002; 159(11):1908–1913.

24. Kranick S, Ekanayake V, Martinez V, et al. Psychopathology and psychogenic movement disorders. *Mov Disord.* 2011; 26(10):1844–1850.

25. Stone J, Sharpe M, Binzer M. Motor conversion symptoms and pseudoseizures: a comparison of clinical characteristics. *Psychosomatics.* 2004; 45(6):492–499.

26. Baslet G. Psychogenic nonepileptic seizures: a treatment review. What have we learned since the beginning of the millennium? *Neuropsychiatr Dis Treat.* 2012; 8:585–598.

27. Anderson G, Yasenik L, Ross CA. Dissociative experiences and disorders among women who identify themselves as sexual abuse survivors. *Child Abuse Negl.* 1993; 17(5):677–686.

28. Ness D. Physical therapy management for conversion disorder: case series. *J Neurol Phys Ther.* 2007; 31(1):30–39.

IV

Surgical Approach to Movement Disorders

16

SURGICAL APPROACH TO MOVEMENT DISORDERS

HISTORY OF SURGERY FOR MOVEMENT DISORDERS

- In the 1950s, Cooper first described ligation of the anterior choroidal artery for the treatment of Parkinson's disease (PD).[1] In his series, tremor and rigidity improved in 70% of patients, while contralateral hemiplegia was noted in 11% and operative mortality occurred in 10%. This has been attributed to the variable vascular distribution of the anterior choroidal artery. This procedure fell out of favor because of its high morbidity rates and the efficacy of emerging treatment options.

- During this time period, Spiegel and colleagues introduced a novel stereotactic method in which intracranial landmarks—in this case, the pineal gland and the foramina of Monro—were used to locate adjacent anatomical structures.[2] In further studies, their stereotactic lesioning techniques were shown to be as effective as open procedures for the treatment of movement disorders, with a lower risk for complications.

- Lars Leksell introduced posteroventral pallidotomy in the 1950s after noting better treatment of all three cardinal symptoms of PD (tremor, rigidity, and bradykinesia) with this technique than with anterodorsal pallidotomy. Outcomes of this procedure were described by Svennilson et al in 1960 and confirmed by Laitinen et al in 1992.[3,4] Posteroventral pallidotomy was considered the standard of care for the treatment of PD before deep brain stimulation (DBS) became available.

- When levodopa was introduced in the 1960s, the surgical treatment of PD declined in favor of medical management. However, the long-term use of levodopa is associated with several side effects, and over time, interest in surgical treatment options was renewed.[5] During this period, significant advances in technology allowed improved imaging studies, microelectrode recording capabilities, and understanding of the underlying anatomy.

■ DBS was pioneered for movement disorders in the 1980s and became a preferred tool because of its reversibility and adjustability. The Food and Drug Administration (FDA) approved thalamic DBS for essential tremor and PD-associated tremor in 1997, followed by subthalamic nucleus (STN) and globus pallidus internus (GPi) DBS for PD in 2003.[6]

■ The remainder of this chapter will provide an overview of the surgical management options currently available for the treatment of movement disorders, with an emphasis on DBS.

SURGERY FOR SPECIFIC MOVEMENT DISORDERS

■ Surgical procedures do not treat the cause of movement disorders, and to date, they have not been shown to alter the natural history of the disease. Surgical procedures are aimed at alleviating the symptoms of some movement disorders in order to improve quality of life.

○ Stereotactic procedures for the symptoms of PD include ablative procedures and DBS of several cerebral targets, predominantly the thalamus, globus pallidus, and subthalamic area.

○ DBS is also currently approved by the FDA for the management of essential tremors and, under a Humanitarian Device Exemption, for the treatment of primary dystonias.[6]

○ The stereotactic methods for probing the brain are similar whether the intent is to produce a radio-frequency thermolesion or to deploy an electrode for chronic electrical stimulation (DBS).

○ In addition, noninvasive techniques, such as radiosurgery, are an option for the ablation of subcortical targets in some cases.

■ Surgical management of some movement disorders can lead to the mitigation of motor symptoms and improvement in daily function for patients with advanced disease, resistance to medication, or unmanageable side effects. When patients are counseled regarding the surgical treatment of movement disorders, it is very important to stress that movement disorders have two distinct categories of symptoms: motor and nonmotor (ie, cognitive and behavioral).

○ The goal of all movement disorder surgery is to attempt to control the motor symptoms and minimize nonmotor adverse effects.

○ It is important to have an open discussion with the patient and family regarding which symptoms are more likely to improve and which symptoms will not or are less likely to improve. It should also be explained that surgery is not curative.

○ **Keep in mind that the appeal of technology and invasive treatment can give some patients the impression that surgical intervention is curative.**

■ As with all surgical procedures, patient selection can influence outcomes. In our experience, we find that multidisciplinary evaluation is helpful in determining candidates who are likely to respond from a motor standpoint with a lower risk for nonmotor complications.

○ The multidisciplinary team may include neurologists, neurosurgeons, neuropsychologists, and physical and/or occupational therapists. A psychiatrist evaluates patients for whom behavioral comorbidities are a significant concern, and a bioethicist is involved as needed.

○ This multidisciplinary evaluation has several goals.

● Although it may sound obvious, confirmation or reevaluation of the diagnosis is an important first goal. It is not rare for patients to be labeled with a diagnosis for several years, and revisiting often leads to a change in the primary diagnosis and treatment plan.

● The team reevaluates the current and past treatment regimens. Some patients may benefit from pharmacologic optimization only and may not require surgery.

● A detailed cognitive evaluation can determine the degree of cognitive decline, which may correlate with risk for postsurgical worsening.

● The risk for negative effects of surgery on nonmotor symptoms is related not only to the procedure and insertion of the leads but also to chronic stimulation of these complex subcortical targets.

Parkinson's Disease

GENERAL INDICATIONS (TABLE 16.1)

■ Advanced movement disorder

■ Poor symptomatic management with drugs

■ Drug-induced side effects

■ Manageable comorbidities

Table 16.1
Typical Surgical Candidates With Parkinson's Disease

Idiopathic Parkinson's Disease
• **Positive response to levodopa:** a response of ~>30% to levodopa in off–on test usually indicates better prognosis[7]
• Tremor-predominant: even levodopa-unresponsive tremor tends to improve with surgery.
• Patient has appendicular symptoms: rigidity, freezing, dystonia, bradykinesia.
• Patient has dyskinesia while on medication.
• On–off surgical fluctuations occur.
• Patient has limited cognitive decline.
• There is no major or severe and unmanaged psychiatric disorder.

Table 16.2
Parkinson Symptoms Likely or Unlikely to Improve With Deep Brain Stimulation

Likely to Improve	Less/Not Likely to Improve
• Tremor	• Gait
• Rigidity	• Sialorrhea/swallowing
• Bradykinesia	• Balance problems/falling
• On–off fluctuations	• Other axial symptoms
• Freezing of gait (±)	• Urinary/gastrointestinal symptoms

▓ Ability of the patient to understand the goals, risks, possible benefits, and limitations of surgery and the available alternatives to surgery

GENERAL CONTRAINDICATIONS (TABLE 16.2)

▓ Dementia, major cognitive decline

▓ Severe or unmanaged psychiatric/behavioral disorder

○ Note: Depression and anxiety are common. They are not contraindications per se if managed.

▓ Poorly controlled medical comorbidities

▓ Clotting disorders that cannot be managed perioperatively

▓ Requirement for anticoagulation or anti-aggregation therapy that cannot be stopped

■ Lack of ability to understand (patient and/or caregiver) the goals, risks, possible benefits, and limitations of surgery

■ Inability to adequately follow-up at the specialized center (greater limitation for DBS than for ablative treatments)

Essential Tremor: General Indications and Contraindications

■ As with other neurological disorders, the first-line treatment is medical management.

■ DBS for essential tremor is generally noted to have good outcomes; the outcomes for secondary tremor are not as good.

■ DBS of the ventral intermediate nucleus (VIM) can be offered to patients with poorly managed tremor.

■ The severity of tremor that "requires" surgery varies from person to person. The goals and needs depend on the patient's occupation, hobbies, and personal interests. Secondary (nonessential) tremor can be treated with DBS (off label), but the outcomes tend to be limited.

■ Patients with distal tremor are thought to have a better prognosis.

Dystonia: General Indications and Contraindications (Table 16.3)

■ Primary generalized dystonia, with or without known genetic mutation (ie, *DYT1*).

■ Primary torticollis.

Table 16.3
Success of Deep Brain Stimulation in Different Types of Dystonia

Primary Dystonia	Secondary Dystonia	Tardive Dystonia
No evident underlying cause	Associated with identifiable brain insult	Associated with long-term neuroleptic administration
Subset known to have *DYT1* mutation	Can be caused by stroke, trauma, toxin exposures	Postsynaptic dopamine striatal receptors sensitized
Potential candidates for bilateral DBS	Mixed results with DBS	May benefit from bilateral DBS

- Surgical treatment for other segmental or focal dystonias possible, but outcomes not as well defined (off label for use of the device in the United States).

- Significant disability related to dystonia.

- Failure of nonsurgical management, including oral drugs, botulinum toxin injections.

SURGICAL TREATMENT OPTIONS AND SYMPTOM MANAGEMENT

- DBS implantation is the most common procedure for the treatment of movement disorders in the United States. DBS has largely supplanted ablative techniques, but some patients are still good candidates for ablative treatment (Table 16.4).

  - The two most common ablative procedures used for movement disorders are radio-frequency (RF) ablation and gamma knife radiosurgery (GKRS).

  - The size of the lesion created with RF ablation can be tailored to a certain extent.

  - Frequent neurological examinations are usually conducted while RF ablation is performed to minimize risk of unforeseen effects due to the lesion created.

- In GKRS, a focused beam of ionizing radiation from multiple locations is used with a high level of precision to create the lesion.

  - Some advantages of GKRS are that patients are discharged home on the day of the procedure and that it can be used for patients who are otherwise not good surgical candidates because of comorbidities.

  - Because of the nature of the ionizing radiation that creates the lesion, the clinical results associated with GKRS are not immediately visible to the patient and may take weeks to become apparent.

- Although ablative procedures are not as commonly performed as DBS, they do have some advantages that should be considered in certain situations.

  - Patients do not have any implanted hardware that can be susceptible to erosion or infection.

  - Patients do not require as frequent follow-up for the adjustment of stimulation (but continue to require medication adjustments and follow-up). This is especially useful when patients are not able to follow up regularly with the movement disorder team.

- DBS has largely replaced ablative procedures like thalamotomy and pallidotomy as standard of care for the treatment of movement disorders because DBS is reversible and does not create a permanent lesion. In addition, the stimulation can be modulated, and the location of the lead can be revised if necessary.[7] On the other hand, implanted hardware is associated with risks. It is important to note that the goal for each of the preceding procedures is similar. Each technique has specific benefits and limitations.

Deep Brain Stimulation

- DBS is the procedure most commonly performed for the treatment of movement disorders in the United States.

- The implanted device has three components: lead, connecting cable, and implantable pulse generator (IPG).

- A risk for cognitive decline has been noted in some patients, although it is usually not clinically significant in selected candidates.

- DBS is associated with improvement in quality of life and a reduction in motor symptoms, including tremor, rigidity, bradykinesia, dyskinesia, and off–on fluctuations.

- Levodopa challenge is a good indicator of symptomatic improvement.

- Complications can be related to surgery (eg, hemorrhage, infection, misplaced lead); hardware (eg, lead migration or failure, erosion through skin); or stimulation (eg, dyskinesia, freezing, speech disturbance, muscle contraction)[7]

Table 16.4
Deep Brain Stimulation Versus Ablative Procedures

Deep Brain Stimulation	Ablative Procedures
Reversible, nonablative Possible to revise location	Irreversible, tissue permanently changed Not possible to revise location
Possible to adjust parameters to modulate effects of stimulation	Reoperation required to increase effects but cannot reverse effects
Increased cost associated with equipment management postoperatively	No further surgical cost after uncomplicated procedure performed
Possibility of equipment failure, infection, erosion	No issues related to implanted equipment
Less risk for bilateral surgery	Greater risk for speech, cognitive, or other deficits with bilateral ablations

Radio-Frequency Ablation

■ Lesions are created with insulated leads that have exposed tips. An RF generator is used to perform the ablation.

■ The lesion size depends on the size of the exposed tip, the temperature, and the duration of RF.

■ Before the lesion is created, electrical stimulation is performed through the lead to assess the effects. The lesion size can be titrated, and multiple small lesions can be used to "stack" a larger lesion shape.

■ Controversy exists regarding lesion site and size and regarding the safety of bilateral lesions.[8]

■ Serial intraoperative neurological examinations are performed to assess for efficacy and adverse effects as a lesion is created.

Gamma Knife Radiosurgery

■ GKRS is considered mostly for patients with medical comorbidities that preclude other surgical procedures.

■ There is a minimal risk for complications such as hemorrhage, infection, and other perioperative medical issues. A delay of weeks to months before the appearance of clinical improvement (or adverse effects) is expected after the procedure.

■ There is a risk for delayed enlargement of lesion into normal tissue secondary to radiation necrosis or cyst formation.

■ Another disadvantage is the inability to perform intraoperative physiologic testing before the target is treated.

■ Results of GKRS have been mixed. Some studies show good safety and efficacy, whereas other studies show limited or no improvement.[9,10]

■ Doses from 100 to 160 Gy for stereotactic radiosurgery thalamotomy have been described.[10]

Frameless Versus Frame-Based Stereotactic Surgery (Table 16.5)

■ Frame-based systems are thought to be the "gold standard" for stereotactic surgery because they are precise and reliable, and they have been used for many years with good results. Head frames are usually placed under local anesthesia. When the head frame is placed, the line between the lateral canthus and the tragus is observed, and the head frame is placed approximately parallel to the anterior commissure–posterior commissure (AC-PC) line.

Table 16.5
Differences Between Frame-Based and Frameless Systems

Feature	Frame-Based	Frameless
Reference point	Frame	Fiducials/frameless system
Benefits	Solid metal construction Stable even with tremor Good support for surgical instrumentation	Greater mobility of head, easy access to airway
Drawbacks	More discomfort or pain at placement Head fixed and immobile	Nonreusable, possibly less secure fixation to head, predetermined penetration points in some systems, less adjustable
Preoperative imaging	CT/MRI performed, images co-registered with frame (fiducial box)	CT/MRI performed, images co-registered with fiducials

- Some groups use frameless systems. These may improve patient comfort, facilitate image acquisition, and increase efficiency in surgical planning. Both systems have been shown to be safe and effective, so the decision is often based upon surgeon preference.[11]

FRAME-BASED SYSTEM

- The stereotactic frame is placed over the patient's head and secured with pins. It remains in place for the entire procedure.

- CT/MRI is performed, and the stereo imaging (containing the fiducial data) is co-registered with the preoperative imaging. The target is selected and trajectories are based upon anatomical structures, coordinates, or atlases.

- The clinical workstation helps calculates coordinates for the frame and arc.

- The entry point is marked and a burr hole placed.

- A microdrive is mounted to the frame for microelectrode recording and/or DBS lead implantation or RF lesion creation.

FRAMELESS SYSTEM

- Skull fiducials are placed before the procedure, sometimes several days in advance of image acquisition.

- A lightweight disposable "frameless system" is affixed to the head.

- A disposable microdrive is mounted over the frameless system for recording or lead placement.

- Frameless surgery is today considered an equivalent choice to the headframe at many centers.

Microelectrode Recording

- The image-based target localization can be physiologically verified and refined with microelectrode recording techniques. Fine, high-impedance electrodes are placed through the target area while recording is performed.

- Anatomical structures are identified by characteristic electrophysiological activity.

- Single or multiple passes may be required to delineate anatomical boundaries. Once the target area is determined, the DBS lead is inserted.

Intraoperative, Real-Time MRI Stereotaxis

- A diagnostic MRI suite prepared for surgery or an intraoperative MRI system is required.

- Intraoperative real-time MRI is used to guide DBS lead implantation.

RESULTS

STN and GPi Deep Brain Stimulation for Parkinson's Disease

- STN DBS allows a greater decrease in postoperative medication requirements.

- A large, double-blinded study showed significant improvements in motor scores with bilateral GPi and STN stimulation, with a trend for superior outcomes with STN stimulation.[12]

- Another large multicenter, randomized, blinded trial showed that STN and GPi targets are associated with similar improvements in motor function after bilateral implantation, and that target selection should take into account the constellation of symptoms and the physician's preference.[13]

- Some evidence indicates that STN DBS is more strongly associated with cognitive and behavioral dysfunction.[14,15]

- Advanced age and levodopa-equivalent dose were found to be correlated with a postoperative decline in neuropsychology test results in one study.[15]

VIM Deep Brain Stimulation for Tremor

■ VIM DBS is used for the treatment of tremor from PD and for essential tremor. However, it is not commonly used for PD because STN and GPi targets can also manage other cardinal symptoms.

■ DBS is the procedure of choice for essential tremor because it has been shown to have efficacy similar to that of thalamotomy and a lower risk profile.

■ Bilateral DBS implantation is considered for patients with bilateral symptoms, although it is often staged. It is not as effective for axial tremors. Bilateral thalamic DBS may carry an increased risk for dysarthria.

■ One study showed a mean reduction in contralateral limb tremor of 79% after 3 months.[16]

GPi Deep Brain Stimulation for Dystonia

■ Pallidotomy can be effective, but bilateral procedures can be associated with lethargy and other complications.

■ Improvement after bilateral DBS can be seen up to 3 years after the initial DBS procedure.

■ Patients with primary dystonia (including those positive for the *DYT1* mutation) had a greater improvement on the Dystonia Rating Scale.[7,17]

COMPLICATIONS

Surgical Complications

■ Intracranial hemorrhage is reported in 0.5% to 5% of DBS procedures. In one series, 0.5% of cases were asymptomatic and 0.5% were symptomatic.[18]

■ Subdural, epidural, and intracortical hemorrhages may occur.

○ Some techniques are commonly used to minimize complications, although their efficacy is not proven: avoid hypertension, limit microelectrode recording, use contrasted imaging studies to assess trajectories.

■ Lead misplacement may require surgical revision.

Infection

■ One large study showed an overall infection rate of 4.2%.[19]

■ Most commonly presents within the first three months after surgery.[19]

- If hardware is exposed or if there is pus in contact with the hardware, partial or complete explantation of the system is usually recommended.

- Partial explantation may be possible if the infection is localized, but the remaining parts of the system may already be contaminated.

Hardware-Related Complications

- These include electrode fracture, extension wire failure, skin erosion, hardware-related pain, and IPG malfunction (Table 16.6). One study showed a 4.3% overall rate of hardware-related complications.[20]

- Erosion through the skin is thought to be more common in slim patients implanted with bulkier hardware.

Stimulation-Related Complications

- Ocular symptoms, worsening dyskinesia and axial symptoms, speech dysfunction, and corticospinal stimulation may be noted.

- Lack of or less than expected change in motor symptoms postoperatively.

- Cognitive decline develops after implantation and chronic stimulation.

- Involuntary muscle contractions.

- Typically, all patients will have stimulation-induced "side" effects at the first programming visits. These define the threshold for stimulation-related side effects. Programming is then set to lower settings.

- Stimulation-related side effects are usually corrected with adjustments to stimulation.

Table 16.6
Hardware-Related Complications

Lead Failure	Extension Wire Failure	IPG Malfunction
Fractures, sometimes after trauma	Erosion through skin	Erosion through skin
Migration	Fractures at the neck	Shocking sensation
Short Circuits	Tightness ("bowstringing") or pain along site	Migration of the implantable pulse generator

SAFETY ISSUES

Electrocautery

■ A monopolar electrocautery device (Bovie) can be used with caution in patients after DBS implantation. The tip and plate of the Bovie device should be away from the DBS system, and the neurostimulator should be turned off preoperatively.

■ Medtronic package instructions:[21] When electrocautery is necessary, following these precautions may reduce electromagnetic interference effects:

○ Disconnect any cable connecting the lead or extension to a screener or external neurostimulator.

○ Use only bipolar cautery.

○ If unipolar cautery is necessary:

● Use only a low-voltage mode.

● Use the lowest possible power setting.

● Keep the current path (ground plate) as far from the neurostimulator, extension, and lead as possible.

● Do not use full-length operating room table grounding pads.

● Keep the implanted neurostimulator and lead system out of the conductive path.

● Keep the electrocautery current flow perpendicular to a line drawn between the neurostimulator case and the lead electrodes.

MRI

After implantation of a DBS, a patient **CANNOT** undergo MRI with body coils. In some cases, MRI of the head may be performed only with transmit–receive head coils and limited sequences. For information regarding safety guidelines, consult the manufacturer's information. At the time of this publication, information for the only marketed system can be found at http://professional.medtronic.com/dbsmri

■ It is important to counsel patients regarding these safety issues so that they are aware of the dangers associated with these devices.

Diathermy

Medtronic safety labeling for diathermy:[21]

■ Do not use shortwave diathermy, microwave diathermy, or therapeutic ultrasound diathermy (all now referred to as diathermy) on patients implanted with a neurostimulation system. Energy from diathermy can be transferred through the implanted system and can cause tissue damage at the location of the implanted electrodes, resulting in severe injury or death.

- Diathermy can also damage the neurostimulation system components, resulting in loss of therapy and requiring additional surgery for system explantation and replacement.

- Advise your patients to inform all their health care professionals that they should not be exposed to diathermy treatment.

- Injury to the patient or damage to the device can occur during diathermy treatment when:

  ○ The neurostimulation system is turned on or off.

  ○ Diathermy is used anywhere on the body—not just at the location of the neurostimulation system.

  ○ Diathermy delivers heat or no heat.

  ○ Any component of the neurostimulation system (lead, extension, neurostimulator) remains in the body.

REFERENCES

1. Cooper IS. Ligation of the anterior choroidal artery for involuntary movement of parkinsonism. *Psychiatr Q.* 1953; 27(2):317–319.
2. Spiegel EA, Wycis HT, Marks M, Lee AJ. Stereotaxic apparatus for operations on the human brain. *Science.* 1947; 106(2754):349–350.
3. Svennilson E, Torvik A, Lowe R, et al. Treatment of parkinsonism by stereotactic thermolesions in the pallidal region. A clinical evaluation of 81 cases. *Acta Psychiatr Neurol Scand.* 1960; 35:358–377.
4. Laitinen LV, Bergenheim AT, Hariz MI. Leksell's posteroventral pallidotomy in the treatment of Parkinson's disease. *J Neurosurg.* 1992; 76(1):53–61.
5. Ludin HP, Bass-Verrey F. Study of deterioration in long-term treatment of parkinsonism with L-dopa plus decarboxylase inhibitor. *J Neural Transm.* 1976; 38(3-4):249–258.
6. Miocinovic S, Somayajula S, Chitnis S, Vitek JL. History, applications, and mechanisms of deep brain stimulation. *JAMA Neurol.* 2013; 70(2):163–171.
7. Machado AG, Deogaonkar M, Cooper S. Deep brain stimulation for movement disorders: patient selection and technical options. *Cleve Clin J Med.* 2012; 79(suppl 2):S19–S24.
8. Okun MS, Vitek JL. Lesion therapy for Parkinson's disease and other movement disorders: update and controversies. *Mov Disord.* 2004; 19(4):375–389.
9. Barbarisi M, Pantelis E, Antypas C, Romanelli P. Radiosurgery for movement disorders. *Comput Aided Surg.* 2011; 16(3):101–111.
10. Frighetto L, Bizzi J, Annes RD, et al. Stereotactic radiosurgery for movement disorders. *Surg Neurol Int.* 2012; 3(suppl 1):S10–S16.

1. Rezai AR, Machado AG, Deogaonkar M, et al. Surgery for movement disorders. *Neurosurgery.* 2008; 62(suppl 2):809–838, discussion 838–839.

2. Deep-Brain Stimulation for Parkinson's Disease Study Group. Deep-brain stimulation of the subthalamic nucleus or the pars interna of the globus pallidus in Parkinson's disease. *N Engl J Med.* 2001;345(13):956–963.

3. Follett KA, Weaver FM, Stern M, et al. Pallidal versus subthalamic deep-brain stimulation for Parkinson's disease. *N Engl J Med.* 2010; 362(22):2077–2091.

4. Funkiewiez A, Ardouin C, Caputo E, et al. Long-term effects of bilateral subthalamic nucleus stimulation on cognitive function, mood, and behaviour in Parkinson's disease. *J Neurol Neurosurg Psychiatry.* 2004; 75(6):834–839.

5. Heo JH, Lee KM, Paek SH, et al. The effects of bilateral subthalamic nucleus deep brain stimulation (STN DBS) on cognition in Parkinson disease. *J Neurol Sci.* 2008; 273(1-2):19–24.

6. Mandat T, Koziara H, Rola R, et al. Thalamic deep brain stimulation in the treatment of essential tremor. *Neurol Neurochir Pol.* 2011; 45(1):37–41.

7. Panov F, Gologorsky Y, Connors G, et al. Deep brain stimulation in DYT1 dystonia: a 10-year experience. *Neurosurgery.* 2013; 73(1):86–93.

8. Zrinzo L, Foltynie T, Limousin P, et al. Reducing hemorrhagic complications in functional neurosurgery: a large case series and systematic literature review. *J Neurosurg.* 2012; 116(1):84–94.

9. Piacentino M, Pilleri M, Bartolomei L. Hardware-related infections after deep brain stimulation surgery: review of incidence, severity and management in 212 single-center procedures in the first year after implantation. *Acta Neurochir (Wien).* 2011; 153(12):2337–2341.

20. Boviatsis EJ, Stavrinou LC, Themistocleous M, et al. Surgical and hardware complications of deep brain stimulation. A seven-year experience and review of the literature. *Acta Neurochir (Wien).* 2010; 152(12):2053–2062.

21. Medtronic DPS therapy. Implanted neurostimulators. http://manuals.medtronic.com/wcm/groups/mdtcom_sg/@emanuals/@era/@neuro/documents/documents/contrib_148347.pdf. Accessed April 14, 2014.

V

Nonpharmacologic Approach to Movement Disorders

17

PHYSICAL AND OCCUPATIONAL THERAPY

Patients with movement disorders can develop motor, cognitive, and behavioral impairments that can lead to a loss of functional ability and independence in activities of daily living and result in decreased quality of life. Physical and occupational therapy can help to prevent and treat these symptoms, and to rehabilitate patients in order to restore maximum movement, functional mobility, and participation in work, family, and society. The aim of therapy is to maximize independence and quality of life at the time of the diagnosis and throughout the course of the disorder.

This chapter is designed to focus on the role of physical and occupational therapists in the care and management of patients with movement disorders. We first discuss the emerging role of exercise in the management of Parkinson's disease (PD). We subsequently discuss the roles of physical and occupational therapists as part of a multidisciplinary team. Finally, we discuss the specific issue of falls in people with movement disorders.

Movement disorders are grouped together on the basis of the similarity of the clinical presentation. Many movement disorders represent progressive, multisystem neurodegenerative processes that can result in increased disability over time. A few important conceptual points are relevant to the clinical care of patients:

- Forms of parkinsonism such as progressive supranuclear palsy (PSP), multiple systems atrophy (MSA), dementia with Lewy bodies (DLB), and corticobasal ganglionic degeneration (CBDG) result in relatively rapid rates of decline.[1–4]

- Idiopathic PD usually has a relatively slower rate of progression, but disabling deficits that are unresponsive to medication will develop over time in a majority of patients.[5]

■ Hereditary choreas, ataxias, and dystonias similarly result in progressive decline at a variable rate, which depends on the disease process.[6-8]

THE ROLE OF EXERCISE IN THE MANAGEMENT OF PARKINSON'S DISEASE

Exercise is an important part of healthy living for everyone, regardless of the presence of any movement disorder. Regular exercise is a vital component to maintain balance, mobility, and activities of daily living in people with movement disorders. Upon diagnosis, people with movements disorders have already reduced their overall level of physical activity and often have withdrawn from recreational and leisure activities despite minimal reports of disability. Individuals with PD show a significant decline in their levels of physical activity in the first year after their diagnosis. Inactivity can accelerate the degenerative process and result in multiple preventable secondary impairments.

Evidence-Based Benefits of Exercise in People With Parkinson's Disease

■ Improved physical function

■ Improved quality of life

■ Increased strength

■ Improved balance

■ Increased walking speed and stride length

■ Increased flexibility and posture

Potential Motor and Nonmotor Targets of Exercise

■ Prevention of cardiovascular complications

■ Reduced risk for osteoporosis

■ Improved cognitive function

■ Prevention of depression

■ Improved sleep

■ Decreased constipation

■ Decreased fatigue

■ Improved functional motor performance

■ Improved drug efficacy

■ Optimization of the dopaminergic system

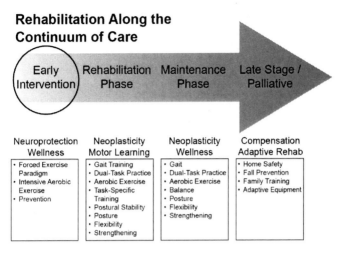

Figure 17.1

Summary of the rehabilitation approach across the continuum of Parkinson's disease.

Disease Modification

Animal models have shown that physical activity may directly impact the neurodegenerative process, likely mediated by brain neurotrophic factors and neuroplasticity. Potential mechanisms include angiogenesis, synaptogenesis, reduced oxidative stress, decreased inflammation, and improved mitochondrial function. Vigorous aerobic exercise has been associated with a reduced risk for developing PD and improved cognitive function. This type of exercise has been shown to increase the volume of gray matter in the brain, and to improve functional connectivity and cortical activation related to cognition. There is also emerging evidence that exercise can improve corticomotor excitability in people with PD.[9–12] With the potential benefit of neuroplasticity and neuroprotection, exercise is an important part in the medical management in people with PD (Figure 17.1).

Ingredients to Promote Neuroplasticity and Neuroprotection

- Exercises based on motor learning
- High level of repetition
- Task-specific training
- "Forced" aerobic exercise
- "Forced-use" exercise
- Complexity: dual tasking

Evidence-Based Approach to Exercise for Parkinson's Disease

- Progressive aerobic training

- Treadmill training

- Pole walking

- High-effort, whole-body, large-amplitude movements (eg, Lee Silverman Voice Therapy–BIG [LSVT-BIG])

- Spinal flexibility

- Agility (coordination and balance training)

- Augmentation of proprioceptive feedback

- Kinesthetic awareness training

- High-effort rate or strength training

- Dual-task training

- Dancing, tai chi, music, boxing[12–22]

PHYSICAL THERAPY AND OCCUPATIONAL THERAPY IN A MULTIDISCIPLINARY APPROACH TO MANAGEMENT

The management of movement disorders is best approached with a patient-centered multidisciplinary team (Figure 17.2 and Table 17.1).

Differentiating the Roles of the Physical Therapist and the Occupational Therapist

Physical therapists and occupational therapists have different areas of expertise (Figure 17.3), and a physician referring a patient to one of these specialists should be familiar with the domains of expertise of each.[23,24]

THE ROLE OF THE PHYSICAL THERAPIST. Postural instability and dysfunction of gait and balance are common symptoms in many movement disorders. The goal of physical therapy is to partner with patients to develop exercises and strategies that maintain or increase activity levels, decrease rigidity and bradykinesia, optimize gait, improve balance and motor coordination, and develop an individualized exercise program to prevent secondary impairments (Figures 17.4 and 17.5; Table 17.2).

WHEN TO REFER TO A PHYSICAL THERAPIST. Upon diagnosis, referral to a physical therapist for an early intervention exercise program is vital in the management of most people with movements disorders. The benefits of early referral include the following:

Multidisciplinary Team

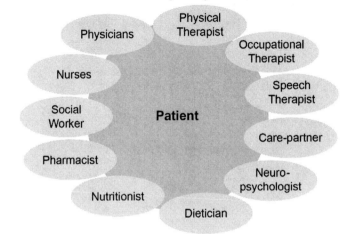

Figure 17.2
The multidisciplinary team providers.

Table 17.1
Members of the Management Team and Their Respective Roles

Function or Problem to Be Addressed	Specialist
Dexterity, gait, balance	Physical and occupational therapists, physiatrists
Swallow function, dysarthria, hypophonia	Speech and swallow clinicians, laryngologists, gastroenterologists
Cognitive decline	Neurologists, geriatricians, neuropsychologists, pharmacists, occupational therapists
Mood disorders	Neurologists, primary care physicians, clinical psychologists, sex therapists, psychiatrists

- Establish baseline physical functional status with the use of standardized outcome tools

- Develop an individualized exercise program

- Identify motor dysfunction as well as impairments that can be addressed through exercise and behavioral modification

- Develop effective gait and balance strategies, which is more easily done before significant disease progression ensues

Dysfunctions appropriate for referral to an **Occupational Therapist**	Dysfunctions appropriate for referral to a **Physical Therapist**

Fine motor function
- Handwriting
- Feeding
- Dressing
- Bathing
- Household tasks
- Ergonomics (Work Site Modification)

Pain
Posture
Strength
Range of Motion
Proprioception
Coordination

Gross motor function
- Gait
- Balance/Falls
- Transfers
- Decrease Endurance
- Flexibility

Figure 17.3

Differentiating the roles of the physical therapist and occupational therapist.

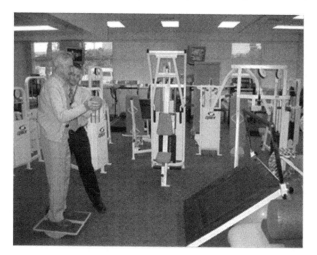

Figure 17.4

Example of balance training. The patient is standing on a "wobble board."
The upper extremities are occupied with a task to mimic the multitasking necessary in many activities of daily living.

- Educate patients and care partners about the disease process and its motor and nonmotor consequences

- Reduce the risk for and fear of falling

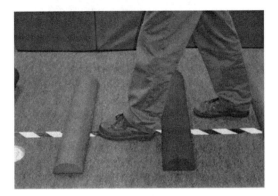

Figure 17.5

Example of a stepping exercise. A patient with gait freezing develops a motor program of stepping by using visual cues.

Table 17.2
Physical Therapy Interventions

Deficit	Treatment
Physical capacity	Cardiovascular endurance training
Rigidity (axial extension and rotation)	Range of motion and flexibility exercises
Weakness (trunk and lower extremity extensors)	Resistance and functional strength training
Postural instability (anticipatory and reactive postural responses)	Balance training (see Figure 17.4), postural adjustment exercises, cognitive strategies training
Gait dysfunction (bradykinesia, freezing, festination)	Whole-body activation Retraining in acceleration and large-amplitude functional movement Treadmill training Adaptive stepping techniques • Visual cues (ie, stepping over an object or caregiver's foot, inverted cane, using a laser pointer to create a dot on floor as a target; see Figure 17.5) • Auditory cues (ie, metronome, counting aloud, walking with music) • Internal cues (for patients with mild disability who are able to concentrate on step-by-step activity rather than continuous gait). Patients can stop/pause to regroup/reset and start again with one good step.
Declining ability to perform activities of daily living	Exercises to improve bed mobility and transfer Exercises to improve performance in leisure and recreational activity

- Monitor changes in functional status and ability to sustain an optimal exercise program

- Delay the onset of activity limitations and prevent secondary impairments

- Evaluate functional or work capacity

The role of the physical therapist in current practice is to harness available circuitry to re-learn skills that have been lost due to deficiencies in striatal function, whether this is due to dopamine deficiency or to other degenerative processes affecting the basal ganglia.

THE ROLE OF THE OCCUPATIONAL THERAPIST. Deficits in dextrous movements, as well as gait and balance deficits affecting performance of the activities of daily living, are common in movement disorders. The primary goal of the occupational therapist is to improve the patient's quality of life throughout the disease process by increasing functional movement and by prescribing adaptive devices to assist in maintaining independent function (Figures 17.6 and 17.7; Table 17.3).[25–29]

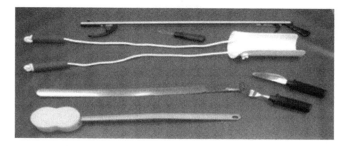

Figure 17.6
Examples of adaptive devices.

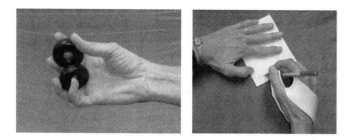

Figure 17.7
Examples of writing exercises.

Table 17.3
Occupational Therapy Interventions

Deficit	Treatment
Poor gait rhythm affecting activities of daily living	Multisensory cueing, cognitive cueing strategies
Poor motor dexterity	Coordination drills
Fatigue	Energy conservation techniques
Declining ability to perform activities of daily living	*Self-care:* Devices and techniques are provided to reduce dependence. Practice in a monitored setting with devices is necessary for devices to be incorporated in patient's activity routines. *Home management:* Lightweight vacuum cleaners and dust mops, jar openers, long-handled scrub brushes, and other devices are used to facilitate independence. Home assessments may be performed to evaluate for safety hazards such as throw rugs, and to provide adaptive devices such as handicap bars, shower seats, ramps, and other devices designed to improve function in the home.
Handwriting	Exercises to improve hand manipulation skills and independent finger movements (see Figure 17.7).

WHEN TO REFER TO AN OCCUPATIONAL THERAPIST. Early referral to an occupational therapist will address the following:

- Baseline evaluations of the severity of the motor disorder, active functional movement, passive joint movement, dependence level in activities of daily living, speed of performance of self-care activities, handwriting skills, and ability to perform simultaneous and sequential tasks

- Cognitive rehabilitation

- Instructions in accommodation principles that can be used throughout the progression of the disease

- Prevention of musculoskeletal deficits

- Instructions in grading of activities so that function can be facilitated despite changing symptoms

- Early initiation of environmental adaptations

- Driver evaluation and rehabilitation

- Caregiver instructions in the disease process and the process of rehabilitation

The occupational therapist uses a different set of strategies from the physical therapist to improve function, and the best outcomes usually develop when the two disciplines work together.

Physical and Occupational Therapy in Parkinsonism and Other Movement Disorders

The overall strategy for physical and occupational therapy in forms of parkinsonism and other movement disorders is similar to the strategy in PD; however, the initial functional disability at diagnosis may be greater, responsiveness to medication may be less, and the rate of decline in function can be steeper. Cases must be treated individually, depending on specific needs.

THE FALLING PATIENT

Falls are a leading cause of morbidity and mortality in the elderly population and frequently contribute to the need for nursing home placement.[30,31] This is a particular issue in patients with movement disorders, which often result in deficits of gait and balance. For example, parkinsonism is a major risk factor for falls in surveys of the elderly.[31,32] Dystonia, chorea, and ataxia can similarly result in gait disturbances that predispose to falls.

The following factors in movement disorders predispose to falling or increase the risk for falls in individuals with movement disorders:

- Older age
- Longer duration of disease
- Advanced stage of disease
- Rigidity or dystonia of the lower limbs
- Freezing or festination
- Severe chorea or dyskinesia
- Ataxia
- Symptomatic orthostatic hypotension
- Other medical or neurological conditions
- Local environmental factors

The clinician confronted with a patient who is falling should not assume that all the causes of falls are the same. Because the basis of falls may not be readily detected on physical examination, the clinician must take a careful history to determine the true frequency of falling and the potential causes and contributing factors. Identification of the probable cause is important for developing an effective treatment plan. Table 17.4 lists some common causes of falls in different movement disorders, and strategies for evaluating the risk for falls.

Table 17.4
Evaluating Falls in Movement Disorders

Source of Fall	Associated Disease Processes	Evaluation
Postural instability	Parkinson's disease and forms of parkinsonism	Mini-best test, timed up and go, five times sit to stand, retropulsion pull test.
Freezing/start hesitation	Parkinson's disease and forms of parkinsonism	Freezing of gait questionnaire, gait observation. Freezing can frequently be observed in enclosed spaces (eg, a small examination room), during turns (turn hesitation), or when the patient starts from a standing position (start hesitation).
Ataxia	Ataxia, Huntington's disease	Evaluate gait. Ataxic gait is wide-based. Patients may weave. Tandem walking is impaired. Individuals are frequently not able to stand with feet together.
Medications	All	Medication history should be obtained. Drugs can contribute to falls, particularly psychoactive drugs, hypotensive medications, and alcohol.
Environmental sources	All	Environmental causes of falls may interact with any of the above sources of falling.

Managing Falls

The festination, freezing, and postural instability related to parkinsonism may respond to drug therapy early in the disease. However, ataxia does not usually respond to multiple-modality therapy, and patients with more advanced disease often fail to improve with pharmacologic therapy. Surgical therapy is only occasionally useful in patients with PD in which falls result from motor fluctuations, and surgical therapies such as deep brain stimulation rarely provide satisfactory results in patients with PD when postural stability cannot be improved (even if only temporarily) with medical management.[33] Surgical intervention is ineffective for reducing falls in other forms of parkinsonism or in ataxic disorders. In most patients who begin to fall because of postural instability, a few principal interventions are prudent:

- Physical therapy can assist in recognizing risk and improving strength. Strategies for turning or providing a more stable base of support during activities may also be taught in this environment. Motor and sensory tricks may be taught to reduce freezing and festination.

- Occupational therapy: environmental modifications may be necessary.

- Home safety: environmental factors leading to falls should be evaluated.

- Table 17.5 details some specific strategies for managing falls.

Table 17.5
Management of Falls in Movement Disorders

Source of Fall	Management Strategy
Postural instability	• Medical therapy: Increasing the levodopa dose may improve postural stability. • Surgical therapy: If motor fluctuations in Parkinson's disease are the source of falls, then deep brain stimulation may be useful. • Physical therapy: Strategies for turning and for improving the base of support may be taught. Strengthening can improve the capacity to resist postural challenge in some patients.
Freezing/festination	• Medical therapy: Increasing the levodopa dose may improve postural stability. • Surgical therapy: If freezing is related to motor fluctuations, then deep brain stimulation may be useful. • Physical therapy: Teaching patients to develop internal cueing, such as counting or focusing on a single action (eg, stepping over a crack in the floor), may be useful, and some individuals may use strategies such as stepping sideways or rocking the trunk backward and forward to break an episode of freezing; however, care must be taken to avoid inducing a fall.
Ataxia	• Both physical therapy and occupational therapy may be useful to improve balance and adaptation to disability.
Medications	• Medications that may be contributing to falls should be adjusted or discontinued.

Environmental causes	• Evaluation of the home environment is the purview of occupational therapists. Specific interventions may be useful:
	  o Footwear: Poorly fitting or nonsupportive footwear may result in falls. Nonskid shoes may augment freezing. An occupational therapist working in concert with a podiatrist may be able to suggest appropriate footwear.
	  o Home visits may be useful to define safety hazards, such as the following:
	    ■ Loose throw rugs or torn carpeting
	    ■ Slippery surfaces
	    ■ Poor lighting conditions
	    ■ Unsafe stairways

Prevention is the best strategy for managing falls.[33] The underlying cause of falling should be determined and corrected if possible. In patients with postural instability or freezing, establishing the relationship between dopaminergic treatment and falls is crucial, as alterations in treatment may decrease alls. In all cases, an underlying medical or neurological condition should be dentified. Physical therapy can improve strength, cardiovascular fitness, and balance. Educating the patient and caregiver is also important. Environmental risk factors must be evaluated.

CONCLUSION

A multidisciplinary team approach is optimal to appropriately manage disability in patients with movement disorders.

- Physical and occupational therapists are important allies on the health care team.

- Immediate referral at diagnosis to a movement disorder–specific early intervention program will promote the benefit of exercise-induced neuroplasticity and prevent functional limitation for most patients.

- There is growing evidence that ongoing moderate to vigorous exercise beyond a self-selected pace (ie, "forced" aerobic exercise, such as pedaling a stationary bike at a consistent rate and pattern) may be necessary to promote neuroplastic changes.

- Studies have shown improved walking, balance, strength, flexibility, and fitness in people with PD who participate in a regular exercise program. However, these studies also indicate that people with PD gradually lose the gains they have made when they are not able to sustain their exercise program.

- Neurological physical and occupational therapists with experience in treating people with PD and other movement disorders can help develop good long-term exercise habits and decrease the risk for falls.

- Continued access to therapy service is important for people with movement disorders to sustain the benefits of exercise and monitor changes in physical funtional status.

- With optimal medication management and a sustained, disorder-specific, individualized exercise program, people with movement disorders can maintain and improve their independence and quality of life.

SELECTED WEBSITES

American Physical Therapy Association
http://www.apta.org
National Center on Physical Activity and Disability
http://www.ncpad.org
National Parkinson Foundation
http://www.parkinson.org

REFERENCES

1. Nath U. Clinical features and natural history of progressive supranuclear palsy: a clinical cohort study. *Neurology.* 2003; 60(6):910–916.
2. Wenning GK. Multiple system atrophy. *Lancet Neurol.* 2004;3(2):93–103.
3. Christine CW. Clinical differentiation of parkinsonian syndromes: prognostic and therapeutic relevance. *Am J Med.* 2004; 117(6):412–419.
4. Thanvi B, Lo N, Robinson T. Vascular parkinsonism—an important cause of parkinsonism in older people. *Age Ageing.* 2005; 34(2):114–119.
5. Hauser RA. Current treatment challenges and emerging therapies in Parkinson's disease. *Neurol Clin.* 2004; 22(3):S149–166.
6. Anderson KE. Huntington's disease and related disorders. *Psychiatr Clin North Am.* 2005; 28(1):275–290.
7. Mariotti C. An overview of the patient with ataxia. *J Neurol.* 2005; 252(5):511–518
8. Defazio G. Epidemiology of primary dystonia. *Lancet Neurol.* 2004; 3(11):673–678
9. Ahlskog JE. Does vigorous exercise have a neuroprotective effect in Parkinson's disease? *Neurology.* 2011; 77(3):288–294.
10. Fisher BE, Wu AD, Salem GJ, et al. The effect of exercise training in improving motor performance and corticomotor excitability in people with early Parkinson's Disease. *Arch Phys Med Rehabil.* 2008; 89(7):1221–1229.
11. Petzinger GM, Walsh JP, Akopian G, et al. Effects of treadmill exercise on dopaminergic transmission in the 1-methyl-4-phenyl-1,2,3,6-tetrahydropyridine-lesioned mouse model of basal ganglia injury. *J Neurosci.* 2007; 27(20):5291–5300.
12. KNGF guidelines for physical therapy in patients with Parkinson's disease. *Supplement to the Dutch Journal of Physical Therapy.* 2004; 114(3).
13. Schenkman M, Ellis T, Christiansen C, et al. Profile of functional limitations and task performance among people with early- and middle-stage Parkinson's disease. *Phys Ther.* 2011; 91:1339–1354.
14. Allen NE, Sherrington C, Paul SS, Canning CG. Balance and falls in Parkinson's disease: a meta-analysis of the effect of exercise and motor training. *Mov Disord.* 2011; 26:1605–1615.
15. Morris ME, Martin CL, Schenkman M. Striding out with Parkinson's disease: evidence-based physical therapy for gait disorders. *Phys Ther.* 2010; 90:280–288.
16. Morris ME, Iansek R, Kirkwood B. A randomized controlled trial of movement strategies compared with exercise for people with Parkinson's disease. *Mov Disord.* 2009; 24:64–71.
17. Thacker EL, Chen H, Patel AV, et al. Recreational physical activity and risk of Parkinson's disease. *Mov Disord.* 2008; 23:69–74.
18. Ellis T, de Goede CJ, Feldman RG, et al. Efficacy of a physical therapy program in patients with Parkinson's disease: a randomized controlled trial. *Arch Phys Med Rehabil.* 2005; 86:626–632.
19. Tillerson JL, Cohen AD, Philhower J, et al. Forced limb-use: effects on the behavioral and neurochemical effects of 6-hydroxydopamine. *J Neurosci.* 2001; 21:4427–4435.
20. Alberts JL, Linder SM, Penko AL, et al. It is not about the bike, it is about the pedaling: forced exercise and Parkinson's disease. *Exerc Sport Sci Rev.* 2011; 39(4):177–186.
21. Dibble L, Ellis T. A comprehensive approach to evidence-based rehabilitation of patients with Parkinson's disease across the continuum of disability. Paper presented at: American Physical Therapy Association Combined Sections Meeting; 2012; Chicago, IL.

22. Farley B. *PWR Clinician Training*. Exercise4BrainChange workshop. 2011.

23. American Physical Therapy Association. *Guide to Physical Therapist Practice*. 2nd ed. Alexandria, VA: American Physical Therapy Association; 2003.

24. Trombly C, Radomski M. *Occupational Therapy for Physical Dysfunction*. 5th ed. Philadelphia, PA: Lippincott Williams & Wilkins; 2002.

25. Byl NN, Melnick ME. The neural consequences of repetition: clinical implications of a learning hypothesis. *J Hand Ther*. 1997; 10:160–172.

26. Cornhill M. In-hand manipulation: the association to writing skills. *Am J Occup Ther*. 1996; 50:732–739.

27. Gauthier L, Dalziel S, Gauthier S. The benefits of group occupational therapy for patients with Parkinson's disease. *Am J Occup Ther*. 1987; 41(6):360–365.

28. Murphy S, Tickle-Degnen L. The effectiveness of occupational therapy-related treatments for persons with Parkinson's disease: a meta-analytic review. *Am J Occup Ther*. 2001; 55(4):385–392.

29. Pedretti LW. *Occupational Therapy Practice Skills for Physical Dysfunction*. 4th ed. St. Louis, MO: Mosby; 1996.

30. Smallegan M. How families decide on nursing home admission. *Geriatr Consult*. 1983; 1:21–24.

31. Tinetti ME, Speechley M, Ginter SF. Risk factors for falls among elderly persons living in the community. *N Engl J Med*. 1988; 319:1701–1707.

32. Nevitt MC, Cummings SR, Kidd S, Black D. Risk factors for recurrent nonsyncopal falls. A prospective study. *JAMA*. 1989; 261: 2663–2668.

33. Olanow CW, Watts RL, Koller WC. An algorithm (decision tree) for the management of Parkinson's disease: treatment guidelines. *Neurology*. 2001; 56(11):S1–S88.

18

SPEECH AND SWALLOWING THERAPY

SPEECH AND SWALLOWING ABNORMALITIES ASSOCIATED WITH MOVEMENT DISORDERS

Speech and swallowing abnormalities occur frequently in patients with movement disorders. The evaluation and treatment of motor speech disorders (ie, dysarthria and apraxia of speech [AOS]) and of oropharyngeal dysphagia are typically performed by speech–language pathologists. These evaluations and treatments can accomplish the following:

- Determine whether speech and swallowing are affected

- Determine the severity of speech and swallowing involvement and the patient's prognosis

- Assist in the formulation of a treatment plan

- Improve the patient's functioning and quality of life

- Assist the medical team in making the differential diagnosis

This chapter summarizes the procedures that speech–language pathologists use to evaluate speech and swallowing. The Mayo classification system of motor speech disorders is introduced, with an emphasis on its relevance for physicians and other health care providers. Finally, speech and swallowing disorders and their treatment in a variety of movement disorders are discussed.

EVALUATION OF SPEECH

- Speech–language pathologists use primarily auditory–perceptual methods to evaluate speech disorders, although the use of instrumental assessment techniques, such as direct laryngoscopy, acoustic analysis of speech, and kinematic measurement, is becoming increasingly common.

- A traditional clinical motor speech evaluation consists of four components

  ○ History

  ○ Examination of the speech mechanism with nonspeech activities

History of the speech problem	Examination of the speech mechanism with nonspeech activities	Examination of the speech mechanism with nonspeech activities	Evaluation of the speech mechanism with speech tasks
Onset and course Insidious or acute, fluctuations over time, effects of medication **Associated deficits** Difficulty with swallowing, cognition, language, and/or changes in affect or emotions, physical function **Patient perception** Patient describes change in speech and strategies to improve speech **Consequences of speech disorder** Changes in ability to participate in vocational or social activities **Overall health care** Other professionals involved, services provided, current medications, utilization of community resources[1,2]	**Respiratory mechanism** Observe for posture, breathing at rest, and with physical exertion. Elicitation of brisk sniff and rapid pant determines strength and coordination of the respiratory mechanism **Larynx** Laryngial integrity assessed by eliciting volitional coughs and grunts. Direct visualization of the larynx via flexible fiberoptic endoscopy or rigid oral laryngoscopy may be necessary in some patients. **Velopharynx (VP)** Evaluate VP at rest for symmetry, involuntary movements, or structural abnormalities **Orofacial mechanism (face/lips, jaw, tongue)** Determines symmetry, strength, range of motion, and coordination. Observe for involuntary movements, structural abnormalities and abnormal posturing[1]	**Respiratory mechanism** Access range of loudness and maximum loudness during phonation. Measure maximum phonation duration **Larynx** Access vocal quality during 3 seconds of the optimal phonation. Assess pitch range with glide from lowest to highest pitch **Velopharynx (VP)** Assess resonance during assimilative nasality task. ("Make me a Hong Kong cookie") and during production of a standard sentence ("Buy Bobby a poppy") with the names open and occluded. **Orofacial mechanism** Assess alternating motion rate by instructing patients to repeat 'puh,' 'tuh,' 'kuh' as quickly, precisely, and regularly as they are able. To isolate the tongue for 'kuh,' have patient put thumb between teeth and bite down lightly[3]	**Connected speech** Considered the most critical part of the evaluation. Used to determine how components of an individual's speech mechanism work together. Used to assess speech characteristics including rate, intonation, stress, rhythm, and naturalness. Elicited during history or conversation (ie, "Tell me about your family") **Repeating words/sentences:** 1. Snowball 2. Impossibility 3. Catastrophe 4. Please put the groceries in the refrigerator 5. The valuable watch was missing 6. The shipwreck washed up on the shore[4] **Reading a standard passage** Use a passage with known number of words, frequency of sounds, and established rate norms, such as the Grandfather Passage[1] (See Appendix A.)

Figure 18.1

Key components of a traditional clinical motor speech evaluation.

- ○ Maximum performance testing of the speech mechanism

- ○ Evaluation of speech performance during a variety of speaking tasks (See Appendix A for a typical paragraph that a patient is asked to read to evaluate speech.)

■ Figure 18.1 reviews the components of typical assessment procedures for speech disorders in greater detail.[1-4]

The Mayo Classification of Speech Disorders

■ Darley et al[5-7] refined the auditory–perceptual method of classifying speech disorders in a series of seminal works. This classification system, now known as the Mayo system, is based on several premises:

- ○ Speech disorders can be categorized into different types.

- ○ They can be characterized by distinguishable auditory–perceptual characteristics.

- ○ They have different underlying pathophysiologic mechanisms associated with different neuromotor deficits.

■ Therefore, the Mayo system has value for localizing neurological disease and can assist the medical team in formulating a differential diagnosis.[1]

■ The Mayo system also provides guidance for treatment planning.[8]

■ Table 18.1 details the types of motor speech disorders, their localization, and their neuromotor basis.

Table 18.1
Types of Motor Speech Disorders With Their Localization and Neuromotor Basis

Type	Localization	Neuromotor Basis
Flaccid dysarthria	Lower motor neuron	Weakness
Spastic dysarthria	Bilateral upper motor neuron	Spasticity
Ataxic dysarthria	Cerebellar control circuit	Incoordination
Hypokinetic dysarthria	Basal ganglia control circuit	Rigidity or reduced range of movements
Hyperkinetic dysarthria	Basal ganglia control circuit	Abnormal movements
Mixed dysarthria	More than one	More than one
Apraxia of speech	Left (dominant) hemisphere	Motor planning and programming

Behavioral Treatment of Speech Disorders

- Most of the approaches to the treatment of speech abnormalities in patients with movement disorders are presented later in this chapter under the sections on specific medical diagnoses. However, regardless of the medical or speech diagnosis, certain therapeutic principles apply:

  - Treatment should be aimed at maximizing intelligibility and naturalness.

  - For maximum benefit, patients and families must be committed to rehabilitation.

  - In many instances, treatment will need to be intensive.

- For further details regarding the principles of treatment for motor speech disorders, see Rosenbek and Jones.[9]

EVALUATION OF SWALLOWING

- Swallowing function is typically considered to comprise three stages:

  - Oral stage

  - Pharyngeal stage

  - Esophageal stage

- The assessment and treatment of the oral and pharyngeal stages of swallowing are within the scope of practice of speech–language pathologists as part of an interdisciplinary team that includes physicians, surgeons, occupational therapists, dieticians, nurses, dentists, and other health care professionals. Esophageal dysphagia is managed primarily by physicians (ie, gastroenterologists).

- The evaluation of oropharyngeal swallowing typically begins with a clinical swallowing evaluation. The traditional components include the following:

  - History

  - Oral motor examination, often with sensory testing

  - Physical examination to assess voice quality and strength of cough, and palpation of laryngeal excursion during swallowing

  - Observation of how foods and liquids are swallowed

- Instrumental assessment techniques may also be necessary, such as videofluoroscopic swallowing evaluation (VFSE) and/or fiber-optic endoscopic evaluation of swallowing (FEES), which allow a skilled clinician to accomplish the following:

  - Assess the integrity of the oropharyngeal swallowing mechanism

○   Establish the biomechanical abnormalities causing dysphagia

○   Make appropriate recommendations with regard to oral intake, therapeutic intervention, and consultations with other health care professionals

■ VFSE and FEES also allow the assessment of penetration and aspiration, which are often critical because of their potential negative effects on health.

■ Penetration occurs when material enters the larynx but does not pass into the trachea. Figure 18.2 shows penetration during VFSE.

■ Aspiration occurs when material passes through the larynx and into the trachea. Figure 18.3 shows aspiration during VFSE.

○   Both aspiration and penetration can be measured during VFSE with the penetration–aspiration scale, an 8-point scale to quantitatively measure the depth of airway entry and whether or not the material is expelled.[10]

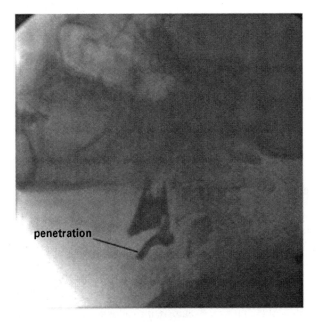

Figure 18.2
Penetration, or entry of material into the larynx but not the trachea, during videofluoroscopic swallowing evaluation.

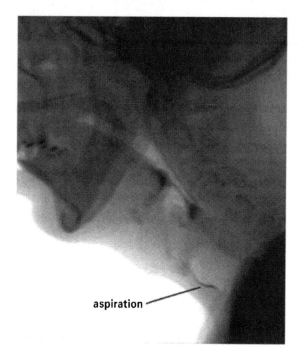

aspiration

Figure 18.3

Aspiration, or entry of material into the trachea, during videofluoroscopic swallowing evaluation.

○ Penetration and aspiration can both occur without overt signs and symptoms (ie, coughing, throat clearing, wet vocal quality). This is referred to as silent penetration and silent aspiration.

Behavioral Treatment of Swallowing Disorders

▪ Behavioral treatments for dysphagia in patients with movement disorders are based primarily on the biomechanical abnormalities observed during evaluation. Treatments for dysphagia tend to be less condition-specific than those for speech. Therefore, the most common methods are discussed next, and this list is referenced in subsequent sections. Specific treatment approaches with application to particular patient populations follow later in this chapter.

▪ Regardless of the medical diagnosis, if swallowing (a) remains unsafe, (b) is inadequate to maintain hydration and nutrition, or (c) requires more effort than the patient can tolerate, a variety of behavioral treatments should be considered.

■ Appropriate behavioral treatments can be most effectively determined with an instrumental assessment of swallowing, which allows a biomechanical analysis of swallowing to be completed.

■ Behavioral treatments can be categorized into rehabilitative and compensatory approaches. General behavioral treatments for patients with dysphagia are described below.

■ Rehabilitative treatments include the following:

○ *Supraglottic swallow* is an airway protection technique in which forceful laryngeal adduction is followed by throat clearing/coughing and a repeated swallow.[11]

○ *Super-supraglottic swallow* is airway protection technique similar to the supraglottic swallow, but in which the patient bears down while holding his or her breath.[11,12]

○ *Effortful swallow* is used to increase posterior tongue base movement and improve bolus clearance from the vallecula by squeezing the muscles forcefully during swallowing.[13]

○ The *Mendelsohn maneuver* is primarily a technique to prolong upper esophageal sphincter (UES) opening.[14] The larynx is held for 1 to 3 seconds in its most anterior–superior position, followed by completion of the swallow.[11]

○ *Shaker head raise* is an exercise for increasing UES opening in which the patient lies supine and repetitively raises and lowers his or her head.[15,16]

○ *Lee Silverman voice treatment* (LSVT) is a series of maximum performance exercises primarily associated with dysarthria rehabilitation. LSVT may also have a general therapeutic effect on swallowing movements.[17]

○ *Expiratory muscle strength training* (EMST) is an exercise in which a pressure threshold device is used to overload the muscles of expiration. EMST may have a general therapeutic effect on speech and swallowing movements.[18]

○ The *Showa maneuver* requires forceful elevation of the tongue against the palate followed by a long, hard swallow, during which the patient is instructed to squeeze all the muscles of the face and neck. This technique appears to influence oral and pharyngeal movements during swallowing.

○ The *Masako technique* is an exercise to increase posterior pharyngeal wall movement. The patient protrudes and holds the tongue while executing a forceful dry swallow.[19]

○ In the *falsetto exercise*, the patient elevates the larynx by sliding up a pitch scale and holding the highest note for several seconds with as much effort as possible.[11]

- ○ Various *lingual strengthening techniques* involve moving the tongue against resistance, which may improve oral stage function and swallow initiation.[20]

- ○ *Sensory therapies* include stimulation with cold, sour, and electrical current. These treatments may improve oral and pharyngeal stage function.[21,22]

- ○ *Intention/attention treatment* is a new type of treatment with no formal protocols established.[23]

- ■ If rehabilitative treatments are unsuccessful or impractical, a variety of compensatory treatments can be considered.

  - ○ General postural stabilization

  - ○ Postural adjustments to the swallowing mechanism, including the chin tuck and head turn

  - ○ Throat clearing or coughing to clear the airway after swallowing

  - ○ Repeated swallows to clear oropharyngeal residue

  - ○ Use of a "liquid wash" to clear oropharyngeal residue

  - ○ Controlling bolus size with instruction or adaptive equipment

  - ○ Increasing the frequency and reducing the size of meals to optimize nutritional intake and swallowing function, especially if swallowing is effortful or causes fatigue

  - ○ Eliminating troublesome foods from the diet or preparing them in a softer, moister form

  - ○ Using dietary supplements

  - ○ Timing eating and drinking to coincide with maximal medication effects

  - ○ Thickening liquids and pureeing foods as a last resort

- ■ If rehabilitative and compensatory strategies are inadequate, decisions about enteral nutrition may become necessary.

SPEECH AND SWALLOWING IN PARKINSON'S DISEASE

Speech Disorders

- ■ *Hypokinetic dysarthria* occurs in most individuals with Parkinson's disease (PD) at some point in the progression of the disease, with approximately 90% of patients with PD having dysarthria in some series.[24,25] See Appendix B for a description of the perceptual features of hypokinetic dysarthria.

- Hypokinetic dysarthria may be the presenting symptom of neurological disease in some patients with PD.

- The term *hypophonia* is often used to describe the decreased vocal loudness of patients with PD.

- Inappropriate silences may occur frequently and be associated with difficulty initiating movements for speech production.

- *Neurogenic stuttering*, consisting most often of sound and word repetitions, may also be observed in some patients with PD.

- Patients with PD appear to have a perceptual disconnect between their actual loudness level and their own internal perception of loudness.

- When patients have insight into their speech problem, they often describe the presence of a "weak" voice. They may report avoiding social situations that require speech.

- The severity of dysarthria may not correspond to the duration of PD or the severity of other motor symptoms.

- *Hyperkinetic dysarthria*, rather than hypokinetic dysarthria, may also be encountered. This most often occurs in the presence of dyskinesia, particularly after prolonged levodopa therapy. Other "communication disorders" commonly encountered in patients with PD include cognitive impairments, masked facies, and micrographia.

TREATMENT

- Although a variety of medical and surgical approaches have been attempted to improve the speech of patients with PD, behavioral treatments have shown the most sustained beneficial effect.[26]

- LSVT has a robust literature supporting its beneficial effects and is considered the treatment of choice for individuals with PD and hypokinetic dysarthria.[27-30]

- Other maximum performance treatments, such as EMST, may also be beneficial.[31]

- A variety of other behavioral techniques may be indicated.

  ○ Speaker-oriented treatments focus on compensatory strategies to improve intelligibility.[32]

  ○ Communication-oriented strategies are often used along with speaker-oriented strategies to improve understanding between speaker and listener.[32]

  ○ Rate control techniques, such as delayed auditory feedback (DAF), pitch-shifted feedback, and pacing boards, may be used.

○ Augmentative–alternative communication (AAC) treatment approaches, such as the use of voice amplifiers or speech-generating computers, may be appropriate, particularly as the severity of dysarthria progresses.

■ **For many patients with PD, pharmacologic treatment does not appear to have a significant beneficial impact on speech production,** although speech function may be improved in some patients.

■ **Surgical treatments for PD also do not appear to have a consistently significant benefit for the speech disorders encountered in PD.** Although speech performance may be improved in some patients after surgery, this is not considered an expected outcome. Speech may be unchanged or worsened following surgery.

Swallowing Disorders

■ Oropharyngeal dysphagia has been reported in up to 90% to 100% of people with PD. However, dysphagia is often unrecognized or underestimated by patients.[33–35]

■ Oropharyngeal dysphagia may be the initial symptom, and a particular pattern of lingual fenestration characterized by repetitive tongue pumping motions is considered a pathognomic sign of PD.[11]

■ The severity of dysphagia may not correspond to the duration of PD or the severity of other motor symptoms.

■ All stages of swallowing function can be affected in patients with PD.

○ Oral stage deficits may include drooling, increased oral transit time, repetitive tongue pumping motions, and premature spillage of the bolus.

○ Pharyngeal stage function may be remarkable for a pharyngeal swallow delay, post-swallow pharyngeal residue, penetration, and aspiration.

○ Esophageal stage swallowing problems are also common and most frequently include abnormalities in esophageal motility.

TREATMENT

■ General treatment strategies can be found in the earlier section on the behavioral treatment of swallowing disorders.

■ Patients with PD often respond well to active range-of-motion and falsetto exercises, effortful swallow, Mendelsohn maneuver, and effortful breath-hold.[11]

■ Maximum performance techniques typically used in the rehabilitation of speech disorders in PD, such as LSVT and EMST, may also improve oropharyngeal swallow function.[17]

■ Referral to an occupational therapist may be beneficial to determine the appropriateness of adaptive utensils and equipment to promote independence with meals and reduce the effects of motor symptoms (ie, tremor) on self-feeding skills.

■ Although dopaminergic medications are not typically associated with significant improvements in swallow function, in some patients these medications may provide benefit. In these selected cases, "on" effects can be timed to coincide with meals.

■ The surgical treatment of PD does not appear to improve swallowing function for most patients, and postoperative dysphagia has been described in the literature as an adverse event.

■ Although dysphagia is common in PD, it rarely is severe enough that patients require an alternative means of nutritional support.

PEECH AND SWALLOWING DISORDERS IN MULTIPLE SYSTEM ATROPHY

peech Disorders

■ Dysarthria is a common symptom of multiple system atrophy (MSA) and has been reported in up to 100% of unselected patients in some studies.[36]

■ Dysarthria in MSA is usually more severe than in PD and often emerges earlier in the course of the disease.[1]

■ Because of the involvement of multiple brain systems in MSA, the presentation of dysarthria can be expected to be heterogeneous and complex.

■ A mixed dysarthria with features of hypokinetic, ataxic, and spastic types of dysarthria is described most frequently in patients with MSA.[1] See Appendix B for a description of the perceptual features of these dysarthria types.[1]

   ○ In patients with prominent features of parkinsonism (ie, MSA-P subtype), features of hypokinetic dysarthria may be expected to predominate.

   ○ In patients with prominent features of cerebellar dysfunction (ie, MSA-C subtype), features of ataxic dysarthria may be most notable.

   ○ In patients with prominent features of autonomic failure and ataxia, hypokinetic, and/or spastic dysarthria, alone or in combination, have been described.[37]

■ Stridor may occur in patients with MSA. This may result in respiratory ataxia and even necessitate a tracheostomy in severe cases. Stridor in MSA has usually been attributed to vocal cord paralysis, but some data suggest that the cause is laryngeal–pharyngeal dystonia.[36]

TREATMENT

■ Some data suggest that patients with MSA may benefit from LSVT.[39]

■ Other maximum performance treatments, such as EMST, may be a sensible approach in some patients.

Swallowing Disorders

■ Dysphagia is a well-known symptom of MSA.

■ Dysphagia is often more severe in MSA than in PD.[40]

■ Results of VFSE in patients with MSA reveal deficits in both the oral and pharyngeal stages.

  ○ Oral stage dysphagia in patients with MSA is often present even early in the disease and may become severe with disease progression. Oral deficits may include difficulty with holding and transporting the bolus.

  ○ Pharyngeal stage function may also be impaired, but much less so than the oral stage, especially early in the disease. Pharyngeal deficits may include decreased pharyngeal clearance, reduced laryngeal elevation, and incomplete relaxation of the UES.[41,42]

■ Not surprisingly, dysphagia has also been reported in the literature, which uses the old terminology for MSA subtypes—striatonigral degeneration (SND), olivopontocerebellar atrophy (OPCA), and Shy-Drager syndrome (SDS)—although it has received little systematic attention.

■ Dysphagia has been reported in 44% of patients with SND and has been described infrequently as the initial symptom.[2,43]

■ In patients with OPCA, dysphagia has been reported in 24% to 33% of cases and has been described infrequently as the initial symptom.[44]

■ Dysphagia in SDS has received little attention, and it can be hypothesized that oropharyngeal dysphagia may be relatively uncommon in "pure" autonomic failure. Of course, with disease progression and the additional involvement of the extrapyramidal and cerebellar systems, oropharyngeal dysphagia becomes increasingly likely.

TREATMENT

■ General treatment strategies can be found in the earlier section on the behavioral treatment of swallowing disorders.

■ Intention treatment and attention treatment may be good approaches if akinesia dominates or if attention is disturbed.[23]

- Depending on the biomechanical cause of the swallowing deficit, other strengthening exercises may be beneficial.[23]

- Maximum performance techniques, such as LSVT and EMST, may benefit oropharyngeal swallow function in patients with MSA.

SPEECH AND SWALLOWING IN PROGRESSIVE SUPRANUCLEAR PALSY

Speech Disorders

- Dysarthria is common in patients with progressive supranuclear palsy (PSP). Some series of unselected patients demonstrate the presence of dysarthria in 70% to 100% of cases.[24,45,46]

  - The dysarthria of PSP is a mixed dysarthria with features of hypokinetic, spastic, and ataxic types.[1,36] Appendix B details the perceptual features of these types of dysarthria.

  - Recognizing the presence of a mixed dysarthria in PSP can help to distinguish it from PD.

  - Dysarthria in PSP occurs early, often within the first 2 years of the onset of disease.[1]

  - Dysarthria is more frequently an initial symptom of neurological disease in PSP than in PD.[1,24]

  - Dysarthria may be severe, even relatively early in the disease. Anarthria or mutism may be exhibited in the later stages of the disease.[47]

- Cognitive–linguistic deficits and other problems that affect communication, such as apathy and disinhibition, may also be present.

TREATMENT

- Although the data are limited, maximum performance treatments, such as LSVT and EMST, may be beneficial in the treatment of dysarthria in PSP.[39] This approach may be most sensible when prominent features of hypokinetic and ataxic dysarthria are present.

- DAF has been reported to slow the speech rate, increase vocal intensity, and improve intelligibility in PSP.[48]

- The rapid nature of decline in patients with PSP and the frequent cognitive deficits are negative prognostic indicators for treatment. Thus, speech treatments in PSP may be more effective if implemented early in the course of the disease, before speech and cognition become severely impaired.

Swallowing Disorders

- When swallowing function has been assessed with VFSE, dysphagia has been reported in more than 95% of patients with PSP.[49]

  - In contrast to patients with PD, those with PSP and dysphagia are often aware of their difficulty in swallowing, even when they present with cognitive impairments.[21]

  - The onset of swallowing difficulties in individuals with PSP may be a negative prognostic indicator of survival.[24,45]

  - Oral stage deficits are often more frequent and severe than pharyngeal deficits in patients with PSP.[23]

TREATMENT

- General treatment strategies can be found in the earlier section on the behavioral treatment of swallowing disorders.

- Intention treatment may benefit patients with prolonged inactivity during the oral stage or inefficient swallowing.[23]

- When long delays in the oral initiation of the swallow are present, thermal tactile application may help.[23]

- Strengthening exercises may also be indicated.

- Maximum performance techniques, such as LSVT and EMST, may benefit oropharyngeal swallow function in patients with PSP.

SPEECH AND SWALLOWING IN CORTICOBASOGANGLIONIC DEGENERATION

Speech Disorders

- The frequency of dysarthria in corticobasoganglionic degeneration (CBGD) has been reported to be as high as 85%.[50]

- Hypokinetic, spastic, and ataxic types of dysarthria, presenting either in isolation or together as a mixed dysarthria, occur most frequently.[1,50] Appendix B details the perceptual features of these types of dysarthria.

- Dysarthria in CBGD may be less severe than other motor impairments.[51]

- AOS has also been reported in cases of CBGD[1,52,53] and may be the earliest symptom.[1,54–57] The presence of AOS can be important to the differential diagnosis. See Appendix B for a description of the perceptual features of AOS.

- Although rarely, the degenerative nature of CBGD may eventually lead to the complete inability to produce speech.[58–60]

- Cognitive–linguistic impairments, including aphasia, often coexist with speech disorders in CBGD.[7]

TREATMENT

- Maximum performance treatments, such as LSVT or EMST, may be sensible when prominent features of hypokinetic and ataxic dysarthria are present.

- Additional targets for treatment of dysarthria in CBGD may include the following:

  - The use of compensatory strategies to increase speech intelligibility, such as reducing the rate of speech, using an alphabet card to identify the first letter of a word, or saying something in a different way when misunderstood.

  - The patient and communication partners can be trained to use compensatory strategies to achieve successful communication.[61]

- The treatment of AOS with intensive drill of sounds, syllables, words, and phrases may also be useful.

- Advance planning for the acquisition and use of an AAC device is recommended, particularly when cognitive and language skills are relatively intact.[47,62]

Swallowing Disorders

- Swallowing disorders may occur in CBGD.

- No distinctive pattern of swallowing difficulty has been reported in patients with CBGD.

- The onset of swallowing difficulties in individuals with CBGD may be a negative prognostic indicator for survival.[24,50]

TREATMENT

- General treatment strategies can be found in the earlier section on the behavioral treatment of swallowing disorders.

- Treatment may include strength training exercises and intention/attention treatment.[23]

- Maximum performance techniques, such as LSVT and EMST, may benefit oropharyngeal swallow function in patients with CBGD.

SPEECH AND SWALLOWING IN SYNDROMES OF PROGRESSIVE ATAXIA

Speech Disorders

- Dysarthria is a common symptom in syndromes of progressive ataxia.

- Ataxic dysarthria is the type of dysarthria most frequently associated with these conditions. See Appendix B for a description of the perceptual features of ataxic dysarthria.

- Mixed dysarthria may also be encountered when neurological involvement is not restricted to the cerebellum. A description of the perceptual features of the following types of dysarthria may be found in Appendix B.

  - Dysarthria in the spinocerebellar ataxias, such as Friedreich ataxia, may present with components of ataxia and spasticity.[1,36]

  - Mixed dysarthria, with features of the ataxic, hypokinetic, spastic, and flaccid types of dysarthria, may be encountered in patients with OPCA (see the section on MSA for further details).[1,36]

TREATMENT

- The literature on the treatment of dysarthria in syndromes of progressive ataxia is noticeably sparse.

- The literature on the treatment of patients with ataxic dysarthria due to a variety of etiologies may provide guidance.

  - Rate control strategies can be beneficial in improving intelligibility in patients with ataxic dysarthria.[63] Appropriate strategies may include DAF or the use of a pacing board.

  - Maximum performance treatments, such as LSVT and EMST, may have benefit in patients with ataxic dysarthria.[64,65]

Swallowing Disorders

- Dysphagia appears to occur less frequently than dysarthria in patients with progressive ataxia.

  - However, VFSE results have shown oral and pharyngeal stage dysphagia, including premature spillage of the bolus, piecemeal deglutition, pharyngeal residue, and aspiration.[66]

  - A likely explanation for dysphagic signs is the discoordination of oral, pharyngeal, and respiratory movements.

TREATMENT

- General treatment strategies can be found in the earlier section on the behavioral treatment of swallowing disorders.

- Dietary modifications, such as thickened liquids, and therapeutic techniques, such as the chin tuck and the supraglottic swallow, have been reported to be beneficial in preventing aspiration in patients with degenerative ataxia.[66]

SPEECH AND SWALLOWING IN HUNTINGTON'S DISEASE[67]

Speech Disorders

- The chorea of Huntington's disease (HD) also manifests in the speech mechanism and results in a hyperkinetic dysarthria. The perceptual features of hyperkinetic dysarthria in chorea are shown in Appendix B.

- Dementia in HD may result in a variety of cognitive–linguistic impairments that have a negative influence on communication.[61]

TREATMENT

- Yorkston et al recommend a treatment approach for patients with HD that depends on the severity of their dysarthria and coexisting cognitive–linguistic deficits.[61]

  - In patients with mild dysarthria, drills to target prosody, techniques to reduce hyperkinesia in the larynx, and rate control activities may be beneficial.

  - In patients with moderate dysarthria, the behavioral techniques used in patients with mild dysarthria may continue, with the addition of patient and family training in strategies used to address communication breakdown.

  - In patients with HD and severe dysarthria, speech may no longer be understandable. Therapy may focus on techniques such as natural speech with supportive partners, alphabet boards, calendars and memory aids, making choices, yes–no questions, and conversation starters.

Swallowing Disorders

- In patients with HD who have primarily hyperkinetic symptoms, swallowing difficulties may include uncontrolled tachyphagia, darting lingual chorea, uninhibited swallow initiation, and impaired inhibition of respiration with swallowing (ie, respiratory chorea).[68,69]

- Tachyphagia, or rapid uncontrolled swallowing, occurs often in patients who have HD with hyperkinetic symptoms.[68,69]

- In patients with HD who have primarily symptoms of rigidity and bradykinesia, dysphagia is characterized by mandibular rigidity, inefficient mastication, and slow oral transit.

  ○ Post-swallow vallecular residue occurs frequently in patients with HD.[68,69]

- Laryngeal penetration and aspiration occur infrequently in patients who have HD with hyperkinetic symptoms, but they are more frequently reported in patients with prominent rigidity and bradykinesia.[68,69]

- Esophageal dysphagia occurs relatively infrequently, but eructation (excessive belching), aerophagia (swallowing air), vomiting, and esophageal dysmotility have been noted in some patients.[69]

- Often, patients with HD do not report symptoms of dysphagia despite the presence of clinical symptoms.[69] Aspiration pneumonia, asphyxiation due to choking on food, cachexia, and severe unintentional weight loss are the most common causes of death in those with long-standing HD.[70]

TREATMENT

- General treatment strategies can be found in the earlier section on the behavioral treatment of swallowing disorders.

- Exercises may include effortful swallow and Showa maneuver as well as intention treatment.[23]

- Management approaches often used in patients with HD and dysphagia include postural and position changes, assistive devices, supervision of meals to control rate of consumption and bolus size, dietary changes, and tube feeding.[65]

- Bracing by having the patient rest his or her head against a wall or other supportive surface may aid swallowing during the early stage of the disease.

- Successful implementation of these approaches generally requires a great deal of caregiver assistance owing to the cognitive deficits in patients with HD, but they have been reported to be of considerable benefit.[71]

- Patients with HD are at increased nutritional risk because of a multitude of factors, which include dysphagia, difficulty with food preparation due to chorea and cognitive deficits, impaired self-feeding skills, and increased calorie consumption due to chorea. Dietary supplements and consultations with dieticians may be beneficial in patients with HD.[72]

SPEECH AND SWALLOWING IN WILSON'S DISEASE

Speech Disorders

- Dysarthria occurs commonly in patients with Wilson's disease[1] and has been reported in more than 90% of unselected patients with neurological manifestations of the disease.[73,74]

- Wilson's disease is most commonly associated with a mixed dysarthria that has features of the hypokinetic, spastic, and ataxic types.[1] Appendix B details the perceptual features of these types of dysarthria.

- Dysarthria has been described to be the most frequent neurological manifestation of Wilson's disease.[75]

- Dysarthria may be the presenting symptom of Wilson's disease.[73]

- Lingual abnormalities, such as tremor, involuntary transverse and bilateral movements at rest and with action, and protrusion of the tongue, have been described in selected cases of Wilson's disease.[76–78]

- Speech involvement in Wilson's disease may be complicated by coexisting dementia.

TREATMENT

- Very few data on the behavioral treatment of dysarthria in Wilson's disease are available, although the benefit of speech therapy has been described.[79]

- Although pharmacologic treatment with D-penicillamine (with or without zinc sulfate) has been shown to mitigate many neurological symptoms of Wilson's disease, dysarthria may be resistant to this treatment.[80]

- Improvement or elimination of dysarthria following liver transplant has been described.[74]

Swallowing Disorders

- Dysphagia in Wilson's disease has received little attention, although swallowing difficulties, including drooling, may occur.[1] Dysphagia appears to be a less frequent neurological manifestation of the disease than dysarthria.

- Aspiration may be expected as disease severity increases.

- Pharyngeal and esophageal dysmotility has been reported.[14,81]

- Sialorrhea, or an excessive secretion of saliva, has been reported in some cases.[74] This problem is likely related to oropharyngeal dysphagia and decreased frequency of swallowing rather than to a true excess in the production of saliva.

TREATMENT

- General treatment strategies can be found in the earlier section on the behavioral treatment of swallowing disorders.

- Because of the likelihood of behavioral, psychiatric, and cognitive abnormalities, strengthening exercises may be difficult for persons with Wilson's disease.[23]

- The effect of dietary changes, pharmacologic treatment, and liver transplant on swallowing has received little attention.

SPEECH AND SWALLOWING DISORDERS IN DYSTONIA

Speech Disorders

- When the locus of dystonia targets any of the components of the speech mechanism, hyperkinetic dysarthria may result. See Appendix B for a description of the perceptual features of the hyperkinetic dysarthria associated with dystonia.

  - *Generalized dystonia* may negatively affect respiratory function and be associated with decreased speech intelligibility.[82]

  - *Neck dystonia* (*cervical dystonia* or *spasmodic torticollis*) may have a negative influence on laryngeal function, with lower habitual pitch, restricted pitch range, and decreased phonatory reaction time described in the literature.[83] Speech differences in patients with neck dystonia are likely due to the effect of postural abnormalities on speech muscle activity and/or changes in the shape of the vocal tract.[1]

  - *Laryngeal dystonia* or *spasmodic dysphonia* (*adductor, abductor,* or *mixed* type) results in prominent laryngeal abnormalities. Adductor spasmodic dysphonia, the most common type, results in a strained, strangled vocal quality, whereas abductor spasmodic dysphonia presents with a voice that is intermittently breathy or aphonic.[1]

  - *Mouth and face dystonia* or *oromandibular dystonia* (OMD) may involve the masticatory, lower facial, and tongue muscles in a variety of combinations. When coupled with blepharospasm, this condition is often known as *Meige syndrome* or *Brueghel syndrome*. OMD can severely disrupt the function of the orofacial mechanism. Speech in OMD has been described as having imprecise consonants, a slow rate, inappropriate pauses, and abnormalities in stress.[84,85]

  - *Lingual dystonia* may also occur in isolation, although rarely. This has been described as unilateral tongue puckering, ridging, and bulging.[86] Lingual dystonia with tongue protrusion in isolation[87] and combined with OMD[88] has also been reported. Lingual dystonia frequently causes dysarthria owing to involvement of the orofacial mechanism.[88] Lingual dystonia coupled with palatal dystonia may also occur in rare cases.[89] In a case such as this, involvement of both the orofacial mechanism and the velopharynx during speech may be expected.

○ *Jaw dystonia* can result in either jaw-opening or jaw-closing OMD. Jaw-opening dystonia has been reported to be associated with cervical dystonia in some patients.[90,91] Either jaw-opening or jaw-closing OMD can be expected to disrupt the orofacial mechanism component of speech production, and speech difficulties have been reported in patients with this condition.[90,91]

■ In dystonias that are considered focal, there may be more widespread involvement than expected. For example, respiratory involvement has been described in patients with cervical dystonia and blepharospasm.[92] Dystonia of the soft palate has been reported in a high percentage of cases with laryngeal involvement (spasmodic dysphonia or essential voice tremor).[93]

TREATMENT

■ Sensory tricks (*geste antagoniste*), such as a light touch to the affected area, may be beneficial for the speech of many patients with dystonia.[1]

■ The use of a bite block, a custom-fitted prosthesis placed between the upper and lower lateral teeth, has been reported to be beneficial in patients with OMD. Such a device may help to inhibit jaw movements during speech.[94,95]

■ The most widely used and accepted therapy for dystonia is local intramuscular injections of botulinum toxin type A, which may have a beneficial influence on speech.[16,96,97]

■ Lesion surgery and deep brain stimulation (DBS) are being increasingly used in the management of dystonia. The effects of surgical treatments on speech function are largely unexplored. Dysarthria may occur as a consequence of stimulation-related muscle contractions in patients who have dystonia treated with DBS.[98]

Swallowing Disorders

■ When the locus of dystonia targets any of the components of the swallowing mechanism, dysphagia may result.

○ *Generalized dystonia* may be associated with dysphagia. Coordination of respiration with swallowing may be more difficult in patients with respiratory involvement.

○ *Neck dystonia* (*cervical dystonia* or *spasmodic torticollis*) has been reported to be associated with dysphagia in approximately 50% of unselected patients is some series. Most frequent swallowing abnormalities include a delay in swallow initiation and vallecular residue.[99]

○ *Laryngeal dystonia* or *spasmodic dysphonia* (*adductor, abductor,* or *mixed* type) may result in dysphagia, but swallowing is usually relatively preserved in comparison with speech.

○ *Mouth and face dystonia* or *oromandibular dystonia* (also known as *Meige syndrome* or *Brueghel syndrome*) may have a negative effect on swallow function. In a series of unselected patients, 90% presented with swallowing abnormalities, which included premature spillage of the bolus and vallecular residue.[100] Swallowing abnormalities in OMD may also include chewing difficulties and other deficits in oral preparation of the bolus.[101]

○ *Lingual dystonia* often results in dysphagia. In patients with tongue protrusion lingual dystonia with or without OMD, tongue biting and pushing food out of the oral cavity with the tongue have been described.[88]

○ *Jaw dystonia* may result in a variety of oral and pharyngeal stage deficits, which can be severe.

TREATMENT

■ General treatment strategies can be found in the earlier section on the behavioral treatment of swallowing disorders.

■ Postural adjustments and sensory tricks may have a beneficial effect on swallowing.[23]

○ Dysphagia may occur after or be exacerbated by treatments such as botulinum toxin injections[102] and selective denervation.[3]

○ Lesion surgery and DBS are being increasingly used in the management of dystonia. The effects of surgical treatments on swallowing function are largely unexplored. Dysphagia may occur as a result of stimulation-related muscle contractions in patients who have dystonia treated with DBS.[98]

SPEECH AND SWALLOWING DISORDERS IN TARDIVE DYSKINESIA

Speech Disorders

■ Hyperkinetic dysarthria is the type of dysarthria associated with tardive dyskinesia (TD).[1]

■ Dysarthria in TD is most often due to orobuccal and lingual dyskinesia, but laryngeal and respiratory dyskinesia has also been reported.[1,4,103,104]

■ Hyperkinetic dysarthria may also be the presenting symptom of TD.[104]

TREATMENT

■ Medical management of TD appears to be the most appropriate treatment for dysarthria associated with this condition.

■ The literature on behavioral treatments for TD is very limited. Appropriate treatments for patients who have hyperkinetic dysarthria associated with other etiologies may include postural adjustments and the use of a bite block.

Swallowing Disorders

■ Dysphagia in TD most commonly consists of difficulty containing foods and liquids in the mouth, as well as inefficient bolus formation and movement.

■ The discoordination of oral and pharyngeal swallowing may result in delayed initiation of the swallow, post-swallow pharyngeal residue, and aspiration.

■ Dysphagia can be severe enough to cause weight loss.[105]

TREATMENT

■ General treatment strategies can be found in the earlier section on the behavioral treatment of swallowing disorders.

■ The medical management of TD appears to be the most appropriate treatment for dysphagia associated with this condition.

REFERENCES

1. Duffy JR. *Motor Speech Disorders: Substrates, Differential Diagnosis, and Management.* 2nd ed. Philadelphia, PA: Elsevier; 2005.
2. Kurihara K, Kita K, Hirayama K, et al. Dysphagia in olivopontocerebellar atrophy [in Japanese]. *Rinsho Shinkeigaku.* 1990; 30(2):146–150.
3. Horner J, Riski JE, Ovelmen-Levitt J, Nashold BSJ. Swallowing in torticollis before and after rhizotomy. *Dysphagia.* 1992; 7(3):117–125.
4. Feve A, Angelard B, Lacau St Guily J. Laryngeal tardive dyskinesia. *J Neurol.* 1995; 242(7):455–459.
5. Darley FL, Aronson AE, Brown JR. *Motor Speech Disorders.* Philadelphia, PA: W.B. Saunders; 1975.
6. Darley FL, Aronson AE, Brown JR. Differential diagnostic patterns of dysarthria. *J Speech Hear Res.* 1969; 12:249–269.
7. Darley FL, Aronson AE, Brown JR. Cluster of deviant speech dimensions in the dysarthrias. *J Speech Hear Res.* 1969; 12:462–496.

8. Duffy JR. Pearls of wisdom—Darley, Aronson, and Brown and the classification of the dysarthrias. *Perspect Neurophysiol Neurogenic Speech Lang Disord.* 2005; 15(3):24–27.

9. Rosenbek JC, Jones HN. Principles of treatment for sensorimotor speech disorders. In: McNeil MR, ed. *Clinical Management of Sensorimotor Speech Disorders.* 2nd ed. New York, NY: Thieme. In press.

10. Rosenbek JC, Robbins J, Roecker EB, et al. A penetration-aspiration scale. *Dysphagia.* 1996; 11:93–98.

11. Logemann JA. *Evaluation and Treatment of Swallowing Disorders.* 2nd ed. Austin, TX: PRO-ED; 1998.

12. Martin BJW, Logemann JA, Shaker R, et al. Normal laryngeal valving patterns during three breath-hold maneuvers: a pilot investigation. *Dysphagia.* 1993;8:11–20.

13. Kahrilas PJ, Logemann JA, Lin S, et al. Pharyngeal clearance during swallow: a combined manometric and videofluoroscopic study. *Gastroenterology.* 1992; 103:128–136.

14. Gulyas AE, Salazar-Grueso EF. Pharyngeal dysmotility in a patient with Wilson's disease. *Dysphagia.* 1988; 2(4):230–234.

15. Shaker R, Easterling C, Kern M, et al. Rehabilitation of swallowing by exercise in tube-fed patients with pharyngeal dysphagia secondary to abnormal UES opening. *Gastroenterology.* 2002; 122(5):1314–1321.

16. Shaker R, Kern M, Bardan E, et al. Augmentation of deglutitive upper esophageal sphincter opening in the elderly by exercise. *Am J Physiol.* 1997; 272(6, pt 1):G1518–G1522.

17. Sharkawi AE, Ramig L, Logemann JA, et al. Swallowing and voice effects of Lee Silverman Voice Treatment (LSVT[R]): a pilot study. *J Neurol Neurosurg Psychiatry.* 2002; 72:31–36.

18. Kim J, Sapienza CM. Implications of expiratory muscle strength training for rehabilitation of the elderly: tutorial. *J Rehabil Res Dev.* 2005; 42(2):211.

19. Fujiu M, Logemann JA. Effect of a tongue-holding maneuver on posterior pharyngeal wall movement during deglutition. *Am J Speech Lang Pathol.* 1996; 5:23–30.

20. Robbins J, Gangnon RE, Theis SM, et al. The effects of lingual exercise on swallowing in older adults. *J Am Geriatr Soc.* 2005; 53(9):1483–1489.

21. Rosenbek JC, Jones HN. Sensorische behandlung oropharyngealer dysphagien bei erwachsenen [Sensory therapies for oroharyngeal dysphagia in adults]. In: Stanschus S, ed. *Rehabilitation von Dysphagien.* Idstein, Germany: Schulz-Kirchner Verlag; 2006.

22. Hamdy S, Aziz Q, Rothwell JC, et al. Recovery of swallowing after dysphagic stroke relates to functional reorganization in the intact motor cortex. *Gastroenterology.* 1998; 115:1104–1112.

23. Rosenbek JC, Jones HN. *Dysphagia in Movement Disorders.* San Diego, CA: Plural Publishing; 2009.

24. Muller J, Wenning GK, Verny N, et al. Progression of dysarthria and dysphagia in postmortem confined parkinsonian disorders. *Arch Neurol.* 2001; 58:259–264.

25. Logemann JA, Fisher HB, Boshes B, Blonsky ER. Frequency and co-occurrence of vocal tract dysfunctions in the speech of a large sample of Parkinson patients. *J Speech Hear Disord.* 1978; 43(1):47–57.

26. Merati AL, Heman-Ackah YD, Abaza M, et al. Common movement disorders affecting the larynx: a report from the neurolaryngology committee of the AAO-HNS. *Otolaryngol Head Neck Surg.* 2005; 133(5):654–665.

27. Ramig LO, Countryman S, Thompson LL, Horii Y. Comparison of two forms of intensive speech treatment for Parkinson disease. *J Speech Hear Res.* 1995; 38(6):1232–1235.

28. Ramig LO, Countryman S, Thompson L, Horii Y. Comparison of two forms of intensive speech treatment for Parkinson disease. *J Speech Hear Res.* 1993; 38(5):1232–1251.

29. Ramig LO, Countryman S, O'Brien C, et al. Intensive speech treatment for patients with Parkinson's disease: short- and long-term comparison of two techniques. *Neurology.* 1996; 47(6):1496–1504.

30. Ramig LO. Voice treatment for patients with Parkinson's disease: development of an approach and preliminary efficacy data. *J Med Speech Lang Pathol.* 1994; 2(3):191–209.

31. Saleem AF, Sapienza CM, Rosenbek JC, et al. The effects of expiratory muscle strength training program on pharyngeal swallowing in patients with idiopathic Parkinson's disease. Paper presented at: 57th Annual Meeting of the American Academy of Neurology; 2005; Miami, FL.

32. Tjaden K. Speech and swallowing in Parkinson's disease. *Top Geriatr Rehabil.* 2008; 24(2):115–126.

33. Leopold NA, Kagel MC. Dysphagia in progressive supranuclear palsy: radiologic features. *Dysphagia.* 1997; 12:140–143.

34. Leopold NA, Kagel MC. Prepharyngeal dysphagia in Parkinson's disease. *Dysphagia.* 1996; 11(1):14–22.

35. Robbins JA, Logemann JA, Kirshner HS. Swallowing and speech production in Parkinson's disease. *Ann Neurol.* 1986; 19(3):283–287.

36. Kluin KJ, L. FM, Berent S, Gilman S. Perceptual analysis of speech disorders in progressive supranuclear palsy. *Neurology.* 1993; 43:563–566.

37. Linebaugh C. The dysarthrias of Shy-Drager syndrome. *J Speech Hear Disord.* 1979; 44(1):55–60.

38. Merlo IM, Occhini A, Pacchetti C, Alfonsi E. Not paralysis, but dystonia causes stridor in multiple system atrophy. *Neurology.* 2002; 58(4):649–652.

39. Countryman S, Ramig LO. Speech and voice deficits in Parkinsonian plus syndromes: can they be treated? *J Med Speech Lang Pathol.* 1994; 2:211–225.

40. Wenning GK, Quinn NP. Parkinsonism. Multiple system atrophy. *Baillieres Clin Neurol.* 1997; 6(1):187–204.

41. Higo R, Tayama N, Watanabe T, et al. Videofluoroscopic and manometric evaluation of swallowing function in patients with multiple system atrophy. *Ann Otol Rhinol Laryngol.* 2003; 112(7):630–636.

42. Higo R, Nito T, Tayama N. Swallowing function in patients with multiple-system atrophy with a clinical predominance of cerebellar symptoms (MSA-C). *Eur Arch Otorhinolaryngol.* 2005; 262(8):646–650.

43. Gouider-Khouja N, Vidailhet M, Bonnet AM, et al. "Pure" striatonigral degeneration and Parkinson's disease: a comparative clinical study. *Mov Disord.* 1995; 10(3):288–294.

44. Berciano J. Olivopontocerebellar atrophy. A review of 117 cases. *J Neurol Sci.* 1982; 53(2):253–272.

45. Nath U, Ben-Shlomo Y, Thomson RG, et al. Clinical features and natural history of progressive supranuclear palsy: a clinical cohort study. *Neurology.* 2003; 60(6):910–916.

46. Diroma C, Dell'Aquila C, Fraddosio A, et al. Natural history and clinical features of progressive supranuclear palsy: a clinical study. *Neurol Sci.* 2003; 24(3):176–177.

47. Yorkston KM, Beukelman DR, Strand EA, Bell KR. *Management of Motor Speech Disorders in Children and Adults.* 2nd ed. Austin, TX: PRO-ED; 1999.

48. Hanson WR, Metter EJ. DAF as instrumental treatment for dysarthria in progressive supranuclear palsy: a case report. *J Speech Hear Dis.* 1980; 45:268–276.

49. Litvan I, Sastry N, Sonies BC. Characterizing swallowing abnormalities in progressive supranuclear palsy. *Neurology.* 1997; 48:1654–1662.

50. Ozsancak C, Auzou P, Jan M, et al. The place of perceptual analysis of dysarthria in the differential diagnosis of corticobasal degeneration and Parkinson's disease. *J Neurol.* 2006; 253:92–97.

51. Frattali CM, Sonies BC. Speech and swallowing disturbances in corticobasal degeneration. In: Litvan I, Goetz CG, Lang AE, eds. *Corticobasal Degeneration. Advances in Neurology.* Philadelphia, PA: Lippincott Williams & Wilkins; 2000:153–160.

52. Kertesz A. Pick complex: an integrative approach to frontotemporal dementia: primary progressive aphasia, corticobasal degeneration, and progressive supranuclear palsy. *Neurology.* 2003; 9(6):311–317.

53. Frattali CM, Grafman J, Patronas N, et al. Language disturbances in corticobasal degeneration. *Neurology.* 2000; 54(4):990–995.

54. Rosenfield DB, Bogatka NS, Viswanath AE, et al. Speech apraxia in cortical-basal ganglionic degeneration [abstract]. *Ann Neurol.* 1991; 30:296–297.

55. Gibb WRG, Luthert PJ, Marsden CD. Corticobasal degeneration. *Brain.* 1989; 112: 1171–1192.

56. Graham NL, Bak TH, Patterson K, Hodges JR. Language function and dysfunction in corticobasal degeneration. *Neurology.* 2003; 61:493–499.

57. Graham NL, Bak TH, Hodges JR. Corticobasal degeneration as a cognitive disorder. *Mov Disord.* 2003; 18(11):1224–1232.

58. Broussolle E, Bakchine S, Tommasi M, et al. Slowly progressive anarthria with late anterior opercular syndrome: a variant form of frontal cortical atrophy syndromes. *J Neurol Sci.* 1996; 144:444–458.

59. Soliveri P, Piacentini S, Carella F, et al. Progressive dysarthria: definition and clinical follow-up. *Neurol Sci.* 2003; 24:211–212.

60. Rosenbek JC. Mutism, neurogenic. In: Kent RD, ed. *The MIT Encyclopedia of Communication Disorders.* Cambridge, MA: MIT Press; 2004.

61. Yorkston KM, Miller RM, Strand EA. *Management of Speech and Swallowing in Degenerative Diseases.* 2nd ed. Austin, TX: PRO-ED; 2004.

62. Beukelman DR, Mirenda P. *Augmentative and Alternative Communication: Management of Severe Communication Disorders in Children and Adults.* 2nd ed. Baltimore, MD: Paul H. Brookes Publishing; 1998.

63. Yorkston KM, Beukelman DR. Ataxic dysarthria: treatment sequences based on intelligibility and prosodic considerations. *J Speech Hear Disord.* 1981; 46(4):398–404.

64. Sapir S, Spielman J, Ramig LO, et al. Effects of intensive voice treatment (the Lee Silverman Voice Treatment [LSVT]) on ataxic dysarthria: a case study. *Am J Speech Lang Pathol.* 2003; 12(4):387–399.

65. Jones HN, Donovan NJ, Sapienza CM, et al. Expiratory muscle strength training in the treatment of mixed dysarthria in a patient with Lance Adams syndrome. *J Med Speech Lang Pathol.* 2006; 14(3): 207–217.

66. Nagaya M, Kachi T, Yamada T, Sumi Y. Videofluorographic observations on swallowing in patients with dysphagia due to neurodegenerative diseases. *Nagoya J Med Sci.* 2004; 67(1-2):17–23.

67. Kronenbuerger M, Fromm C, Block F, et al. On-demand deep brain stimulation for essential tremor: a report on four cases. *Mov Disord.* 2006; 21(3):401–405.

68. Hamakawa S, Koda C, Umeno H, et al. Oropharyngeal dysphagia in a case of Huntington's disease. *Auris Nasus Larynx.* 2004; 31(2):171–176.

69. Kagel MC, Leopold NA. Dysphagia in Huntington's disease: a 16-year retrospective. *Dysphagia.* 1992; 7(2):106–114.

70. Heemskerk AW, Ross RA. Dysphagia in Huntington's disease: a review. *Dysphagia.* 2011; 26(1):62–66.

71. Kagel MC, Leopold NA. Dysphagia in Huntington's disease. *Arch Neurol.* 1985; 42(1):57–60.

72. Trejo A, Tarrats RM, Alonso ME, et al. Assessment of the nutrition status of patients with Huntington's disease. *Nutrition.* 2004; 20(2):192–196.

73. Oder W, Grimm G, Kollegger H, et al. Neurological and neuropsychiatric spectrum of Wilson's disease: a prospective study of 45 cases. *J Neurol.* 1991; 238(5):281–287.

74. Wang XH, Cheng F, Zhang F, et al. Living-related liver transplantation for Wilson's disease. *Transpl Int.* 2005; 18(6):651–656.

75. Stremmel W, Meyerrose K, Niederau C, et al. Wilson disease: clinical presentation, treatment, and survival. *Ann Intern Med.* 1991; 115(9):720–726.

76. Topaloglu H, Gucuyener K, Orkun C, Renda Y. Tremor of tongue and dysarthria as the sole manifestation of Wilson's disease. *Clin Neurol Neurosurg.* 1990; 92(3):295–296.

77. Liao KK, Wang SJ, Kwan SY, et al. Tongue dyskinesia as an early manifestation of Wilson disease. *Brain Dev.* 1991; 13(6):451–453.

78. Kumar TS, Moses PD. Isolated tongue involvement—an unusual presentation of Wilson's disease. *J Postgrad Med.* 2005; 51(4):337.

79. Day LS, Parnell MM. Ten-year study of a Wilson's disease dysarthria. *J Commun Disord.* 1987; 20(3):207–218.

80. Pellecchia MT, Criscuolo C, Longo K, et al. Clinical presentation and treatment of Wilson's disease: a single-centre experience. *Eur Neurol.* 2003; 50(1):48–52.

81. Haggstrom G, Hirschowitz BI. Disordered esophageal motility in Wilson's disease. *J Clin Gastroenterol.* 1980; 2(3):273–275.

82. LaBlance GR, Rutherford DR. Respiratory dynamics and speech intelligibility in speakers with generalized dystonia. *J Commun Disord.* 1991; 24(2):141–156.

83. LaPointe LL, Case J, Duane D. Perceptual-acoustic speech and voice characteristics of subjects with spasmodic torticollis. In: Till J, Yorkston K, Beukelman D, eds. *Motor Speech Disorders: Advances in Assessment and Treatment.* Baltimore, MD: Paul H. Brookes Publishing; 1994; 40–45.

84. Golper LA, Nutt JG, Rau MT, Coleman RO. Focal cranial dystonia. *J Speech Hear Disord.* 1983; 48(2):128–134.

85. Tolosa E. Clinical Features of Meige's disease (idiopathic orofacial dystonia): a report of 17 cases. *Arch Neurol.* 1981; 38:147–151.

86. Edwards M, Schott G, Bhatia K. Episodic focal lingual dystonic spasms. *Mov Disord.* 2003; 18(7):836–837.

87. Baik JS, Park JH, Kim J Y. Primary lingual dystonia induced by speaking. *Mov Disord.* 2004; 19(10):1251–1252.

88. Charles PD, Davis TL, Shannon KM, et al. Tongue protrusion dystonia: treatmen with botulinum toxin. *South Med J.* 1997; 90(5):522–525.

89. Robertson-Hoffman DE, Mark MH, Sage JL. Isolated lingual/palatal dystonia. *Mov Disord.* 1991; 6(2):177–179.

90. Singer C, Papapetropoulos S. A comparison of jaw-closing and jaw-opening idio pathic oromandibular dystonia. *Parkinsonism Relat Disord.* 2006;12(2):115–118.

91. Tan EK, Jankovic J. Bilateral hemifacial spasm: a report of five cases and a literature review. *Mov Disord.* 1999; 14(2):345–349.

92. Lagueny A, Burbaud P, LeMasson G, et al. Involvement of respiratory muscles in adult-onset dystonia: a clinical and electrophysiological study. *Mov Disord.* 1995 10(6):708–713.

93. Lundy DS, Casiano RR, Lu FL, Xue JW. Abnormal soft palate posturing in patients with laryngeal movement disorders. *J Voice.* 1996; 10(4):348–53.

94. Dworkin JP. Bite-block therapy for oromandibular dystonia. In: Cannito MP Yorkston K, Beukelman D, eds. *Neuromotor Speech Disorders: Nature, Assessment and Management.* Baltimore, MD: Paul H. Brookes Publishing; 1998.

95. Dworkin J P. Bite-block therapy for oromandibular dystonia. *J Med Speech Lang Pathol.* 1996; 4:47.

96. Brin MF, Fahn S, Moskowitz C, et al. Localized injections of botulinum toxin for the treatment of focal dystonia and hemifacial spasm. *Mov Disord.* 1987; 2:237–254.

97. Brin M, Blitzer A, Stewart C. Laryngeal dystonia (spasmodic dysphonia): observations of 901 patients and treatment with botulinum toxin. *Adv Neurol.* 1998; 78:237–252.

98. Tagliati M, Shils J, Sun C, Alterman R. Deep brain stimulation for dystonia. *Expert Rev Med Devices.* 2004; 1(1):33–41.

99. Riski JE, Horner J, Nashold BS Jr. NB. Swallowing function in patients with spas modic torticollis. *Neurology.* 1990; 40(9):1443–1445.

100. Cersosimo MG, Juri S, Suarez de Chandler S, et al. Swallowing disorders in patients with blepharospasm. *Medicina.* 2005; 65(2):117–120.

101. Mascia MM, Valls-Sole J, Marti MJ, Sanz S. Chewing pattern in patients with Meige's syndrome. *Mov Disord.* 2005; 20(1):26–33.

102. Holzer SE, Ludlow CL. The swallowing side effects of botulinum toxin type A injection in spasmodic dysphonia. *Laryngoscope.* 1996; 106:86–92.

103. Gerratt BR. Formant frequency fluctuation as an index of motor steadiness in the vocal tract. *J Speech Hear Res.* 1983; 26(2):297–304.

104. Portnoy RA. Hyperkinetic dysarthria as an early indicator of impending tardive dyskinesia. *J Speech Hear Disord.* 1979; 44(2):214–219.

105. Frangos E, Christodoulides H. Clinical observations of the treatment of tardive dyskinesia with haloperidol. *Acta Psychiatr Belg.* 1975; 75(1):19–32.

APPENDIX A

Grandfather Passage

You wish to know all about my grandfather. Well, he is nearly 93 years old, yet he still thinks as swiftly as ever. He dresses himself in an old black frock coat, usually with several buttons missing. A long beard clings to his chin, giving those who observe him a pronounced feeling of the utmost respect. Twice each day, he plays skillfully and with zest upon a small organ. Except in the winter, when the snow or ice prevents, he slowly takes a short walk in the open air each day. We have often urged him to walk more and smoke less, but he always answers, "Banana oil!" Grandfather likes to be modern in his language.

Source: From Ref. 1: Duffy JR. *Motor Speech Disorders. Substrates, Differential Diagnosis, and Management.* 2nd ed. Philadelphia, PA: Elsevier; 2005, with permission.

APPENDIX B

Table Appendix B
Perceptual Features of Motor Speech Disorders

Hyperkinetic Dysarthria–Chorea	Hyperkinetic Dysarthria–Dystonia	Apraxia of Speech	Flaccid Dysarthria	Spastic Dysarthria	Ataxic Dysarthria	Hypokinetic Dysarthria
Imprecise consonants	Imprecise consonants	Consonant distortions	Hypernasality[a]	Imprecise consonants[a]	Imprecise consonants	Monopitch
Prolonged intervals[a]	Distorted vowels[a]	Substitutions		Monopitch	Equal and excess stress	Reduced stress
Variable rate[a]	Harsh vocal quality[a]	Distorted substitutions	Imprecise consonants	Reduced stress	Irregular articulatory breakdowns[a]	Monoloudness
Monopitch	Irregular articulatory breakdowns[a]	Additions	Breathiness (continuous)[a]	Harshness	Distorted vowels[a]	Imprecise consonants
Harsh vocal quality	Strained–strangled voice[a]	Distorted additions	Monopitch	Low pitch[a]	Harsh vocal quality	Inappropriate silences
Inappropriate silences[a]	Monopitch	Omissions	Nasal emission[a]	Slow rate[a]	Prolonged phonemes[a]	Short rushes of speech
Distorted vowels	Monoloudness	Slow overall rate	Audible inspiration[a]	Strained–strangled voice[a]	Prolonged intervals[a]	Harsh vocal quality

Excess loudness variations[a]	Inappropriate silences[a]	Syllable segregation	Harsh vocal quality	Short phrases	Monopitch	Breathy voice (continuous)
Prolonged phonemes[a]	Short phrases	Groping for articulatory postures	Short phrases[a]	Distorted vowels	Monoloudness	Low pitch
Monoloudness	Prolonged intervals	Difficulty with initiation	Monoloudness	Pitch breaks		Variable rate
Short phrases	Prolonged phonemes					Increased rate in segments
Irregular articulatory breakdowns	Excess loudness variations[a]					
Equal and excess stress	Reduced stress					

[a] Indicates features that may be more distinctive or severe than in other types of dysarthria.

Source: From Ref. 1: Duffy JR. Motor Speech Disorders. Substrates, Differential Diagnosis, and Management. 2nd ed. Philadelphia, PA: Elsevier; 2005, with permission.

19

NUTRITIONAL CONSIDERATIONS

Good nutrition is essential to maintain the well-being of individuals with neurological disease. There are several reasons why nutrition is important in movement disorders:

- Nutrition may impact mobility, cognition, and swallowing function. Movement disorders, by definition, result in changes in mobility and may lead to a decreased capacity to perform activities of daily living, such as cooking and shopping.

- Cognitive dysfunction may impact the capacity to plan healthy meals.

- Parkinson's disease (PD), other parkinsonian disorders, and many causes of chorea and ataxia can be associated with dysphagia.

- Poor nutrition in movement disorders may contribute to weight loss. Conversely, decreased levels of activity may lead to a sedentary lifestyle and obesity, exacerbating the underlying neurological disability.

- Finally, individuals with movement disorders often actively pursue both traditional and nontraditional treatment alternatives, vitamin therapies, and herbal remedies, which are frequently proposed for the management of many symptoms.

Patients will often discuss nutrition with their primary neurologist or primary care physician. All of the reasons listed above suggest that physicians caring for individuals with movement disorders should be familiar with appropriate nutritional strategies for these patients. This chapter is structured to discuss the malnourished patient and nutritional issues with respect to the various movement disorders (ie, PD and other parkinsonian disorders, Huntington's disease [HD] and other choreiform disorders, dystonia, and ataxia). These sections are followed by a discussion of nutritional supplements.

THE MALNOURISHED PATIENT: UNINTENDED WEIGHT LOSS IN MOVEMENT DISORDERS

Unintended weight loss is simply defined as a decrease in body weight that is *not* voluntary. Weight loss can occur with decreased food intake, increased metabolism, or both. Individuals with movement disorders should be weighed periodically as part of a routine neurological evaluation. Significant weight loss (<10% of body weight) that is unintended should prompt a discussion of potential causes. Various parkinsonian disorders, choreiform disorders, essential tremor and ataxic disorders can all be similarly associated with weight loss. Weight loss in movement disorders may be due not only to decreased intake but also to changes in energy demands (in some cases, individuals with severe tremor, dyskinesia, or chorea may have associated weight loss).[1,2] Unintentional weight loss can have similar causes across movement disorders (Figure 19.1).

■ *Decreased ability to swallow.* Patients who have trouble swallowing eat more slowly, are satiated (satisfied) more easily, and eat less.

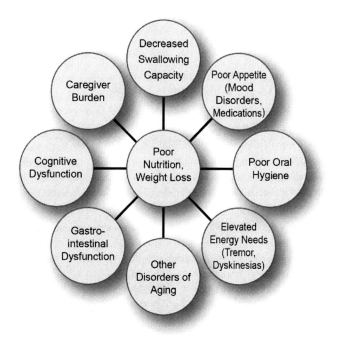

Figure 19.1
Factors leading to poor nutrition in patients with movement disorders.

■ *Decreased appetite.* Apathy, anxiety, or depression frequently accompanies movement disorders such as HD and PD, and any of them may result in a decreased interest in food or food preparation. Drugs such as *levodopa* may cause nausea or decreased appetite. Changes in sensation, such as a decreased sense of smell (a common finding in PD), may result in decreased taste and craving for food.

■ *Poor oral hygiene.* Motor deficits associated with difficulties in performing activities of daily living, such as attending to hygiene needs, may contribute to poor dentition and impact nutrition.

■ *Elevated energy needs.* Patients who have frequent episodes of moderate to marked tremors, dyskinesia, or rigidity may burn calories faster.

■ *Psychosocial factors.* Individuals with advancing disease may progressively burden caregivers, sometimes overwhelming their capacity to provide adequate care.

■ *Gastrointestinal dysfunction.* In many disorders, such as PD and multiple system atrophy (MSA), autonomic dysfunction can affect gut function, causing reflux, constipation, and other problems.

■ *Executive dysfunction.* Cognitive dysfunction, particularly difficulties in planning and coordinating complex activities, can interfere with the capacity of individuals with limited support networks to plan and cook meals.

■ *Other disorders of aging.* Although weight loss may be a unique feature of many movement disorders, unplanned weight loss may also be a sign of other medical illnesses, such as malignancy, gastrointestinal defects, chronic infections, and endocrine defects.

Nutritional assessment and intervention are important components of overall care in individuals with movement disorders. The purpose of this chapter is to discuss factors that may result in poor nutrition in the various movement disorders and strategies for their evaluation and management.

NUTRITION IN PARKINSON'S DISEASE

Helping patients become aware of their dietary habits and energy needs, and educating them about the elements of a balanced diet as well as techniques for altering poor eating habits, can be an important part of the management of nutrition in PD. Patients should eat a balanced diet with sufficient fiber and fluid to prevent constipation. Individuals with PD may have many of the barriers to nutrition identified in Figure 19.1. Management strategies tailored to each assessed need should be formulated.

Dysphagia

Increased oral transit time is a common finding in PD. As discussed in Chapter 18, all phases of swallowing can be involved. The early phases (oral and pharyngeal) of swallowing are most affected. Modified barium swallow examination or videofluoroscopic assessment may be needed. There is no universal approach to the management of dysphagia in PD. **Management can be challenging because dysphagia in PD invariably does not respond well to pharmacologic treatment for the motor symptoms of PD.** Current management includes the following:

- Referral for speech therapy for any patient who experiences choking or problems with swallowing. Alterations in swallowing technique may help with function.

- Changes in food consistency (soft, texture-modified diet and thickening of fluids) may be helpful for some patients.

- Postural adaptations and adjustments may be useful.

- Optimizing dopaminergic medications may be helpful in some patients. Levodopa and apomorphine can improve the early phases of swallowing.

- Gastrostomy feeding tube placement should be considered in patients with advanced disease.

- Botulinum toxin injection, cricopharyngeal muscle resection, and deep brain stimulation (DBS) for dysphagia in PD have been reported in a limited number of cases.

- Currently, there is no clear evidence to recommend to the use of complementary therapies for the treatment of dysphagia in PD.

- Limited reports on the benefits of speech therapy (eg, Lee Silverman voice therapy) suggest that it may mitigate dysphasia because it strengthens not only the speech muscles but the swallowing muscles as well.

Decreased Appetite

Individuals with weight loss should specifically be asked about appetite. Dopaminergic therapy can change appetite. Levodopa, for example, commonly decreases appetite and may cause nausea. Dopamine agonists, on the other hand, may increase appetite. A mood disorder, such as depression or anxiety, may also impact appetite. Management may include the following:

- Taking levodopa with meals. Patients who experience nausea as a side effect of levodopa may take this medication with meals. However, in the presence of wearing-off symptoms, protein competition (large amino acids in particular) can limit levodopa absorption; therefore, it may be best for the patient to take levodopa at least half an hour before meals or 2 hours after eating. The timing of levodopa dosing should be individualized.

- Evaluation for and treatment of anxiety or depression. These may cause a loss of appetite or sometimes overeating.

- Although some nutritional supplements, such as branched-chain amino acids, may stimulate appetite, they may induce wearing off and should be used with extra caution.[3]

Elevated Energy Needs

Treatment should be tailored to the patient.

- Mild dyskinesia may be a necessary compromise to maintain good motor function in levodopa-sensitive patients in the later stages of PD, and it should not automatically be a reason to alter medical therapy. A mild increase in dietary caloric intake may be an appropriate management strategy to replenish calories lost from excessive movement.

- In patients with severe dyskinesia sufficient to alter energy requirements, changes in medication, including lowering the overall dose of levodopa, may help mitigate symptoms.

- Severe tremor can increase energy requirements and can significantly interfere with quality of life. Increasing the levodopa dose or adding an agonist or anticholinergic agent may be helpful.

- If medication alterations are not helpful for severe tremors or dyskinesia, DBS may be considered in selected patients, as discussed in Chapter 16.

Autonomic Dysfunction

Autonomic dysfunction is a common complication of PD. Although overshadowed by motor dysfunction in many patients, a large number of patients with PD experience significant effects of autonomic dysfunction, including constipation, urinary problems, impotence, orthostasis, impaired thermoregulation, and sensory disturbances. Gastrointestinal manifestations may in particular impact nutrition.

- *Gastroesophageal reflux.* Poor transit through the stomach can lead to the reflux of acid into the esophagus. Gastroesophageal reflux is treatable and should not be overlooked as a cause of nausea in PD. If reflux is present, decreasing the size of meals and avoiding trigger foods like caffeine, citrus fruits, tomatoes, and alcohol should be first-line treatment. Numerous small meals and snacks that are nutrient-dense and moderate in fat and fiber may be helpful. The day's final meal should be consumed at least 4 hours before bedtime, so that the stomach is empty before the patient lies down. Herbal remedies for dyspepsia with metallic additives should not be given because they can inhibit levodopa absorption.

■ *Constipation.* There is evidence that the neurodegenerative process may cause constipation. Lewy body deposition has been discovered in the myenteric plexus of patients with PD.[4] Slowed stool transit time may result in constipation, with changes in appetite related to a feeling of fullness and intestinal discomfort. Dietary changes form the keystone of good management for PD. The management of constipation can be conservative, pharmacologic, or both.

   ○ Conservative treatment includes the following recommendations:

      ● Drink at least eight full glasses of water each day.

      ● Include high-fiber raw vegetables in at least two meals per day.

      ● Oat bran and other high-fiber additives may be helpful.

      ● Avoid baked goods and bananas.

      ● Increase physical activity; for example, walking and swimming are good.

      ● Discontinue medications causing constipation if possible.

   ○ Pharmacologic treatment

      ● Consider psyllium (5.1 g twice daily) or polyethylene glycol 3350 (up to 17 mg daily) if conservative management fails.[5]

      ● **Avoid the *chronic* use of laxatives,** including senna and cascara sagrada, as these are less physiologic strategies that may damage the colon with prolonged use.

■ *Defecatory dysfunction.* Some practitioners have suggested that a paradoxical contraction of the pelvic floor musculature consistent with a pelvic floor dystonia may occur in some patients, leading to poor colonic emptying. In one study, defecatory function was improved in eight patients with PD after the administration of apomorphine.[6] Botulinum toxin injections into the puborectalis muscle under ultrasonic guidance have also been reported to improve anorectal function in PD.[7]

■ *Sialorrhea.* Sialorrhea is very common in PD, affecting more than 70% of patients. It may affect nutrition and can be embarrassing in social situations. Recent studies have shown that sialorrhea results from concomitant swallowing difficulties rather than excessive salivation.[8,9] Although the use of sugar-free chewing gum or hard candy may be helpful in patients with mild symptoms, pharmacologic treatment should be considered when more aggressive interventions are warranted. Evidence-based pharmacologic treatment includes the following:

- Glycopyrrolate (1 mg 3 times daily)[10]

- Sublingual administration of ipratropium spray and atropine ophthalmic[11]

- Botulinum toxin type A or B injections into the parotid and submandibular glands[12,13]

- *Xerostomia (dry mouth)*. Some anticholinergic medications, such as benztropine and medications used for bladder dysfunction, can cause dry mouth. The long-term effects of dry mouth include increased dental caries and gingivitis, and dry mouth can be a significant problem in individuals who already have difficulty in performing the activities of daily living, including oral hygiene. Stopping the offending medication, if possible, is usually the only effective therapy.

Cognitive and Psychosocial Factors

Caregivers of individuals with PD, especially spouses, face an increasing burden with time, particularly in the later stages of disease, when the rate of depression for caregivers is higher.[14] Caregivers may themselves be ill or older. Increasing problems with activities of daily living may result in decreased overall hygiene, including decreased oral hygiene, which may affect the patient's capacity to eat. Evidence of malnutrition in a patient with PD should prompt a full psychosocial evaluation, including the following:

- Home physical therapy and occupational therapy evaluation to evaluate the living situation

- Social work interaction to evaluate caregiver resources

- Dental evaluation if there is evidence of dental disease

- Neuropsychological evaluation to gauge the presence of significant dementia interfering with function

Other Disorders

- Individuals with PD are subject to other disorders of aging, and abrupt changes in weight or appetite should prompt a consideration of other potential medical causes, including malignancy and endocrine abnormalities.

- A recent review suggested that overweight in PD seems to be associated with cardiovascular risk factors, such as hypertension, diabetes, and hypercholesterolemia.[15] However, further studies are needed to put forth strong evidence of this association.

Other Nutritional Considerations in Parkinson's Disease

Medical management in PD has significant nutritional ramifications. Dopaminergic medications may cause nausea and vomiting in some patients. Medications may also cause other side effects that impact nutrition. Conversely, protein intake may interfere with medication absorption. The effects of medical therapy on overall nutritional status should be attended to. Specific issues include the following:

■ *Levodopa-related nausea and vomiting.* The initiation of levodopa may cause nausea and vomiting. Management strategies to mitigate levodopa-induced nausea include these:

○ When a patient starts levodopa, an initial dose of half a tablet 3 times daily should be used to decrease the chance of nausea.

○ Initially, patients may need to take levodopa with food.

○ Ginger tea and crystallized ginger, which can be chewed, may help some patients.

○ Extra carbidopa (25- to 50-mg dose, taken with levodopa) may help mitigate the peripheral effects of levodopa (when converted to dopamine outside the central nervous system), including nausea.

○ Domperidone, available in pharmacies outside the United States and occasionally in compound pharmacies, has proved to be effective and safe in PD and can also mitigate nausea.

○ **Prochlorperazine (Compazine) and metoclopramide (Reglan) are to be avoided because they block dopamine receptors and can increase parkinsonian symptoms.**

■ *Levodopa–protein interaction.* Large, neutral amino acids compete with levodopa for uptake, both from the gut and across the blood–brain barrier. Interactions between protein and levodopa usually become evident in patients in the later stages of PD. Management strategies include the following:

○ The immediate-release formulation of levodopa is taken 30 minutes before meals.

○ Protein restriction during the day has been recommended by some practitioners.[16] This strategy works as a short-term solution but may not be as effective as a long-term solution.[4] It is not tolerated by patients and results in a low energy intake.

○ Domperidone can improve both gastric emptying and levodopa absorption. It can combat nausea and vomiting in extreme cases.

○ Recently, levodopa/carbidopa intestinal gel, which is delivered directly to the proximal jejunum via a percutaneous endoscopic gastrojejunostomy tube connected to a portable infusion pump, has been tested in patients with advanced PD, as delayed gastric emptying may contribute to the motor fluctuations seen with oral levodopa.[17]

■ *Unplanned weight gain.* Unplanned weight gain can be an idiosyncratic side effect of dopamine agonists such as pramipexole (Mirapex), rotigotine (Neupro patch), and ropinirole (Requip). They may cause an increased caloric intake, or they may increase fluid retention. Compulsive eating, particularly sweets and carbohydrates, may also occur. Amantadine may also increase fluid retention. Management may include the following:

○ Physical activity can be increased.

○ Decreased salt intake may help in some cases.

○ Discontinuation or alteration of the dose of the offending medication may be necessary.

○ Obsessive behaviors related to dopamine agonists are idiosyncratic and do not appear to be strictly dose-related. Typically, these problems are not treatable except by stopping the offending medication. The observation of obsessive eating should prompt questions about other obsessive behaviors, such as gambling and sexual obsessions.

○ DBS, in particular DBS of the subthalamic nucleus (STN), may result in weight gain for unclear reasons.

NUTRITION IN OTHER PARKINSONIAN DISORDERS

The management of nutrition in other neurodegenerative parkinsonian conditions is similar to the management in PD. In many cases, dysphagia is a more significant cause of poor nutrition. Specific issues relevant to individual disorders are discussed next.

Multiple System Atrophy

Patients with MSA have unique pharmacologic challenges related to nutrition. In many cases, autonomic instability with orthostasis is a significant cause of disability.

Many patients are levodopa-responsive, but levodopa may cause significant side effects, such as lowering blood pressure. Blood pressure fluctuations may also be related to the digestion of meals. Dysphagia clearly impacts nutrition. Issues related to nutrition in MSA may include these:

■ *Dysphagia.* Individuals with MSA may experience choking, difficulties swallowing, and aspiration. Management includes the following:

○ Speech pathologists should be part of the management team and should be consulted early.

○ Because dysphagia can become significant later in the disease process, it is reasonable to ascertain early the patient's wishes with respect to feeding tubes and other supportive nutritional devices.

■ *Gastrointestinal dysfunction.* The autonomic dysfunction impacting the gastrointestinal tract is similar to that found in idiopathic PD but is frequently more severe. Management is similar to the management in PD.

■ *Postprandial hypotension.* This complication commonly occurs 30 to 90 minutes after a meal. Hypotension can be significant and sometimes results in syncope and falls. Management includes the following:

○ Limiting meal size and increasing the frequency of meals.

○ Taking 5 to 10 mg of midodrine before meals to increase adrenergic tone after meals. **Midodrine should not be taken within 4 hours of sleep.**

○ Limiting the levodopa dose. The impact of levodopa on motor function must be balanced against its impact on blood pressure.

■ *Cognitive dysfunction.* Executive dysfunction can become a significant source of disability and caregiver strain later in the disease process, and it should be managed in a multidisciplinary fashion.

■ *Increased energy requirements.* Later in the disease process, patients are less mobile and prone to develop pressure sores, and a catabolic metabolism may develop as the capacity to take food by mouth declines. The management can be challenging, and the strategy should be based on the wishes of the family and patient.

Progressive Supranuclear Palsy

Patients with progressive supranuclear palsy (PSP) are rarely levodopa-responsive, and medications interact less with nutrition than they do in PD or MSA. Dysphagia and executive dysfunction are significant sources of disability. The management of issues related to nutrition includes the following:

■ *Dysphagia.* Aspiration is a common cause of mortality in PSP. A speech pathologist should be consulted early. End-of-life issues should be discussed early, before cognitive dysfunction limits the patient's capacity to make decisions.

■ *Executive dysfunction.* Executive dysfunction is a significant cause of disability in PSP. Significant cognitive changes develop relatively early in the course of the disease, increasing caregiver burden.

■ *Apraxia.* Individuals with PSP and parkinsonism associated with dementia may develop progressive bradykinesia and apraxia of limb movements. This type of apraxia may impact eating behavior. Supranuclear gaze palsy together with neck rigidity frequently interferes with the ability to look down at a plate in the later stages of the disease. Consequently, individuals with PSP develop progressive problems with self-feeding.

■ *Increased energy requirements.* As mentioned, later in the disease process, patients are less mobile and prone to develop pressure sores, and a catabolic metabolism may develop as the capacity to take food by mouth declines. The management of PSP, MSA, and parkinsonism in the end stages is challenging and should respect the wishes of the family and patient.

Other Parkinsonian Syndromes

Corticobasoganglionic degeneration (CBGD) and other causes of parkinsonism, including vascular parkinsonism, typically require management strategies similar to those delineated for PD, MSA, and PSP.

NUTRITION IN CHOREIFORM DISORDERS

Choreiform disorders comprise a vast landscape of disease processes. Although the causes of these disorders vary, phenomenologically, the disorders share similar issues with respect to nutrition.

■ *Increased energy requirements* due to chorea may necessitate an increase in the patient's caloric intake. In HD, chorea is associated with weight loss.[1] Nutrition should be planned to allow for the increased energy demands of individuals who have significant chorea.

■ *Dysphagia* is a common complaint in nearly all choreiform disorders (with the exception of tardive dyskinesia). The speech pathologist is an integral part of the management team for all of these disorders.

■ *Chorea* may occasionally interfere with self-feeding.

■ *Cognitive and mood changes* are common in all of the choreiform disorders and can impact the caregiver burden, as well as the patient's and caregiver's capacity to develop appropriate nutritional plans.

■ Nutritional management in HD may include the following:

○ A thick, pureed, or chopped diet with sufficient energy and protein. Usually, 1 to 1.5 g of protein per kilogram of patient weight is needed. Patients with HD may need up to 5,000 kcal/d.[18]

○ Fluid intake should be sufficient because dehydration is common.

○ Adequate fiber should be provided.

○ The caregiver should be educated about thickening liquids to preven
episodes of choking.

○ Percutaneous gastrostomy tube feeding should be implemented when
necessary.

NUTRITION IN ATAXIA

Genetic causes of ataxia overlap in many cases with genetic causes of chorea
Ataxia brings specific challenges to nutrition, many of which have been discussed in previous sections with respect to other movement disorders.

■ *Dysphagia.* This is a common finding and warrants referral for swallowing
evaluation. As in many of the movement disorders, the speech pathologist
is an integral part of the team.

■ *Ataxia.* Ataxia can significantly interfere with feeding. In some patients, a
cerebellar or rubral tremor may prevent the patient from bringing food to
the mouth. Occupational therapy may be able to assist with weighted utensils or other devices that allow feeding.

NUTRITION IN TARDIVE DYSKINESIA

Tardive dyskinesia may occur in patients taking dopamine receptor blockers,
including neuroleptics and antiemetics. Tardive dyskinesia primarily involves
the tongue, lips, and jaw. Nutrition may be affected because these patients
mostly have psychiatric conditions, are often elderly, and are not uncommonly
institutionalized. Difficulty with self-feeding often leads to weight loss. Nutritional management may include the following:

■ Offer a soft diet for some patients to reduce chewing as needed.

■ Assess weight status. Increase energy intake in case of increased energy demands
due to severe dyskinesia. Decrease energy intake if the patient is obese.

■ Carbohydrate craving is common. Watch overall intake of sweets, or offer
nutrient-dense varieties to reduce hyperglycemia.[18]

■ Self-feeding practices may be needed.

NUTRITIONAL DERANGEMENTS AS A CAUSE OF MOVEMENT DISORDERS

Although rare, a limited number of movement disorders are caused by aberrant
nutritional absorption. Wilson's disease is caused by aberrant copper metabolism. Vitamin E deficiency can cause ataxia. Disorders of iron storage can cause
chorea and ataxia. Specific nutritional requirements may be required for some
diseases based on the diagnosis.

SWALLOWING DYSFUNCTION IN PATIENTS WITH MOVEMENT DISORDERS

It is appropriate to close our discussion of barriers to nutrition in movement disorders by briefly discussing swallowing dysfunction. Swallowing dysfunction is a common feature of many movement disorders.[19]

- Oropharyngeal dysphagia (abnormal swallowing) may result in many complications, including dehydration, malnutrition, bronchospasm, and airway obstruction, as well as aspiration pneumonia and chronic chest infection.

- Secondary consequences of poor swallowing function may include increased caregiver strain, social isolation, and depression,[20] and swallowing dysfunction may therefore become a substantial component of disability.

- Evidence of aspiration, such as coughing or choking during meals, should be elicited during routine history.

- The management of dysphagia in movement disorders is covered elsewhere in this textbook; however, prompt referral to a speech pathologist is mandatory for any patient with swallowing dysfunction. In later stages of disease, the insertion of a percutaneous endoscopic gastrostomy (PEG) tube for nutrition may be warranted.

EVIDENCE ON NUTRITIONAL SUPPLEMENTS

A large body of literature has been developed in support of the hypothesis that oxidative stress is a contributing factor in the pathophysiology of many neurodegenerative diseases.[20,21] This literature led to the hypothesis that nutritional supplements that are antioxidant "scavengers" of free radicals might alter the progression of neurodegenerative disease. Multiple nutritional supplements have been proposed. Well-designed studies are lacking for any but a few nutritional supplements, owing in part to the large number of contenders in the field and to a lack of consensus on appropriate trial design. No nutritional agent has been shown to date to have the capacity to alter the course of any neurodegenerative disease.[22] As nutrition is a subject that is frequently brought up by patients, it is appropriate for clinicians to have some familiarity with research in this area. A discussion of the nutritional supplements that have been formally evaluated in well-designed clinical studies follows.

Vitamin Therapy

- **Vitamins C and E**

  ○ Vitamins C and E both have antioxidant properties, which has prompted some practitioners to tout them as potential neuroprotective agents. Moreover, vitamin C can elevate levodopa levels, theoretically leading to potential symptomatic effects.[23] Epidemiological studies have shown that consuming foods rich in vitamins C and E is associated with a lower risk for developing PD.[24] A nonrandomized, unblinded study suggested that combining vitamins E and C might slow the rate of progression in patients with early PD;[25] however, DATATOP (Deprenyl And Tocopherol Antioxidative Therapy of Parkinsonism), a randomized, blinded study of high-dose vitamin E alone by the Parkinson Study Group, in which the initiation of levodopa was used as a surrogate marker, did not show any difference between the vitamin E group and a placebo group.[26] In addition, a meta-analysis of observational studies assessing high dietary intake of vitamin E and risk for PD suggested an overall decreased risk for PD.[27] Vitamin C supplementation was not found to reduce the risk for incident PD in this meta-analysis. As a result of these studies, the American Academy of Neurology Quality Standards Subcommittee reported that vitamin E probably does not delay the need for levodopa therapy and recommended that treatment with 2,000 units of vitamin E not be considered for neuroprotection in PD.[22]

○ Vitamin E has also been tried in other movement disorders. A trial of vitamin E in HD showed no improvement in the primary outcome variable (neuropsychological change).[28] Although it has been suggested, there is no clear evidence of the beneficial effect of vitamin E in Friedreich ataxia in the literature because of the lack of controlled studies, the variable doses used, and the association with other antioxidant medications. Some researchers have proposed vitamin E as a treatment for tardive dyskinesia. However, current data from small trials of limited quality suggest that the beneficial effect of vitamin E seems restricted, at best, to the prevention of deterioration of tardive dyskinesia rather than relief of symptoms.[29]

○ A fairly large literature exists on vitamins E and C in the prevention or treatment of Alzheimer dementia; however, randomized, well-controlled studies are lacking, and there is currently no clear evidence in the dementia literature that either vitamin alone or the two in combination affect neurological function in the dementias.[30]

○ **There is therefore no evidence to recommend vitamin E treatment to patients with movement disorders. The evidence is currently insufficient to evaluate if vitamin C may have disease-modifying effects.**

■ **Vitamin D**

○ Vitamin D deficiency can cause osteoporosis in elderly people. Patients with PD may be at particular risk. Because of postural instability, increased risk for falling, and bone fractures, the prevention of osteoporosis is essential in patients with PD. **Vitamin D insufficiency is common among patients with PD.** It has been proposed that vitamin D deficiency has a significant role in the development and progression of PD.[31] A recent longitudinal study with a cohort of 3,173 individuals and a 29-year follow-up period also showed that subjects with higher serum levels of vitamin D had a significantly lower risk for the development of PD.[32] Although it is not clear whether vitamin D insufficiency contributes to the development of PD or is a result of reduced physical activity and exposure to sunlight resulting from the nature of the disease, recent studies support the possible link between vitamin D intake and the pathogenesis of PD.

○ **Vitamin D levels should be analyzed regularly in patients with PD to maintain bone health.** Vitamin D can be obtained through exposure to sunlight, diet, or nutritional supplements. The diet of patients who live in a region with limited sunshine or who have difficulty getting outdoors should include calcium and vitamin D. Milk, yogurt, fish, and breakfast cereals are the richest sources of calcium. The recommended dietary allowance of vitamin D is 200 to 600 IU per day.[33]

Vitamin B_6, Vitamin B_{12}, and Folate

○ It has been documented that elevated homocysteine, which is a modestly independent predictor of risk for ischemic heart disease and stroke, occurs in patients with PD who are taking levodopa.[34,35] Because the B vitamins, including folate, vitamin B_6, and vitamin B_{12}, are important cofactors for homocysteine, a deficiency of B vitamins can lead to elevated homocysteine. A double-blinded study showed that B-vitamin supplementation can lower this elevation.[36] Therefore, it has been suggested that B-vitamin supplements may be warranted for patients who have PD with levodopa-related elevated homocysteine to overcome the possibly related risk for ischemic heart disease and stroke. However, no studies have shown an increased risk for vascular diseases in patients with PD and elevated homocysteine.[37]

○ The effects of homocysteine and B vitamins on the motor and non-motor symptoms of PD also have been studied. In a recent study, the homocysteine level did not correlate with global measures of cognition, mood, or parkinsonism in PD or with dyskinesia fluctuations, or freezing, whereas higher levels of vitamin B_{12} were associated with a lower risk for dyskinesia risk.[38] Because it has also been demonstrated that elevated homocysteine levels are more likely in patients with PD who have depression and worse cognition, it has been suggested that the benefits of folate, vitamin B_6, and vitamin B_{12} may be more evident for the nonmotor symptoms of PD than for the motor symptoms.[39,40]

○ In terms of the neuroprotective effects of B vitamins, studies have shown that folate and vitamin B_{12} intake does not reduce the risk for incident PD, whereas vitamin B_6 intake may lower the risk for PD among smokers only, probably through mechanisms unrelated to homocysteine metabolism.[3,41–43]

○ Although some researchers suggest that supplementation with B vitamins is important for managing elevated homocysteine levels in patients with PD, the effects of B vitamins on PD are still unclear, and further studies evaluating the effects of B vitamins on motor and non-motor function in patients with PD are needed.

○ Vitamin B_{12} supplementation should be considered in PD because its deficiency is very common in elderly people and may cause neuropathy, cognitive changes, and vision loss. Cognitive decline is often the most limiting nonmotor feature of PD. **Patients with PD taking high doses of levodopa may also present with peripheral neuropathy due to vitamin B12 deficiency.** On the other hand, patients with PD may avoid meat and other foods that contain vitamin B_{12} because protein intake among patients with PD may interfere with the clinical benefit of levodopa. **Therefore, patients with PD should be assessed for possible vitamin B12 deficiency and treated as needed.**

○ The effect of B vitamins on other movement disorders is not clear. A double-blinded, placebo-controlled, crossover study of 15 patients showed that symptoms of tardive dyskinesia were reduced in those taking vitamin B_6 by the third week of treatment. However, the duration of the benefit is uncertain.[44]

■ Coenzyme Q

○ Mitochondrial dysfunction has been demonstrated in idiopathic PD. Coenzyme Q is an important intermediary in the respiratory chain. A single randomized, blinded study of the safety and efficacy of coenzyme Q showed a positive trend ($P = .09$) in individuals given a higher (1,200-mg) dose of coenzyme Q, with less disability as shown by a decreased change from baseline in the Unified Parkinson's Disease Rating Scale (UPDRS).[45] Subsequently, a randomized, double-blinded, placebo-controlled trial of coenzyme Q10 evaluating its symptomatic effects in PD showed no significant difference between treatment and placebo, although patients in both groups showed significant improvements from baseline in UPDRS scores.[46] In a multicenter, randomized, double-blinded, placebo-controlled study of coenzyme Q10, it was found that the mean changes in total UPDRS scores were not significantly greater than the predetermined futility threshold value.[47]

○ A multicenter, randomized, double-blinded, placebo-controlled trial of coenzyme Q10 at a dosage of 600 mg/d in patients with HD showed no change in the rate of decline.[48] Because this study noted a trend toward slowed progression of HD without statistical significance among subjects treated with coenzyme Q10, a study evaluating the safety and tolerability of high-dose coenzyme Q10 in HD was recently conducted to assess the possibility of beneficial effects of a higher dose of coenzyme Q.[49] The study showed that high doses of coenzyme Q10 were well tolerated, and further studies examining the efficacy of 2,400 mg/d are planned. Currently, the American Academy of Neurology guideline recommends that clinicians may choose not to prescribe coenzyme Q10 for moderate improvements in HD chorea; however, modest antichoreic benefits cannot be excluded.[50]

- Coenzyme Q10 was also studied in PSP in a randomized, placebo-controlled trial, which has shown that coenzyme Q10 is safe and tolerable, leads to mild clinical amelioration, and improves cerebral energy metabolism.[51] A study of coenzyme Q10 in PSP is now ongoing.[52]

- As a result, there is no strong evidence thus far to recommend coenzyme Q10 treatment to patients with any movement disorder.

Diet and Dietary Supplements

Diet

- Although some studies have suggested that low-protein diet, ketogenic diet, high-urate diet, and "prudent" diet may lower the risk for incident PD, currently there are insufficient data to recommend any specific diet for patients with PD.[3]

Creatine

- Recent studies have shown creatine to be safe in HD and to reduce some of the laboratory biomarkers proposed to reflect progressive neuronal damage.[53,54] Doses of 8 g/d were well tolerated. Based on one randomized clinical trial, which showed no difference in any 16-week Unified Huntington's Disease Rating Scale (UHDRS) outcome, the American Academy of Neurology guideline recommends that clinicians may choose not to prescribe creatine for very important improvements in HD chorea; however, moderate antichoreic benefits cannot be excluded.[50]

- Creatine has also been studied in a randomized, double-blinded fashion in a "futility trial" designed to evaluate if further studies of the supplement are warranted in PD.[55] No definitive evidence of alteration of clinical function has been demonstrated. A 2-year, randomized, placebo-controlled study also reported that creatine did not improve UPDRS motor scores in patients with PD, whereas creatine can improve mood scores and reduce the doses required for dopamine replacement therapy.[56]

- A large multicenter, double-blind, parallel group, placebo-controlled, long-term study of creatine for treatment of early stage Parkinson's disease (NET-PD LS-1) has been terminated recently, since the interim analysis showed that it was "futile" to complete the study because longer patient follow-up was not likely to demonstrate a statistically significant difference between creatine and placebo.[57] Another study of creatine in both disorders is ongoing based on preliminary work.[58]

■ S-Adenosylmethionine

○ S-Adenosylmethionine (SAM) is an over-the-counter dietary supplement. Although an open-label study showed that SAM may reduce depression in patients with PD patients, it may increase the metabolism of levodopa over time and lead to wearing off.[59] So far, there is no clear evidence for recommending SAM in PD, and further studies are needed.

■ Iron

○ **Iron supplements can interfere with the absorption of levodopa.** Patients with PD should be informed about this interaction. Some patients with restless legs syndrome may have iron deficiency. In this case, iron supplementation should be initiated.

■ Medical food

○ A small, nonblinded study reported that Tarvil, a medical food with a high level of branched-chain amino acids, is beneficial for male patients with tardive dyskinesia.[60] Tarvil targets excess phenylalanine, which has been speculated to be the cause of tardive dyskinesia. However, this study does not provide strong evidence for Tarvil as a treatment for tardive dyskinesia.

Herbal Supplements

■ Herbal supplements have been used in traditional medicine, especially in China and India. *Mucuna pruriens* and *Vicia faba*, which are natural sources of levodopa, have been studied and suggested to be therapeutic in PD; however, it is difficult to measure the amount of levodopa in these herbs, and taking them with medications may cause significant side effects.

■ A recent systematic review of randomized clinical trials of herbal medicines for PD concluded that there is no conclusive evidence about the effectiveness of herbal medicines in PD.[61]

■ Although a study with only four patients with HD taking traditional Chinese medicines showed a decrease in UHDRS-m (motor subscale) scores, placebo-controlled studies with a large population of patients with HD are lacking.[62]

■ A recent randomized, double-blinded, placebo-controlled trial of extract of *Ginkgo biloba* for tardive dyskinesia has shown beneficial effects in reducing symptoms of tardive dyskinesia in people with schizophrenia.[63] Choline, lecithin, and manganese supplements and evening primrose oil have also been suggested as possible treatments for tardive dyskinesia; however, there is currently insufficient evidence to recommend any herbal supplement for tardive dyskinesia. Moreover, because herbs and supplements may interact adversely with drugs used to treat schizophrenia, they should not be taken without a physician's supervision.

Caffeine and Nicotine

- Epidemiologic studies show that smoking may offer neuroprotection in PD. An inverse association between caffeine intake and risk for PD has also been shown. A recent meta-analysis showed that a history of smoking reduces the risk for PD by about 36%, with coffee and alcohol consumption also reducing risk.[64] Because smoking and alcohol consumption cannot be recommended for patients, caffeine- and nicotine-containing edibles have lately become the center of interest in studies.

- A large, prospective study that included both men and women found a markedly lower risk for the development of PD among individuals who regularly consume caffeine, particularly in men but also in women, with an attenuating influence of hormone replacement therapy.[65]

- A new population-based study including 490 patients with newly diagnosed idiopathic PD has evaluated the association between the consumption of nicotine-containing edibles, such as peppers, tomatoes, and potatoes, and the risk for PD. The study has shown that eating peppers 2 to 4 times per week is "consistently" associated with a 30% reduction in risk for PD. However, these findings are preliminary and need to be further demonstrated in prospective studies evaluating the association.[66]

- Currently, there is no evidence of an association between caffeine and HD. However, in a retrospective study evaluating the relationship between caffeine consumption and age at onset of HD, the consumption of more than 190 mg of caffeine per day was significantly associated with an earlier age at onset.[67]

Melatonin

- Melatonin is an endogenous hormone that promotes sleep in humans. Melatonin can also be taken as a supplement.

- Melatonin has been studied mainly for sleep problems in patients with PD, and it has been shown that melatonin may improve sleep time and quality, although no statistically significant change in motor scores was observed. Based on these findings, the evidence-based review of the Movement Disorder Society reported that there is insufficient evidence regarding the efficacy of melatonin for the treatment of insomnia in PD.[68]

- So far, studies of melatonin in HD are limited to animals. The efficacy of melatonin has also been studied in tardive dyskinesia; however, there is no clear evidence, and further studies are warranted.[69]

CONCLUSION

- Movement disorders often cause barriers to appropriate nutrition.

- Decreased ability to swallow, poor appetite, elevated energy needs, and psychosocial and cognitive factors may all impact the ability of affected individuals to maintain proper nutrition.

- Clinical attention to nutrition in patients with these disorders is useful for preventing further disability.

- Including a speech pathologist and a nutritionist on the multidisciplinary team caring for individuals with these neurodegenerative diseases will improve outcomes.

REFERENCES

1. Mahant N, McCusker EA, Byth K, et al. Huntington's disease: clinical correlates of disability and progression. *Neurology.* 2003; 61(8):1085–1092.
2. Uc EY, Struck LK, Rodnitzky RL, et al. Predictors of weight loss in Parkinson's disease. *Mov Disord.* 2006; 21(7):930–936.
3. Zesiewicz TA, Evatt ML. Potential influences of complementary therapy on motor and non-motor complications in Parkinson's disease. *CNS Drugs.* 2009; 23(10):817–835
4. Olanow CW, Watts RL, Koller WC. An algorithm (decision tree) for the management of Parkinson's disease (2001): treatment guidelines. *Neurology.* 2001; 56(11):S1–S88.
5. Cloud LJ, Greene JG. Gastrointestinal features of Parkinson's disease. *Curr Neurol Neurosci Rep.* 2011; 11(4):379–384.
6. Edwards LL, Quigley EM, Harrned RK, et al. Defecatory function in Parkinson's disease: response to apomorphine. *Ann Neurol.* 1993; 33(5):490–493.
7. Albanese A, Maria G, Bentivoglio AR, et al. Severe constipation in Parkinson's disease relieved by botulinum toxin. *Mov Disord.* 1997; 12:764–766.
8. Tumilasci OR, Cersosimo MG, Belforte JE, et al. Quantitative study of salivary secretion in Parkinson's disease. *Mov Disord.* 2006; 21:660–667.
9. Nobrega AC, Rodrigues B, Torres AC, et al. Is drooling secondary to a swallowing disorder in patients with Parkinson's disease? *Parkinsonism Relat Disord.* 2008; 14:243–245.
10. Arbouw ME, Movig KL, Koopmann M, et al. Glycopyrrolate for sialorrhea in Parkinson disease: a randomized, double-blind, crossover trial. *Neurology.* 2010; 74:1203–1207.
11. Thomsen TR, Galpern WR, Asante A, et al. Ipratropium bromide spray as treatment for sialorrhea in Parkinson's disease. *Mov Disord.* 2007; 22:2268–2273.
12. Ondo W, Hunter C, Moore W. A double-blind placebo-controlled trial of botulinum toxin B for sialorrhea in Parkinson's disease. *Neurology.* 2004; 62:37–40.
13. Lagalla G, Millevolte M, Capecci M, et al. Botulinum toxin type A for drooling in Parkinson's disease: a double-blind, randomized, placebo-controlled study. *Mov Disord.* 2006; 21:704–707.
14. Carter JH, Stewart BJ, Archbold PG, et al. Living with a person who has Parkinson's disease: the spouse's perspective by stage of disease. *Mov Disord.* 1998; 13(1):20–28.

15. Barichella M, Cereda E, Pezzoli G. Major nutritional issues in the management of Parkinson's disease. *Mov Disord.* 2009; 24(13):1881–1892.

16. Pincus JH. Influence of dietary protein on motor fluctuations in Parkinson's disease. *Arch Neurol.* 1987; 44(3):270–272.

17. Fernandez HH, Vanagunas A, Odin P, et al. Levodopa-carbidopa intestinal gel in advanced Parkinson's disease open-label study: interim results. *Parkinsonism Relat Disord.* 2013; 19(3):339–345.

18. Escott-Stump SA. *Nutrition and Diagnosis-Related Care.* 7th ed. Philadelphia, PA: Lippincott Williams & Wilkins; 2012.

19. Hammond CA, Goldstein LB. Cough and aspiration of food and liquids due to oral-pharyngeal dysphagia. ACCP Evidence-Based Clinical Practice Guidelines. *Chest.* 2006; 129(1 suppl):186S–196S.

20. Olanow CW. A radical hypothesis for neurodegeneration. *Trends Neurosci.* 1993; 16:439–444.

21. Simonian NA, Coyle JT. Oxidative stress in neurodegenerative disease. *Ann Rev Pharmacol Toxicol.* 1996; 36:53–106.

22. Suchowersky O, Gronseth G, Perlmutter J, et al. Practice parameter: neuroprotective strategies and alternative therapies for Parkinson's disease (an evidence-based review): report of the Quality Standards Subcommittee of the American Academy of Neurology. *Neurology.* 2006; 66:976–982.

23. Ferry P, Johnson M, Wallis P. Use of complementary therapies and non-prescribed medication in patients with Parkinson's disease. *Postgrad Med J.* 2002; 78:612–614.

24. Anderson C, Checkoway H, Franklin GM, et al. Dietary factors in Parkinson's disease: the role of food groups and specific foods. *Mov Disord.* 1999; 14:21–27.

25. Fahn S. A pilot trial of high-dose alpha-tocopherol and ascorbate in early Parkinson's disease. *Ann Neurol.* 1992; 32(suppl):S128–S132.

26. The Parkinson Study Group. Effects of tocopherol and deprenyl on the progression of disability in early Parkinson's disease. *N Engl J Med.* 1993; 328(3):176–183.

27. Etminan M, Gill SS, Samii A. Intake of vitamin E, vitamin C, and carotenoids and the risk of Parkinson's disease: a meta-analysis. *Lancet Neurol.* 2005; 4(6):362–365.

28. Peyser CE, Folstein M, Chase GA, et al. Trial of d-alpha-tocopherol in Huntington's disease. *Am J Psychiatry.* 1995; 152(12):1771–1775.

29. Soares-Weiser K, Maayan N, McGrath J. Vitamin E for neuroleptic-induced tardive dyskinesia. *Cochrane Database Syst Rev.* 2011; (2):CD000209.

30. Boothby LA, Doering PL. Vitamin C and vitamin E for Alzheimer's disease. *Ann Pharmacother.* 2005; 39(12):2073–2080.

31. Newmark HL, Newmark J. Vitamin D and Parkinson's disease—a hypothesis. *Mov Disord.* 2007; 22(4):461–468.

32. Knekt P, Kilkkinen A, Rissanen H, et al. Serum vitamin D and the risk of Parkinson disease. *Arch Neurol.* 2010; 67:808–811.

33. Evatt ML. Nutritional therapies in Parkinson's disease. *Curr Treat Options Neurol.* 2007; 9(3):198–204.

34. O'Suilleabhain PE, Bottiglieri T, Dewey RB, et al. Modest increase in plasma homocysteine follows levodopa initiation in Parkinson's disease. *Mov Disord.* 2004; 19:1403–1408.

35. Miller JW, Selhub J, Nadeau MR, et al. Effect of L-dopa on plasma homocysteine in PD patients: relationship to B-vitamin status. *Neurology.* 2003; 60:1125–1129.

36. Postuma RB, Espay AJ, Zadikoff C, et al. Vitamins and entacapone in levodopa induced hyperhomocysteinemia: a randomized controlled study. *Neurology.* 2006 66:1941–1943.

37. Barichella M, Cereda E, Pezzoli G. Major nutritional issues in the management o Parkinson's disease. *Mov Disord.* 2009; 24(13):1881–1892.

38. Camicioli RM, Bouchard TP, Somerville MJ. Homocysteine is not associated with global motor or cognitive measures in nondemented older Parkinson's disease patients. *Mov Disord.* 2009; 24(2):176–182.

39. O'Suilleabhain PE, Sung V, Hernandez C, et al. Elevated plasma homocysteine leve in patients with Parkinson disease: motor, affective, and cognitive associations. *Arch Neurol.* 2004; 61(6):865–868.

40. Triantafyllou NI, Nikolaou C, Boufidou F, et al. Folate and vitamin B12 levels ir levodopa-treated Parkinson's disease patients: their relationship to clinical manifes tations, mood and cognition. *Parkinsonism Relat Disord.* 2008; 14(4):321–325.

41. Chen H, Zhang SM, Schwarzschild MA, et al. Folate intake and risk of Parkinson's disease. *Am J Epidemiol.* 2004; 160(4):368–375.

42. de Lau LM, Koudstaal PJ, Witteman JC, et al. Dietary folate, vitamin B12, and vita min B6 and the risk of Parkinson disease. *Neurology.* 2006; 67(2):315–318.

43. Murakami K, Miyake Y, Sasaki S, et al. Dietary intake of folate, vitamin B6, vitamir B12 and riboflavin and risk of Parkinson's disease: a case-control study in Japan. *Br J Nutr.* 2010; 104(5):757–764.

44. Lerner V, Miodownik C, Kaptsan A, et al. Vitamin B6 in the treatment of tardive dys kinesia: double-blind, placebo-controlled, crossover study. *Am J Psychiatry.* 2001 158:1511–1514.

45. Shults CW, Oakes D, Kieburtz K, et al. Effects of coenzyme Q10 in early Par kinson's disease: evidence of slowing of functional decline. *Arch Neurol.* 2002 59(10):1541–1550.

46. Storch A, Jost WH, Vieregge P, et al. Randomized, double blind, placebo-controlled trial on symptomatic effects of coenzyme Q10 in Parkinson disease. *Arch Neurol.* 2007; 64(7):938–944.

47. NINDS NET-PD Investigators. A randomized clinical trial of coenzyme Q10 and GPI-1485 in early Parkinson disease. *Neurology.* 2007; 68(1):20–28.

48. Huntington Study Group. A randomized, placebo-controlled trial of coenzyme Q10 and remacemide in Huntington's disease. *Neurology.* 2001; 57(3):397–404.

49. Huntington Study Group Pre2CARE Investigators. Safety and tolerability of high dosage coenzyme Q10 in Huntington's disease and healthy subjects. *Mov Disord.* 2010; 25(12):1924–1928.

50. Armstrong MJ, Miyasaki JM; American Academy of Neurology. Evidence-based guideline: pharmacologic treatment of chorea in Huntington disease: report of the guideline development subcommittee of the American Academy of Neurology. *Neurology.* 2012; 79(6):597–603.

51. Stamelou M, Reuss A, Pilatus U, et al. Short-term effects of coenzyme Q10 in pro gressive supranuclear palsy: a randomized, placebo-controlled trial. *Mov Disord.* 2008; 23(7):942-949.

52. Effects of coenzyme Q10 in progressive supranuclear palsy (PSP). http://clinicaltri als.gov/ct2/show/NCT00382824. Accessed April 14, 2014.

53. Hersch SM, Gevorkian S, Marder K, et al. Creatine in Huntington disease is safe, tolerable, bioavailable in brain and reduces serum 8OH2'dG. *Neurology.* 2006; 66(2):250–252.

44. Bender A, Auer DP, Merl T, et al. Creatine supplementation lowers brain glutamate levels in Huntington's disease. *J Neurol.* 2005; 252(1):36–41.

45. NINDS NET-PD Investigators. A randomized, double-blind, futility clinical trial of creatine and minocycline in early Parkinson disease. *Neurology.* 2006; 66(5):664–671.

46. Bender A, Koch W, Elstner M, et al. Creatine supplementation in Parkinson disease: a placebo-controlled randomized pilot trial. *Neurology.* 2006; 67(7):1262–1264.

47. NET-PD LS-1 Creatine in Parkinson's Disease. http://clinicaltrials.gov/show/ NCT00449865

48. Creatine safety, tolerability, & efficacy in Huntington's disease (CREST-E). http:// clinicaltrials.gov/show/NCT00712426. Accessed April 14, 2014.

49. Di Rocco A, Rogers JD, Brown R, et al. S-Adenosylmethionine improves depression in patients with Parkinson's disease in an open-label clinical trial. *Mov Disord.* 2000; 15(6):1225–1229.

50. Richardson MA, Bevans ML, Read LL, et al. Efficacy of the branched-chain amino acids in the treatment of tardive dyskinesia in men. *Am J Psychiatry.* 2003; 160(6):1117–1124.

51. Kim TH, Cho KH, Jung WS, Lee MS. Herbal medicines for Parkinson's disease: a systematic review of randomized controlled trials. *PLoS One.* 2012; 7(5):e35695.

52. Satoh T, Takahashi T, Iwasaki K, et al. Traditional Chinese medicine on four patients with Huntington's disease. *Mov Disord.* 2009; 24(3):453–455.

53. Zhang WF, Tan YL, Zhang XY, et al. Extract of ginkgo biloba treatment for tardive dyskinesia in schizophrenia: a randomized, double-blind, placebo-controlled trial. *J Clin Psychiatry.* 2011; 72(5):615–621.

54. Noyce AJ, Bestwick JP, Silveira-Moriyama L, et al. Meta-analysis of early nonmotor features and risk factors for Parkinson disease. *Ann Neurol.* 2012; 72(6):893–901.

55. Palacios N, Gao X, McCullough ML, et al. Caffeine and risk of Parkinson's disease in a large cohort of men and women. *Mov Disord.* 2012; 27(10):1276–1282.

56. Nielsen SS, Franklin GM, Longstreth WT, et al. Nicotine from edible Solanaceae and risk of Parkinson disease. *Ann Neurol.* 2013; 74(3):472–477.

57. Simonin C, Duru C, Salleron J, et al. Association between caffeine intake and age at onset in Huntington's disease. *Neurobiol Dis.* 2013; 58:179–182.

58. Seppi K, Weintraub D, Coelho M, et al. The Movement Disorder Society Evidence-Based Medicine Review Update: Treatments for the non-motor symptoms of Parkinson's disease. *Mov Disord.* 2011; 26(suppl 3):S42–S80.

59. Shamir E, Barak Y, Shalman I, et al. Melatonin treatment for tardive dyskinesia: a double-blind, placebo-controlled, crossover study. *Arch Gen Psychiatry.* 2001; 58(11):1049–1052.

INDEX